Medical Radiology

Diagnostic Imaging

Series Editors

Hans-Ulrich Kauczor
Paul M. Parizel
Wilfred C. G. Peh

The book series *Medical Radiology – Diagnostic Imaging* provides accurate and up-to-date overviews about the latest advances in the rapidly evolving field of diagnostic imaging and interventional radiology. Each volume is conceived as a practical and clinically useful reference book and is developed under the direction of an experienced editor, who is a world-renowned specialist in the field. Book chapters are written by expert authors in the field and are richly illustrated with high quality figures, tables and graphs. Editors and authors are committed to provide detailed and coherent information in a readily accessible and easy-to-understand format, directly applicable to daily practice.

Medical Radiology – Diagnostic Imaging covers all organ systems and addresses all modern imaging techniques and image-guided treatment modalities, as well as hot topics in management, workflow, and quality and safety issues in radiology and imaging. The judicious choice of relevant topics, the careful selection of expert editors and authors, and the emphasis on providing practically useful information, contribute to the wide appeal and ongoing success of the series. The series is indexed in Scopus.

More information about this series at https://link.springer.com/bookseries/174

Douglas P. Beall • Peter L. Munk
Michael J. DePalma
Timothy Davis • Kasra Amirdelfan
Corey W. Hunter
Editors

Intrathecal Pump Drug Delivery

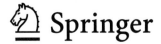
Springer

Editors
Douglas P. Beall
Comprehensive Specialty Care
Edmond, OK
USA

Michael J. DePalma
Virginia iSpine Physicians, PC
Richmond, VA
USA

Kasra Amirdelfan
IPM Medical Group, Inc.
Walnut Creek, CA
USA

Peter L. Munk
Department of Radiology
Vancouver General Hospital
Vancouver, BC
Canada

Timothy Davis
Source Healthcare
Santa Monica, CA
USA

Corey W. Hunter
Ainsworth Institute of Pain Management
New York, NY
USA

ISSN 0942-5373   ISSN 2197-4187   (electronic)
Medical Radiology
ISSN 2731-4677   ISSN 2731-4685   (electronic)
Diagnostic Imaging
ISBN 978-3-030-86246-6   ISBN 978-3-030-86244-2   (eBook)
https://doi.org/10.1007/978-3-030-86244-2

This Springer imprint is published by the registered company Springer Nature Switzerland AG
The registered company address is: Gewerbestrasse 11, 6330 Cham, Switzerland

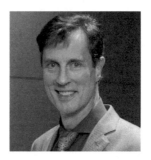

Douglas P. Beall, MD, FIPP, FSIR, DAAPM
Director Interventional Spine Care, Comprehensive Specialty Care,
Chief of Radiology Services and Director of Fellowship Programs,
Oklahoma City, OK, USA

This book is dedicated to all the practitioners who are willing to tackle complex therapies in order to ease their patient's pain and improve their lives. My hope is that a comprehensive single source of information will help to optimize IDD therapy and improve your patient's outcomes.

Preface

Intrathecal drug delivery (IDD) has been one of my very favorite treatments since I saw my first case performed in fellowship in the early 2000s and saw the incredibly good and immediate results. After transitioning from academia and into private practice I found myself inheriting 67 intrathecal baclofen patients from two physicians who were transitioning from managing this patient population to being employed hospitalists. As an Interventional Radiologist, my staff was unfamiliar and somewhat hesitant to accept this service line but did so anyway without hesitation and this patient population quickly became their favorite group.

Intrathecal medication delivery has since become an essential part of our medical and interventional practice. In patients who have certain conditions this therapy is absolutely essential including patients who have severe spasticity, multi-site pain, severe degenerative conditions without a surgical solution, patients with chronic pain on high-dose systemic narcotics, and metastatic cancer pain especially from a pancreatic source or those with bony metastases. I have found that IDD is often the only solution for some of the most complex patients and without it they simply do not receive optimal care.

As useful and essential as this therapy is it is, in my opinion, tremendously underutilized. I think there are two primary reasons for this. The first is that IDD has had its reputation tarnished in the early days of therapy where it was commonplace to provide oral opioid medication along with intrathecal opioids. As we now know, providing oral or systemic medication is a self-defeating strategy as it causes an upregulation of the cytochrome P-450 system to the point that there is no amount of intrathecal opioid that can be provided that can overcome the patient's upregulated metabolic activity that eliminates the opioid very quickly and results in a very high tolerance to these medications. During the peak of the opioid epidemic, we were seeing patients with chronic pain that were on 500–1000 MME of morphine or more for IDD trials. One of these patients was on an incredible 1200 MME of morphine daily and refused to taper his medication dose before the trial. We typically use a 1:100 ratio of intrathecal to oral MME of opioids for a bolus trial and keep the patients overnight with continuous monitoring of the pulse oximetry and cardiac activity and multiple vital signs measurements. In this patient, however I was very reluctant to give that amount of intrathecal morphine and settled on 8 mg of morphine injected as a bolus into the lumbar spine cerebrospinal fluid. We were prepared for treatment of an overdose of intrathecal medication but what happened was exactly the opposite with the patient receiving

2–3 h of excellent pain relief followed by a return of his pain to the point where he was unhappy, wanted to take his oral medication and checked out of the hospital against medical advice. This scenario permanently etched in my mind the absolute requirement not to use a combination of systemic and intrathecal medication as there is no amount of opioid that can be given intrathecally to overcome the hypermetabolism that results from systemic opioid administration.

The second reason for underutilization of TDD relates to the perceived complicated nature of this therapy. In my opinion this is nothing more than a perception and confusion of what is complicated verses what is complex. The term complicated refers to a high level of difficulty and the pragmatic application of TDD is certainly not that. It is, however, complex which means that it utilization of this therapy has many components but it is not necessarily difficult and can be learned in a manner that is logical and straightforward. There are some useful guides to the delivery of TDD including the comprehensive consensus-based guidelines on IDD systems in the treatment of pain caused by cancer and the Polyanalgesic Consensus Guidelines but, surprisingly, there is no book that provides a comprehensive guide to the wide variety of clinical applications of IDD…that is until now.

This book was designed to be a comprehensive guide, and it has certainly accomplished that discussing all aspects of IDD including the various applications in cancer pain, nonmalignant pain, acute and chronic pain, and in severe spasticity. The information provided expands on the typical patient histories, the diagnostic processes, the surgical techniques and approaches, IDD system troubleshooting, preoperative and postoperative assessments, electronic analysis and reprogramming, different on and off-label intrathecal medications, and the management of pain or baclofen pumps. We have even included conditions and concepts that are frequently encountered clinically but never before described in the medical literature. It has certainly been a pleasure and a privilege to be involved in the writing of this book. I would like to thank all of my editors, authors, coauthors, and all others who have made this work possible. From an early observational start to a sudden immersion in intrathecal baclofen therapy to an ongoing comprehensive and diversified program, IDD just keeps getting better and just like any other tool that is have found to be optimal; it first becomes useful and then becomes essential.

Oklahoma City, OK   Douglas P. Beall

Acknowledgements

Bradley Philips for his tireless and continuing contribution to Intrathecal Drug Delivery

Contents

Introduction and Background for Intrathecal Pumps Used for Pain and Spasticity

Brent Earls, Matt Sullivan, and Paul J. Christo

Contents

B. Earls · P. J. Christo (✉)
Division of Pain Medicine, Department of
Anesthesiology and Critical Care Medicine,
Johns Hopkins University School of Medicine,
Baltimore, MD, USA
e-mail: pchristo@jhmi.edu

M. Sullivan
Division of Pain Medicine, Department of
Anesthesiology and Critical Care Medicine and
Emergency Medicine, Johns Hopkins University
School of Medicine, Baltimore, MD, USA

Abstract

Intrathecal drug delivery has expanded since the inception of this technology in the 1980s and is utilized for a number of different conditions for the purposes of pain control and the management of spasticity. The use of intrathecal pumps is less common than many other techniques for interventional pain management but is essential in such conditions as refractory pain, cancer pain, multifocal pain, severe spasticity, and in patients who are not candidates for surgical correction of their underlying condition. Intrathecal drug delivery is usually considered when analgesics or antispasmodics administered via the oral, transdermal, or intravenous routes are ineffective or are associated with unacceptable side effects. The intrathecal delivery of medications bypasses the blood-brain barrier, which produces much higher concentrations of medication within the cerebrospinal fluid. This higher concentration can serve to dramatically reduce the effective dose of the medication and can be associated with higher rates of pain and spasm reduction as compared to other routes of medication delivery. Although intrathecal drug delivery has been shown to be clinically effective and cost-effective, this pain and spasticity management tool is less well understood regarding its implantation and management than other implantable technologies. This chapter will serve to highlight the proper clinical use and appropriate management of intrathecal pumps for the management of spasticity and pain.

Abbreviations

BBB	Blood-brain barrier
CMM	Conventional medical management
CP	Cerebral palsy
CSF	Cerebrospinal fluid
CT	Computed tomography
CVA	Cerebrovascular accident
FDA	Food and drug administration
ITB	Intrathecal baclofen
MRI	Magnetic resonance imaging
MS	Multiple sclerosis
PSS	Poststroke spasticity
ROM	Range of movement
SCI	Spinal cord injury
SCS	Spinal cord stimulator
TBI	Traumatic brain injury
TDD	Targeted drug delivery

1 Introduction and Background for Intrathecal Pumps Used for Pain and Spasticity

Chronic pain is exceedingly common with prevalence estimates ranging from 13 to 51% and is more common than other chronic conditions such as diabetes or chronic obstructive pulmonary disease, and more common than diabetes, cancer, and heart disease combined (Breivik et al. 2006; Craig et al. 2011; Fayaz et al. 2016; Gupta et al. 2010; Manchikanti et al. 2009; Tsang et al. 2008). There are more than 100 million Americans suffering from chronic pain and estimates from the Institute of Medicine place the annual healthcare cost of treating this pain at nearly \$635 billion annually (Institute of Medicine (US) Committee on Advancing Pain Research, Care, and Education 2011).

In addition to the economic costs, chronic pain is a significant burden causing substantial reduction in patients' quality of life. A national pain audit found that the average quality of life score in people suffering from chronic pain was lower than that reported by people suffering from progressive neurological disorders such as Parkinson's disease (Price et al. 2019). Common chronic pain disorders such as migraine headaches and neck pain cause significant disruptions in quality of life, and low back pain causes more disability worldwide than any other single condition (Hoy et al. 2014). Patients suffering from chronic pain are also less productive in their work and are seven times more likely to quit their jobs due to ill health than the general population (Donaldson 2009).

2 Historical Background and Perspectives of Intrathecal Drug Delivery

Understanding and treating pain has been a challenge to humanity as far back as 5000 BC when the first records of using opium for analgesia were etched on clay tablets. For over 6000 years, humankind continued this practice with similar treatments while making relatively little advancement in understanding. Even the earliest theories of anatomy by Hippocrates, who although he recognized the brain as the place of the mind and the seat of thought, sensation, emotion, and cognition still believed that the heart was responsible for pain's sensation (Linton 2005). During the Roman Empire, the Greek anatomist Galen dissected a variety of mammalian brains and posited that the cerebrum processed sensations and that certain spinal nerves control muscles. Despite anatomic advancements, the perception of pain prior to the Renaissance remained vague and largely spiritual or mystical, with the majority of theories arguing for the appeasement of God as the best treatment. With the publication of Descartes' *Treatise of Man* in 1664, the French philosopher provided the first physical and mechanical descriptions of pain pathways and laid a foundation for modern neuroanatomy (Hadjistavropoulos and Craig 2004). Descartes proposed his theory through illustrations of a hand being struck with a hammer and a foot being held near a flame, both of which resulted in pain traveling up "a fine thread" to the brain, where it would cause a variety of responses such as flinching away from or turning toward the stimulus (Hadjistavropoulos and Craig 2004).

It was not until the nineteenth century that pain as a "specific sensation" emerged and with this notion came a cascade of discoveries to characterize pain at a fundamental level. In 1811, Scottish anatomist Charles Bell published his findings from human cadaveric dissections. He discovered the existence and discrete function of the spinocerebellar tracts by demonstrating motor functions via nerve fibers exiting the ventral roots from the spine. Eleven years later, while performing his notorious public experiments on dogs, French Physiologist Francois Magendie verified the sensory function of dorsal root ganglia by exciting the anterior nerve roots of the spinal cord to cause pain. Brown-Sequard furthered this research with his findings on the decussation of pain fibers in 1880 (Laporte 2006), which was succeeded in 1889 by Edinger's discovery of the spinothalamic tracts. Edinger's implication that superficial long tracts in the lateral spinal cord were the carriers of afferent pain signal helped to complete the basic understandings of neuroanatomy enough for successful interventions and treatments.

With the invention of the hollow needle and the glass syringe by Scottish surgeon (and soon-to-be the Royal College of Physicians' President) Alexander Wood in 1853, the medical community had the tools it needed to conduct more targeted analgesic interventions. Nonetheless, the targets themselves were as of yet unknown. A contemporary and rival of Wood, fellow-surgeon Charles Hunter proved that pain relief could be achieved by injecting narcotics anywhere in the body and not just at the area of pain, as Wood had argued (Brunton 2000). Despite these advancements in neuroanatomy and medical technology, little progress had been made in the field of pharmacology, and morphine remained the primary, if not the only, analgesic available to most physicians until the late nineteenth century. Though South American Indians had been chewing coca leaves for over 5000 years, it was not until 1859 that German pharmacists isolated and characterized cocaine as the active compound. This revolutionary discovery added cocaine to a growing list of natural alkaloids that were starting to be used as empiric treatments for a variety of diseases (Holmstedt and Fredga 1981). This was occurring throughout the latter half of the nineteenth century, but the chemical structure of alkaloids would not be revealed until 1898 by the work of Nobel Laureate Richard Willstatter (Willstätter 1898). This all changed in 1884 when a young Viennese neurologist, Sigmund Freud, learned of cocaine's impressive ability to suppress fatigue and ultimately decided to try the drug himself. Inspired by what he called a "magical drug," Freud shared his experience and small samples of cocaine to his scientific contemporaries (Freud and Freud 1992). One of these was Viennese ophthalmologist, Carl Koller, who was disappointed by the failures of general anesthesia for ocular procedures, when he happened to sample the drug himself and noted a surprising numbing effect to his tongue. In late 1884, he applied a cocaine solution to a patient's cornea with excellent anesthetic effect (Koller 1928). Halstead and Hall found that this could be directed even more precisely, at the level of the inferior alveolar and dental nerves, and subsequently pioneered the first peripheral nerve block in 1885 (López-Valverde et al. 2011).

James Leonard Corning, a surgeon in New York City, read of Koller's discovery and decided to translate this to his own neurosurgical studies. In 1885, Corning was the first to discover that cocaine delivered to the epidural space of dogs resulted in "hind limb weakness and ataxia." In 1891, Heinrich Quincke developed a uniquely fine, hollow cutting needle that would allow him to access the subarachnoid space in attempts to relieve the hydrocephalus resulting from tubercular meningitis (Dugacki 1992). Just 14 years after the first clinical application of local anesthetic, on August 16, 1898, German surgeon August Bier, and his assistant, August Hildebrand, performed the first successful intrathecal anesthesia (Pravaz and Gabriel 1853). Despite successful anesthesia after spinal cocainization in just six patients, Bier criticized his own work, stating, "so many complaints had arisen in association with this method (back and leg pain, vomiting, prolonged headache) that they equalled the complaints usually occurring after general anesthesia" (Bier 1899). Naturally, Bier and Hildebrand volunteered to perform similar experiments on each other. While the experiment on Bier resulted in CSF loss after Hildebrand struggled to connect a Prvaz syringe to the Quincke needle, he characterized the first dural puncture headache. The intrathecal anesthesia Bier delivered to Hildebrand was much more successful, as he demonstrated no sensual perception to needle sticks of the thigh, tickling of his feet, pushing a helved needle to the femur, incising his thigh, tamping out a burning cigar, pulling pubic hairs, striking his shins with an iron hammer, and even applying pressure to his testicles. Bier later wrote, "After these experiments on our own bodies, we both went to dinner without any physical complaints," though "Hildebrandt felt very poor the next morning" (Bier 1899).

3 Intrathecal Drug Delivery for Pain Indications

Intrathecal treatment of chronic pain and spasticity has been approved for those patients who experience severe symptoms from their condition and who have proven unresponsiveness to less invasive medical therapy (National Coverage Determination 2004). With such a broad indication, the role of intrathecal drug delivery continues to evolve within the pain treatment continuum. Intrathecal drug delivery had previously been seen as a salvage therapy or last resort measure. New consensus guidelines, however, suggest this modality should be considered in the same line of management as neurostimulation, with important caveats (Deer et al. 2017). These important considerations would include having a clear diagnosis, an appropriate physical examination, and a complete psychosocial evaluation (which may be optional for cancer pain) before undergoing either a trial or an implant (Deer et al. 2017).

In an article by Deer et al., an effort is made to clearly define refractory pain that may then help clinicians better assess patient suitability for neuromodulatory techniques, including intrathecal drug therapy (Deer et al. 2014). This approach helps with three important issues when beginning to consider this line of therapy, first, by preventing unnecessary device implants in inappropriate patients; second, by identifying appropriate patients early in the process, we may improve the therapeutic efficacy of treatment with implanted devices; and third, by early identification of psychosocial comorbidities, there is an opportunity to improve the treatment response by optimizing these factors prior to any device implantation.

4 Goals of Therapy

Evidence for intrathecal drug delivery (ITDD) is strong for short-term and moderate for the long-term management of neuropathic and mixed pain conditions (Smith et al. 2008). De Lissovoy et al. previously demonstrated that ITDD appears cost-effective when compared with alternative (medical) management for selected patients with pain associated with failed back surgery (FBSS) when the duration of therapy exceeds 12–22 months (de Lissovoy et al. 1997). Kumar and colleagues modeled the comparative cost-effectiveness of the ITDD continuum, in which they explicitly addressed costs related to polyanalgesia versus conventional medical management for chronic non-cancer pain. Over 10 years, a patient receiving ITDD would stand to accrue an additional 1.15 quality-adjusted life years (QALY) compared with a patient receiving conventional medical management. Despite the increased price of the device and medication to fill it, the authors concluded that ITDD remains a highly cost-effective treatment strategy with costs of therapy falling well below commonly accepted societal willingness to pay thresholds (Kumar et al. 2013). When making management decisions for patients in chronic pain, it is important to consider factors such as cost, long-term quality of life, and duration of efficacy as they pertain to the chosen therapy.

5 Long-Term Effectiveness

Utilization of intrathecal drug delivery systems (IDDS) in patients with malignancy-related pain has significant support in the literature. Pain is a frequent symptom in patients with cancer, and it often results in substantial detrimental impact. Despite the availability of opioids and updated guidelines from reliable leading societies, undertreatment is still frequent (Greco et al. 2014). Additionally, multiple high-quality studies have shown IDDS to be more efficacious than medical management alone (Baker et al. 2004; Bruel and Burton 2016; Rauck et al. 2003; Zech et al. 1995). The Cancer Pain Trial showed that IDDS could relieve pain more effectively with less toxicity and possibly improve survival in patients with intractable cancer pain after appropriate therapy that followed approved guidelines (Smith et al. 2005). Perhaps more importantly, the patients receiving IDDS in this trial showed substantial reduction in medication side effects with the IDDS group having a 66% decrease versus a 37% decrease in the medical management group as

determined using a baseline adjusted regression model ($p < 0.01$) (Smith et al. 2005).

Intrathecal drug delivery has also been shown to be very efficacious in chronic nonmalignant pain. Ziconotide has presented some challenges in clinical use due to a narrow therapeutic window and a relatively high incidence of adverse events (Hayek et al. 2015; Rauck et al. 2006). There are reports of flexible dosing strategies that may be used to mitigate unwanted adverse effects (Zech et al. 1995). This has been shown to improve the response to the therapy and decrease the need for systemic opioid medications (Pope and Deer 2015). In a study by Duarte and colleagues, they showed that participants receiving intrathecal opioids maintained a significant reduction in pain intensity and an improved quality of life up to 13 years after the initiation of treatment (Duarte et al. 2012). At a follow-up averaging 13 years after the initiation of IDDS therapy, 90% of patients continued to be very satisfied with the treatment. Other reports have shown patients followed even up to 20 years still had significantly reduced pain from their baseline (Sommer et al. 2020).

6 Types of Intrathecal Systems (Pumps)

Broadly speaking, ITDD systems are available in four different configurations and are distinguished by which parts may or may not be implanted under the skin along with their programming capabilities. The least invasive option for the intrathecal system is a percutaneous catheter (tunneled or not tunneled) connected to an external pump. A slightly more invasive option is a totally implanted catheter with a subcutaneous injection port connected to an external pump. These two abovementioned systems are usually used in patients with limited life expectancy. Next is a fully implanted fixed rate ITDD system, which is generally less expensive than programmable systems. The notable drawback is that dosage alteration requires that the pump be emptied and refilled with a new drug formulation or a different drug concentration. Finally, there are the fully implanted and programmable ITDD systems (Duarte et al. 2016). Details about these systems, including a more robust discussion of benefits and drawbacks, will be discussed further in chapter "The Components of Intrathecal Drug Delivery".

7 Initial Drug Therapy

Several factors have been shown to contribute to the distribution of any given medication within the CSF following intrathecal administration. The five main factors include lipid solubility, baricity, regional CSF mixing, flow rate, and residence time within the intrathecal space (Table 1) (Bernards 2002). Compared to hydrophilic medications, lipophilic medications have shorter half-lives, largely due to faster redistribution into fatty tissues and higher volumes of distribution (Jose et al. 2013; Waara-Wolleat et al. 2006). Despite the hydrophilic nature of some medications, like morphine, animal and human models have shown relatively limited distribution in the CSF following continuous infusion (Wallace and Yaksh 2012). In a study by Flack et al., concentrations of morphine beyond 5 cm from the catheter, above or below the origin of infusion, were shown to be about 20% of the concentration at the infusion point itself and drop to about 5% when sampling at 10 cm (Flack et al. 2011). Studies have shown manipulation of the drug concentration or volume delivered can increase the drug spread. Some of these techniques have also shown higher rates of adverse events as well as reduction in quality of life in patients being treated with continuous intrathecal therapy. In a study by Perruchoud and colleagues, higher pump flow rates consistently demonstrated no

Table 1 The five main factors contributing to the intrathecal distribution of medication within the cerebrospinal fluid

1.	Lipid solubility
2.	Baricity
3.	Regional CSF mixing
4.	Pump flow rate
5.	Residence time within the intrathecal space

change in pain VAS (visual analog scale) but worsening of pain and anxiety dimensions on questionnaires. This led the researchers to conclude higher flow rates may increase drug dilution thereby reducing the receptor site effect of the medication (Perruchoud et al. 2011)

8 Choice of Medication

Two medications have been approved by the Food and Drug Administration (FDA) for intrathecal use in treating chronic pain, morphine sulfate (Infumorph® Sterile Solution, Baxter Healthcare Corp., Deerfield, IL, USA and Mitigo™ Pirimal Critical Care, Inc., Mumbai, India) and ziconotide (Prialt® for intrathecal infusion; Jazz Pharmaceuticals, Inc., Dublin, Ireland). While morphine and ziconotide are the only two medications with an FDA indication for intrathecal use for pain, a number of combinations of drugs have been proposed in the literature to improve efficacy and reduce side effects. The methodical use of polyanalgesia may be more effective in addressing painful conditions through the modulation of multiple mechanisms and using multiple mechanisms of action to attenuate the development of tolerance (Kumar et al. 2013). This approach has the distinct potential to provide optimal pain control while reducing the need for opioid dose escalation (Kumar et al. 2013). In cancer pain, evidence would suggest that combination therapy might be warranted as a first-line strategy, which is a different recommendation as compared to the treatment of non-cancer pain (Veizi et al. 2011). It is, therefore, important to understand the patient's pain characteristics, including their pain type and location, expected length of therapy, and the patient's age when choosing a medication or combination of medications (Deer et al. 2017).

9 Adverse Events

Intrathecal therapy is not without its risks, although continued utilization over the years has improved the patients' treatment experience and their safety (Hayek et al. 2011). Adverse events can be broadly categorized as related to the implantation procedure, medication effects, or related to the catheter or the pump itself. Adverse events related to surgical procedures can be many, but the most common are infection and CSF leak. Bleeding is uncommon but can be an emergency and should be monitored closely. Seroma formation in the pump pocket is usually benign but should also be monitored for the development of infection. Hygromas, associated with CSF leaking around the catheter, are usually self-limited but may persist and need either drainage or additional surgical attention (Czernicki et al. 2015).

Due to the number of medications and medication combinations that are used in targeted drug delivery, the potential for medication associated side effects is not insubstantial. Direct delivery at the spinal cord level is helpful to limit adverse effects usually seen with systemic delivery, but it is important to monitor the patient for side effect nevertheless. Intrathecally delivered opioid medications can cause sedation, lightheadedness, nausea, and urinary retention (Prager et al. 2014; Spiegel et al. 2021). Long-term administration has been shown to cause tolerance, hypogonadism, and low bone density (Duarte et al. 2012). In a study by Coffee and colleagues, intrathecal opioid therapy was associated with slightly higher mortality (3.8%) than cohorts of spinal cord stimulator patients and discectomy patients due to medication-related respiratory depression or overdose (Coffey et al. 2009). Alternatively, Smith and colleagues found that ITDD decreased pain intensity and improved survival in cancer patients (Smith and Coyne 2004). Intrathecal ziconotide has most commonly been associated with dizziness, nausea, and confusion. It is also important to note that ziconotide is contraindicated in patients with psychosis (Pope and Deer 2013).

Catheter migration and dislodgement are the most common device-related complications of ITDD and are reported to occur between 0.7 and 1.5% (Deer et al. 2004). Granuloma formation at the catheter tip has also been documented especially at high medication concentrations (Deer et al. 2012). Overt device failure is an extremely rare event, but it should be treated urgently to prevent medication withdrawal. Medication compounding for intrathecal use has been a popular technique to attempt to optimize the therapeutic response to ITDD while minimizing the side effects (Pope et al. 2017). This requires pharmacy compounding, which is not regulated by the FDA but by state boards of pharmacy, incorporating the United States Pharmacopeia (USP) chapters of pharmaceutical compounding for both sterile and non-sterile preparations (Gudeman et al. 2013). Recently, the FDA released a communication sharing information about pump failures, dosing errors, and other safety information so that patients and providers can make informed treatment decisions (Health, Center for Devices and Radiological 2018). A more comprehensive list, including postoperative care, will be discussed in more detail in later chapters.

10 Intrathecal Drug Delivery for Spasticity

Spasticity is defined as an abnormal increase in muscle tone caused by injury of upper motor neuron pathways regulating muscles and may be caused by injury or disease of the central nervous system. There is a velocity-dependent increased resistance to passive stretch, and this may be characterized by exaggerated tendon jerks and accompanied by hyperexcitability of the stretch reflex (Emos and Agarwal 2020). A more encompassing definition is from the 2005 SPASM consortium, which defines spasticity as disordered sensorimotor control resulting from an upper motor neuron lesion that presents as intermittent or sustained involuntary activation of muscles (Pandyan et al. 2005). A multitude of diseases can lead to the development of spasticity. In this chapter, we will introduce some of the more common causes and the principles behind its treatment.

Spasticity of spinal cord origin is most commonly seen in patients with spinal cord disease or traumatic injury. There are about 12,000 new cases of spinal cord injury (SCI) that occur each year, and in the last 20 years, the majority of the injuries have resulted in incomplete tetraplegia (30.1%) and complete paraplegia (25.6%) (Anson and Shepherd 1996). Multiple sclerosis (MS) has shown to be a devastating disease for those who suffer from the condition. Movement disorders can vary greatly in patients with MS depending upon the location of the plaques within the brain and spinal cord, and spasticity is a common feature among patients, with up to 84% of the patients experiencing some degree of spasticity (Wallin et al. 2019). Poststroke syndrome (PSS) can also commonly cause spasticity and has been shown to cause permanent disability in about five million people worldwide every year, with about 38% of those individuals experiencing spasticity (Katan and Luft 2018; Watkins et al. 2002). While most strokes occur in the brain parenchyma, the resulting imbalance of inhibitory and excitatory signals at the spinal level is thought to be the cause of PSS (Trompetto et al. 2014). The functional impairments associated with severe spasticity seen in all of these disease processes include pain, difficulty sleeping, flexion contractures, and bladder and bowel dysfunction (Dvorak et al. 2011; Mandigo and Anderson 2006; Mutch et al. 1992; Rizzo et al. 2004). Patients with spasticity also have difficulty with various activities of daily life such as walking, changing positions, mobilizing from a wheelchair, and other activities (Dvorak et al. 2011; Mandigo and Anderson 2006; Mutch et al. 1992; Rizzo et al. 2004).

Baclofen is a GABA agonist that is thought to selectively bind to presynaptic GABA-B receptors, resulting in hyperpolarization of the motor horn cells and a subsequent reduction in hyperactivity of the muscle stretch reflexes, a decreased amount of clonus, and dampened cutaneous reflexes that elicit muscle spasms (Newman et al. 1982; Stien et al. 1987). Baclofen has been used in the treatment of spasticity since the 1960s but was not introduced as an intrathecal therapy in humans until 1984. In a case series of two patients, intrathecal baclofen was given in small doses (5–25 mcg) and showed improvement of spasticity for up to 8 h (Penn and Kroin 1984). The current literature

supporting the use of baclofen can be difficult to evaluate because there is no single universally accepted standard on spasticity rating, and a large degree of heterogeneity in existing studies. The best available evidence suggests that baclofen offers the optimal efficacy for most clinical outcomes, including decreasing spasms, improving functional status, and scoring high for patient preference in patients with spasticity (Chou et al. 2004). The most common adverse reactions to intrathecal baclofen include hypotonia and somnolence, and both are reported at slightly greater than 5% in study subjects. Nausea, headache, and dry mouth were also noted in approximately 2% of participants at 2 months post implant (Ertzgaard et al. 2017). Overdose may present with sudden coma or in more insidious ways such as drowsiness, lightheadedness, dizziness, somnolence, respiratory depression, seizures, rostral progression of hypotonia, and loss of consciousness that progresses to coma. Sudden withdrawal of the medication is also a major concern as this can lead to severe symptomatology, including death. Signs of withdrawal include high fever, altered mental status, and rebound spasticity that, if severe, can lead to severe rhabdomyolysis. While these events are exceedingly rare, it is important to closely monitor patients at vulnerable times such as after dose adjustments and pump refills.

11   Conclusion

Intrathecal drug delivery as a therapy has increased since its inception due to the contributions of clinicians, pharmacologists, and medical device manufacturers and has been facilitated by the recommendations of various consensus panels (Deer et al. 2017; American Society of Anesthesiologists Task Force on Neuraxial Opioids 2016; Fitzgibbon et al. 2010). There have been algorithms introduced for the appropriate application of clinical therapies for patients with various types of pain and spasticity. There has also been widespread encouragement for continued research and development of new medications, devices, and treatment recommen-

Table 2 Targeted drug delivery important tips: The ten commandments of intrathecal pump placement

1.	Use as large of a pump that the patient's preference and body habitus will allow
2.	Use perioperative and wound antibiotics to reduce risk of infection
3.	Place the pump in the lower quadrant of the abdomen to facilitate patient comfort
4.	Do not place the pump at a depth that will make the refills overly challenging (don't place the pump too deep)
5.	Anchor the pump to the underlying fascia with durable permanent sutures
6.	In morbidly obese patients, place the pump 8–9 cm lateral to the normal midclavicular line location. This will allow for a more superficial placement as the adipose tissue is typically less thick in this location
7.	Remember the blood patch as a treatment for a CSF leak around the catheter
8.	Always calculate the final implanted length of the catheter
9.	Always aspirate the catheter prior to closing the abdominal wound to ensure catheter patency
10.	Use an abdominal binder or the equivalent for 6 weeks following implantation

Table 3 Targeted drug delivery important tips: The ten commandments of intrathecal pump management

1.	Do not use systemic opioids (i.e., oral or transdermal) concurrently with IT opioids
2.	Do not use benzodiazepine medications in patients receiving IT opioid therapy
3.	Start with branded and single medications first then convert to compounded and multiple medications if necessary
4.	Make sure not to exceed the maximum concentrations of the compounded intrathecal medications
5.	Try to achieve the maximum time between refills to maximize patient comfort and convenience
6.	Use as large of a pump that the patient's preference and body habitus will allow
7.	If pump or catheter malfunction is suspected, have a low threshold for conducting a catheter and rotor study
8.	Use the lowest amount of medication possible to accomplish the treatment goals
9.	Use the patient controlled intermittent bolus dosing feature when possible
10.	Reduction of systemic opioids prior to the trial or implantation improves the success of the IT therapy and allows for better control of pain at a lower dose

dations. This chapter has provided an introduction for the appropriate use of IT therapy in patients with chronic nonmalignant and malignancy-associated pain and in patients with spasticity from various origins. This chapter has also presented and explained the various components of IT drug delivery including the IT pump, the catheter, and the supplies for implanting the pump and catheter. In addition, we have given a brief introduction for goals of therapy, medication choice, and common adverse effects associated with IT baclofen. The processes of patient identification, pre-trialing management, IT trialing, preoperative patient management, surgical pump implantation, post-op management, and long-term medication management can be challenging even with the appropriate knowledge and guidelines, and optimal information is certainly necessary to guide treatment and produce the best quality outcomes. In addition to the guidelines discussed above, the authors of this chapter have put forth their best helpful hints in the form of the Ten Commandments for the placement and management of intrathecal pumps (Tables 2 and 3, respectively). These can be combined with other consensus guidelines for determination of optimal strategies for IT medication therapy and which patients are best suited for this treatment paradigm. The application of IT therapy can greatly benefit carefully selected patients, many of whom are otherwise susceptible to undertreatment of their difficult conditions.

References

American Society of Anesthesiologists Task Force on Neuraxial Opioids (2016) Practice guidelines for the prevention, detection, and management of respiratory depression associated with neuraxial opioid administration: an updated report by the American Society of Anesthesiologists Task Force on Neuraxial Opioids and the American Society of Regional Anesthesia and Pain Medicine. Anesthesiology 124:535–552

Anson CA, Shepherd C (1996) Incidence of secondary complications in spinal cord injury. Int J Rehabil Res 19:55–66

Baker L, Lee M, Regnard C et al (2004) Evolving spinal analgesia practice in palliative care. Palliat Med 18:507–515

Bernards CM (2002) Understanding the physiology and pharmacology of epidural and intrathecal opioids. Best Pract Res Clin Anaesthesiol 16:489–505

Bier A (1899) Versuche über cocainisirung des rückenmarkes. Deutsche Zeitschrift für Chirurgie 51:361–369

Breivik H, Collett B, Ventafridda V et al (2006) Survey of chronic pain in Europe: prevalence, impact on daily life, and treatment. Eur J Pain 10:287–333

Bruel BM, Burton AW (2016) Intrathecal therapy for cancer-related pain. Pain Med 17:2404–2421

Brunton D (2000) A question of priority: Alexander Wood, Charles Hunter and the hypodermic method. Proc R Coll Physicians Edinb 30:349–351

Chou R, Peterson K, Helfand M (2004) Comparative efficacy and safety of skeletal muscle relaxants for spasticity and musculoskeletal conditions: a systematic review. J Pain Symptom Manag 28:140–175

Coffey RJ, Owens ML, Broste SK et al (2009) Mortality associated with implantation and management of intrathecal opioid drug infusion systems to treat non-cancer pain. Anesthesiology 111:881–891

Craig R, Hirani V, Mindell J (2011) Health survey for England 2011: health, social care and lifestyles. NHS Information Centre

Czernicki M, Sinovich G, Mihaylov I et al (2015) Intrathecal drug delivery for chronic pain management-scope, limitations and future. J Clin Monit Comput 29:241–249

de Lissovoy G, Brown RE, Halpern M et al (1997) Cost-effectiveness of long-term intrathecal morphine therapy for pain associated with failed back surgery syndrome. Clin Ther 19:96–112; discussion 84–5

Deer T, Chapple I, Classen A et al (2004) Intrathecal drug delivery for treatment of chronic low back pain: report from the National Outcomes Registry for low back pain. Pain Med 5:6–13

Deer TR, Levy R, Prager J et al (2012) Polyanalgesic Consensus Conference—2012: recommendations to reduce morbidity and mortality in intrathecal drug delivery in the treatment of chronic pain. Neuromodulation 15:467–482; discussion 482

Deer TR, Caraway DL, Wallace MS (2014) A definition of refractory pain to help determine suitability for device implantation. Neuromodulation 17:711–715

Deer TR, Pope JE, Hayek SM et al (2017) The polyanalgesic consensus conference (PACC): recommendations on intrathecal drug infusion systems best practices and guidelines. Neuromodulation 20:96–132

Donaldson L (2009) Pain: breaking through the barrier. In: Donaldson L (ed) 150 years of the annual report of the Chief Medical Officer: on the state of public health 2008. Department of Health, London, pp 32–39

Duarte RV, Raphael JH, Sparkes E et al (2012) Long-term intrathecal drug administration for chronic nonmalignant pain. J Neurosurg Anesthesiol 24:63–70

Duarte R, Raphael J, Eldabe S (2016) Intrathecal drug delivery for the management of pain and spasticity in adults: an executive summary of the British Pain Society's recommendations for best clinical practice. Br J Pain 10:67–69

Dugacki V (1992) A hundred years of lumbar puncture. Neurol Croat 41:241–245

Dvorak EM, Ketchum NC, McGuire JR (2011) The underutilization of intrathecal baclofen in poststroke spasticity. Top Stroke Rehabil 18:195–202

Emos MC, Agarwal S (2020) Neuroanatomy, upper motor neuron lesion. [Updated 2020 Jul 31]. In: StatPearls [Internet]. StatPearls Publishing, Treasure Island

Ertzgaard P, Campo C, Calabrese A (2017) Efficacy and safety of oral baclofen in the management of spasticity: a rationale for intrathecal baclofen. J Rehabil Med 49:193–203

Fayaz A, Croft P, Langford RM et al (2016) Prevalence of chronic pain in the UK: a systematic review and meta-analysis of population studies. BMJ Open 6: e010364

Fitzgibbon DR, Rathmell JP, Michna E et al (2010) Malpractice claims associated with medication management for chronic pain. Anesthesiology 112:948–956

Flack SH, Anderson CM, Bernards C (2011) Morphine distribution in the spinal cord after chronic infusion in pigs. Anesth Analg 112:460–464

Freud S, Freud EL (1992) Letters of Sigmund Freud. Dover

Greco MT, Roberto A, Corli O et al (2014) Quality of cancer pain management: an update of a systematic review of undertreatment of patients with cancer. J Clin Oncol 32:4149–4154

Gudeman J, Jozwiakowski M, Chollet J et al (2013) Potential risks of pharmacy compounding. Drugs R D 13:1–8

Gupta A, Mehdi A, Duwell M et al (2010) Evidence-based review of the pharmacoeconomics related to the management of chronic nonmalignant pain. J Pain Palliat Care Pharmacother 24:152–156

Hadjistavropoulos T, Craig KD (2004) Pain: psychological perspectives. Taylor & Francis

Hayek SM, Deer TR, Pope JE et al (2011) Intrathecal therapy for cancer and non-cancer pain. Pain Physician 14:219–248

Hayek SM, Hanes MC, Wang C et al (2015) Ziconotide combination intrathecal therapy for noncancer pain is limited secondary to delayed adverse effects: a case series with a 24-month follow-up. Neuromodulation 18:397–403

Health, Center for Devices and Radiological (2018) Use caution with implanted pumps for intrathecal administration of medicines for pain management: FDA safety communication. FDA. http://www.fda.

gov/medical-devices/safety-communications/use-caution-implanted-pumps-intrathecal-administration-medicines-pain-management-fda-safety

Holmstedt B, Fredga A (1981) Sundry episodes in the history of coca and cocaine. J Ethnopharmacol 3:113–147

Hoy D, March L, Brooks P et al (2014) The global burden of low back pain: estimates from the global burden of disease 2010 study. Ann Rheum Dis 73: 968–974

Institute of Medicine (US) Committee on Advancing Pain Research, Care, and Education (2011) Relieving pain in America: a blueprint for transforming prevention, care, education, and research. National Academies Press (US), Washington. PMID: 22553896

Jose DA, Luciano P, Vicente V et al (2013) Role of catheter's position for final results in intrathecal drug delivery. Analysis based on CSF dynamics and specific drugs profiles. Korean J Pain 26:336–346

Katan M, Luft A (2018) Global burden of stroke. Semin Neurol 38:208–211

Koller C (1928) Historical notes on the beginning of local anesthesia. J Am Med Assoc 90:1742–1743

Kumar K, Rizvi S, Bishop S (2013) Cost effectiveness of intrathecal drug therapy in management of chronic nonmalignant pain. Clin J Pain 29:138–145

Laporte Y (2006) Charles-Édouard Brown-Séquard. An eventful life and a significant contribution to the study of the nervous system. Comptes Rendus Biologies 329:363–368

Linton S (2005) Understanding pain for better clinical practice: a psychological perspective. Elsevier

López-Valverde A, De Vicente J, Cutando A (2011) The surgeons Halsted and Hall, cocaine and the discovery of dental anaesthesia by nerve blocking. Br Dent J 211:485–487

Manchikanti L, Boswell MV, Singh V et al (2009) Comprehensive evidence-based guidelines for interventional techniques in the management of chronic spinal pain. Pain Physician 12:699–802

Mandigo CE, Anderson RC (2006) Management of childhood spasticity: a neurosurgical perspective. Pediatr Ann 35:354–362

Mutch L, Alberman E, Hagberg B et al (1992) Cerebral palsy epidemiology: where are we now and where are we going? Dev Med Child Neurol 34:547–551

National Coverage Determination (2004) National Coverage Determination (NCD) for Infusion Pumps (280.14), CMS. http://www.cms.gov/medicare-coverage-database/details/ncddetails.aspx?NCDId=223&ncdver=2&DocID=280.14&SearchType=Advanced&bc=IAAAABAAAAAA

Newman P, Nogues M, Newman P et al (1982) Tizanidine in the treatment of spasticity. Eur J Clin Pharmacol 23:31–35

Pandyan A, Gregoric M, Barnes M et al (2005) Spasticity: clinical perceptions, neurological realities and meaningful measurement. Disabil Rehabil 27:2–6

Penn RD, Kroin JS (1984) Intrathecal baclofen alleviates spinal cord spasticity. Lancet 1:1078

Perruchoud C, Eldabe S, Durrer A et al (2011) Effects of flow rate modifications on reported analgesia and quality of life in chronic pain patients treated with continuous intrathecal drug therapy. Pain Med 12:571–576

Pope JE, Deer TR (2013) Ziconotide: a clinical update and pharmacologic review. Expert Opin Pharmacother 14:957–966

Pope JE, Deer TR (2015) Intrathecal pharmacology update: novel dosing strategy for intrathecal monotherapy ziconotide on efficacy and sustainability. Neuromodulation 18:414–420

Pope JE, Deer TR, Amirdelfan K et al (2017) The pharmacology of spinal opioids and ziconotide for the treatment of non-cancer pain. Curr Neuropharmacol 15:206–216

Prager J, Deer T, Levy R et al (2014) Best practices for intrathecal drug delivery for pain. Neuromodulation 17:354–372; discussion 372

Pravaz C-G, Gabriel P (1853) Sur un nouveau moyen d'opérer la coagulation du sang dans les arteres applicable a la guerison des aneurismes. Comptes rend Hebd des siances de l'Acad D Sciences 56:88–90

Price C, de C Williams AC, Smith BH et al (2019) The National Pain Audit for specialist pain services in England and Wales 2010–2014. Br J Pain 13: 185–193

Rauck RL, Cherry D, Boyer MF et al (2003) Long-term intrathecal opioid therapy with a patient-activated, implanted delivery system for the treatment of refractory cancer pain. J Pain 4:441–447

Rauck RL, Wallace MS, Leong MS et al (2006) A randomized, double-blind, placebo-controlled study of intrathecal ziconotide in adults with severe chronic pain. J Pain Symptom Manag 31:393–406

Rizzo MA, Hadjimichael OC, Preiningerova J et al (2004) Prevalence and treatment of spasticity reported by multiple sclerosis patients. Mult Scler 10:589–595

Smith TJ, Coyne P (2004) What is the evidence for implantable drug delivery systems for refractory cancer pain? Support Cancer Ther 1:185–189

Smith TJ, Coyne PJ, Staats PS et al (2005) An implantable drug delivery system (IDDS) for refractory cancer pain provides sustained pain control, less drug-related toxicity, and possibly better survival compared with comprehensive medical management (CMM). Ann Oncol 16:825–833

Smith HS, Deer TR, Staats PS et al (2008) Intrathecal drug delivery. Pain Physician 11:S89–S104

Sommer B, Karageorgos N, AlSharif M et al (2020) Long-term outcome and adverse events of intrathecal opioid therapy for nonmalignant pain syndrome. Pain Pract 20:8–15

Spiegel MA, Chen GH, Solla AC et al (2021) Evaluation of an intrathecal drug delivery protocol leads to rapid reduction of systemic opioids in the oncological population. J Palliat Med 24(3):418–422

Stien R, Nordal H, Oftedal S et al (1987) The treatment of spasticity in multiple sclerosis: a double blind clinical trial of a new anti spastic drug tizanidine* compared with baclofen. Acta Neurol Scand 75:190–194

Trompetto C, Marinelli L, Mori L et al (2014) Pathophysiology of spasticity: implications for neurorehabilitation. Biomed Res Int 2014:354906

Tsang A, Von Korff M, Lee S et al (2008) Common chronic pain conditions in developed and developing countries: gender and age differences and comorbidity with depression-anxiety disorders. J Pain 9:883–891

Veizi IE, Hayek SM, Narouze S et al (2011) Combination of intrathecal opioids with bupivacaine attenuates opioid dose escalation in chronic noncancer pain patients. Pain Med 12:1481–1489

Waara-Wolleat KL, Hildebrand KR, Stewart GR (2006) A review of intrathecal fentanyl and sufentanil for the treatment of chronic pain. Pain Med 7:251–259

Wallace M, Yaksh TL (2012) Characteristics of distribution of morphine and metabolites in cerebrospinal fluid and plasma with chronic intrathecal morphine infusion in humans. Anesth Analg 115:797–804

Wallin MT, Culpepper WJ, Campbell JD et al (2019) The prevalence of MS in the United States: a population-based estimate using health claims data. Neurology 92:e1029–e1040

Watkins CL, Leathley MJ, Gregson JM et al (2002) Prevalence of spasticity post stroke. Clin Rehabil 16:515–522

Willstätter R (1898) Ueber die Constitution der Spaltungsproducte von Atropin und Cocaïn. Ber Dtsch Chem Ges 31:1534–1553

Zech DF, Grond S, Lynch J et al (1995) Validation of World Health Organization guidelines for cancer pain relief: a 10-year prospective study. Pain 63:65–76

Intrathecal Drug Delivery for Cancer-Related Pain

Clarisse F. San Juan and Amitabh Gulati

Contents

1 Introduction and Background for Cancer Pain

From 1970 to 2019, the 5-year relative survival rates for all cancers have increased from 49 to 69% (Brogan and Gulati 2020). Breast cancer 5-year relative survival rates have improved even more with an increase from 75 to 91% (Brogan and Gulati 2020). Prostate cancer has also improved substantially with survival rates increasing from 68 to 99% (Brogan and Gulati 2020). The goal of cancer pain management is to preserve or even increase the quality of life of these cancer patients that are now living longer (Brogan and Gulati 2020).

Pain in patients diagnosed with cancer has prevalence rates as high as 66.4% in advanced metastatic or terminal disease, 55% during anticancer treatment, and 39.3% even after curative treatment (van den Beuken-van Everdingen 2016). A recent meta-analysis showed 38% of cancer patients reported pain that was rated as moderate to severe (van den Beuken-van Everdingen 2016). Pain is often the most feared symptom among individuals living with cancer (Bhatia et al. 2014). The treatment of pain is important in improving quality-adjusted life year (QALY) scores as it is usually a component of the health-related quality of life (HRQoL) weight as

C. F. San Juan (✉)
Physical Medicine and Rehabilitation, SUNY Downstate Medical Center, Brooklyn, NY, USA

A. Gulati
Memorial Sloan Kettering Cancer Center, New York, NY, USA
e-mail: Gulatia@mskcc.org

© The Author(s), under exclusive license to Springer Nature Switzerland AG 2022
D. P. Beall et al. (eds.), *Intrathecal Pump Drug Delivery*, Medical Radiology Diagnostic Imaging,
https://doi.org/10.1007/978-3-030-86244-2_2

measured by several methods including EuroQol (EQ-5D) and short form 6D (SF-6D). The EQ-5D questionnaire asks about patients' mobility, self-care, performing usual activities, pain/discomfort, and anxiety/depression (Whitehead and Ali 2010). The use of advanced pain procedures may improve both pain and quality of life in the cancer patient.

Previously, cancer pain management had focused on comfort at end of life with the use of high-dose opioids analgesics (Brogan and Gulati 2020). Recently, there has been a shift away from this practice as the patients have starting living longer and with the increase in cancer life expectancy; the cancer pain management has evolved to become more of a chronic and sustainable long-term issue. Treatment options include oral nonsteroidal anti-inflammatory drugs; neuropathic pain medications; oral, transdermal, and parenteral opioids; peripheral nerve blocks; neurolysis with plexus blocks; local anesthetic injections; spinal cord stimulation; continuous epidural analgesia; and intrathecal medication pumps (Bhatia et al. 2014). This chapter will be focusing on intrathecal drug delivery systems (IDDS) as they are one of the most effective modalities that are used for cancer-related pain.

2 Intrathecal Drug Delivery (IDD) for Cancer-Related Pain

Intrathecal drug delivery (IDD) delivers the analgesic drug of choice intrathecally into the cerebrospinal fluid bypassing systemic circulation and placing it in the location of the end-target receptors in the spinal cord. This is important in reducing unwanted systemic opioid side effects, such as sedation and fatigue that can interfere with the patient's normal functioning and can limit the utility of systemic opioid therapy due to the inability of the patient to tolerate the side effects. Another benefit is the reduced dosage of medication needed to achieve an equivalent level of analgesia as compared to oral and intravenous (IV) route because of the more direct route to the pain processing centers in the spinal cord (Bhatia et al. 2014). Intrathecal drug delivery for the management of cancer-related pain has been shown to have less pain, less drug toxicities especially for those on chemotherapy or radiation, and improved survival (Smith et al. 2002).

2.1 Considerations for Patient Selection

There are certain characteristics that make patients good candidates for IDD (Table 1). The most common characteristic is that the patient is not getting adequate relief on relatively high doses of oral or transdermal opioids especially when these medications produce unacceptable side effects (Bhatia et al. 2014). Intrathecal drug delivery has been shown to reduce adverse events in patients on long-term chemotherapy (Smith et al. 2002), and the therapy is now recommended in the absence of impending death as IDD may indeed improve life expectancy (Deer et al. 2011). Prior to placement, it is recommended that the patient be assessed for psychosocial issues

Table 1 Cancer patients who are considered good candidates for IDD

• Patients on significantly high doses of opioids with inadequate analgesia
• Patients with considerable side effects to oral or IV opiate medications that the dosages cannot be increased to achieve adequate analgesia (Bhatia et al. 2014)
• Patients on long-term chemotherapy regimens to reduce adverse events (Smith et al. 2002)
• Patients whose psychosocial issues are not a hindrance to IDD therapy as determined by a multidisciplinary evaluation from various professionals including oncologists, neurologists, psychiatrists, and social workers (this assessment may be foregone in end-stage cancer) (Gulati et al. 2014)
• It is no longer recommended to only consider patients with >3 months life expectancy as IDD may improve life expectancy (Deer et al. 2011). In the absence of impending death, IDD should be considered
• Timing of IDDS placement dependent upon acceptable white blood cell and platelet counts (Deer et al. 2011)

that would prevent either the placement of the pump or the return visits necessary for refilling the pump. Typically a formal assessment is determined by a multidisciplinary evaluation from various professionals, but this assessment may be waived in patients with end-stage cancer (Gulati et al. 2014). The timing of the pump placement is also dependent upon the patient having an acceptable presurgical evaluation including an adequate cardiopulmonary status and normal blood count and clotting factors (Deer et al. 2011). There are also other nonsurgical considerations that can increase the risk of IDD for the patient including some common comorbidities (Table 2). These should be taken into consideration prior to considering the patient a candidate for IDD as these comorbidities can increase the risk of an adverse event (Prager et al. 2014; Deer et al. 2010; Deer et al. 2012).

2.2 Screening Trial

The opinions regarding the need for a screening trial prior to the placement of IDD have changed through the years with the constantly evolving practices of pain medicine and oncology. Trialing is typically performed before the patient undergoes pump implantation to determine the efficacy of the IDD and to make sure the patient can tolerate the medication. Trialing was considered to be the standard of care and was a critical step prior

to placement of an intrathecal pump (Deer et al. 2012). In the 2012 Polyanalgesic Consensus Conference (PACC) recommendations, Deer et al. posed the question of the need for trialing in cancer or in any of the end-of-life patients (Deer et al. 2012). The PACC 2012 panel members felt that trialing is not necessary if patients have already tolerated the same drug by another route (Deer et al. 2012). A trial period usually leads to an underestimation of the failure rate and side effects of the IDD as a one-time intrathecal trial dose does not take into account the issues of opioid-induced hyperalgesia (OIH) or disease progression (Deer et al. 2012). Following the 2012 PACC recommendations, Prager et al. just 1 year later in 2013 published the best practice guidelines for IDD for pain and considered trialing as part of the clinical path in a patient being considered for treatment with IDD but did not discuss any of the issues surrounding the necessity of this step, nor did the authors discuss trialing specifically in the setting of cancer pain (Deer et al. 2012). In 2016, Bruel and Burton discussed the same issues raised in the 2012 PACC recommendations and stated that trialing may not be necessary in patients with cancer-related pain and a limited life expectancy (Bruel and Burton 2016). In the following year, an updated PACC guidelines are recommended, with a moderate consensus level (50–79% consensus), against a screening trial for cancer patients (Deer et al. 2017).

Table 2 Other considerations and comorbidities that increase the risks for IDD

- Obstructive sleep apnea
- Restricted cardiac or lung capacity
- Venous insufficiency or existing peripheral edema
- Obesity
- Metabolic syndrome
- Hypertension
- Diabetes
- Kidney disease
- Smoking
- Immunosuppression
- Use of certain drugs (e.g., systemic opioids, benzodiazepines, psychotropics, antihistamines) or supplements (e.g., melatonin, valerian)

2.3 Considerations for the Type of Intrathecal Drug Delivery System (IDDS) for Cancer Patients

Intrathecal drug delivery systems (IDDS) may be placed either percutaneously or fully implanted. Some of the factors to be considered for picking the type of IDDS include the patient's life expectancy, the cost of the system, the availability of professional personnel to place and manage the IDDS, the patients preferences and comfort level with the system, the location of the patient's primary tumor or metastatic disease, and the need for access to certain regions of the body for chemotherapy and radiation (Bhatia et al. 2014; Gulati et al. 2014).

2.3.1 Characteristics of Percutaneous Vs Fully Implanted IDDS (Bhatia et al. 2014)

Percutaneous and fully implanted IDDS systems have different characteristics (Table 3), and knowledge of the differences can help with the selection of the appropriate system for each individual patient. Percutaneous systems are easier to place, are less costly but have a smaller reservoir that is external to the patient, and are typically used for patients that have a limited life expectancy or in patients with limited mobility (Bhatia et al. 2014). Fully implanted subcutaneous systems are placed surgically against the anterior abdominal wall in the right or left lower quadrant, are intended for longer-term use in patients who are mobile, can be controlled via a wireless radiofrequency transmitter, and have a larger reservoir that has to be refilled less often than external pump systems (Bhatia et al. 2014).

See chapter "The Components of Intrathecal Drug Delivery" for information on the components and placement of intrathecal drug delivery systems.

2.4 Choice of Intrathecal Drug for Cancer Pain

Morphine and ziconotide are the only pain medications approved by the FDA for intrathecal (IT) use in chronic pain, which includes cancer pain (Deer et al. 2012). Of the two on-label medications, morphine is the more commonly utilized (Bhatia et al. 2014). Despite only two medications approved for intrathecal use and as monotherapy use only, it is common to combine these with other medications like bupivacaine, hydromorphone, clonidine, fentanyl, and sufentanil (Deer et al. 2012). About 1/100th to 1/300th of the amount of oral medication is needed when switching to IDD (Bhatia et al. 2014). The dosage difference is much lower for intrathecal drug delivery as compared to oral, but if the patient has developed a tolerance to a medication by taking it orally, they will be more in the range of a 1–100 dose rather than a 1 to 300 dose of the medication especially if that medication is an opioid. In general, the management of IT drugs for cancer pain is the same as that of non-cancer pain, which is discussed in detail in chapter "Intrathecal Pump Management". A slight difference in the medication-dosing regimen is the earlier use of multiple medications in those with cancer (Deer

Table 3 Characteristics of percutaneous vs fully implanted IDDS

• **Percutaneous IDDS**
– Easier to place via needle puncture of the skin
– Preferred for limited life expectancy
– Preferred for patients with limited mobility due to risk of catheter migration
– Fluoroscopy may be used to confirm catheter placement
– Medication pump is external
– Costs less
– Reservoirs are smaller, more frequent refills
• **Fully implanted IDDS**
– Placement requires the use of operating room with local or general anesthetic
– Preferred for more long-term use
– Preferred for more mobile patients
– Pump is implanted into the subcutaneous tissue of the abdomen
– Comes in fixed rate pump with potential for variable rate delivery with boluses
– Wireless radiofrequency transmitter may be used to control the pumps with bolus function
– Costs more
– Larger reservoirs, less frequent refills

et al. 2012). In support of multiple intrathecal medications, there is level I evidence for the use of a combination of bupivacaine with an opioid or ziconotide for cancer pain (Deer et al. 2017; Staats et al. 2004). There is also evidence for a higher ratio of bupivacaine to morphine (10:1) to achieve significant pain relief while also reducing opioid side effects (Sjoberg et al. 1994). The reduction of opioid side effect is optimal, but that has to be clinically balanced with potential for side effects from bupivacaine, such as urinary retention, paresthesias, gait impairment, and orthostatic hypotension (Sjoberg et al. 1994). A consultation with experienced cancer care professionals is recommended due to the complexity of the treatment of cancer patients (Deer et al. 2012).

Patients at the end of life may receive higher doses or higher concentrations of drugs, or non-standard combinations of drugs (Deer et al. 2012). It is also recommended to weigh the risks and benefits of IDD, including the optimal pain relief versus the necessary surgical placement and the possibility of infection along with the future possibilities of hospice care and palliative measures (Deer et al. 2012).

2.5 Complications

Complications of IDDS in non-cancer pain patients are the same as those for cancer pain patients. The placement of an IDD system has the potential risks of respiratory depression, infection, bleeding, epidural/spinal hematomas, spinal cord injury during initial catheter placement, wound dehiscence, pocket seromas, and pump malfunction (Bhatia et al. 2014). Catheter complications are the most common, in that they can become dislodged or displaced out of the intrathecal location or can develop tears or kinks (Deer et al. 2012). There are rare reports of mechanical or electronic failure of IT pumps, and some of the earlier generation pumps were found to develop corrosion when a particular non-FDA-approved medication was utilized (Deer et al. 2012). Significant radiation exposure may also cause the IDDS to fail (Deer et al. 2011). Another

consideration is the anatomic surroundings in the intrathecal space where the delivery of the medication occurs. For example, in patients with metastatic disease, the presence of epidural metastases can impair diffusion of IT medication throughout the CSF (Deer et al. 2011).

Opioid medications are associated with respiratory depression, granuloma formation, peripheral edema, and hormone imbalances, and the patient can develop substantial tolerance to any opioid medication (Saulino et al. 2014). Smoking, sleep apnea, chronic obstructive pulmonary disease (COPD), obesity, emphysema, and the use of benzodiazepines, systemic opioids, gabapentin, or melatonin increase the risk for respiratory depression (Deer et al. 2012). In the first 24 h after placement of an IDDS, oxygenation, adequate ventilation, and level of consciousness should be monitored if possible (Deer et al. 2012).

Opioid therapy also affects levels of antidiuretic hormone, which can lead to the development of peripheral edema (Deer et al. 2012). If patients develop peripheral edema that fails other treatments and the edema has no renal or cardiovascular causes, they may be considered for switching the IT medication to ziconotide or other non-opioid medications (Deer et al. 2012). Mechanical treatment for the peripheral edema such as sequential compression, diuretics, or compression stockings may also be used (Deer et al. 2012).

Intrathecal opioids may also cause hormonal changes such as changes in growth hormone, follicle-stimulating hormone, luteinizing hormone, and testosterone (Deer et al. 2012). The potential of opioids to affect hormones should be known as the changes in these hormones may be manifested by a wide variety of symptoms from excessive fatigue to infertility. Risks and benefits of weaning the patient from IT opioids versus treatment with hormone replacement should be discussed prior to selecting the appropriate therapy (Deer et al. 2012).

Intrathecal morphine, hydromorphone, sufentanil, and tramadol have all been associated with granuloma formation (Deer et al. 2012). Using adjuvant therapy with non-opioids can allow for a lower dose of IT opioids to be used and can reduce the risk of granuloma formation (Deer et al. 2012). Switching to other agents such as ziconotide or fentanyl may also be effective as these agents, thus far, have not been associated with granuloma formation (Deer et al. 2012).

Opioid-induced hyperalgesia (OIH) should be suspected in those patients with nociceptive pain that have inadequate pain control on multiple opioids or high-dose opioids (Deer et al. 2012). Weaning the patient off the opioid medication(s) can confirm or refute the presence of OIH (Deer et al. 2012). Weaning the patient down or off of systemic opioids has been shown to be effective in reducing their tolerance and can decrease their degree of OIH (Deer et al. 2012; Hamza et al. 2012). After the weaning process, IT opioids can be started at very low doses and microdosing with doses as low as 12.5 mcg/day may help to prevent or lessen the recurrence of their OIH (Deer et al. 2012; Hamza et al. 2012).

One of the most common complications of IDDS placement is a post-dural puncture headache caused by a cerebrospinal fluid (CSF) leak, usually around the catheter that has been placed into the CSF. This type of headache can be treated with hydration, caffeine, and bed rest (Deer et al. 2012). If it does not resolve with these conservative measures, the patient may be admitted and treated with IV dexamethasone, analgesics, and an epidural blood patch (Deer et al. 2012). Other treatment options include reanchoring of the catheter or placement of fibrin glue around the catheter's dural entry point (Deer et al. 2012). A subdural hematoma is also a potential complication that can contribute to the patient's morbidity and even mortality (Deer et al. 2012).

3 Conclusion

Intrathecal drug delivery has the potential to improve pain and quality of life in the cancer pain patient. Given the recent increasing longevity of the oncologic patient, the use of intrathecal drug delivery may help to reduce the side effects from systemic opioids and from the long-term use of opioids. Moreover, in addition to the proven ben-efits of pain reduction, less medication toxicity, and improved patient survival, advances in intra-thecal medications and technology may continue to improve clinical outcomes in this patient population.

References

Bhatia G, Lau ME, Koury KM, Gulur P (2014) Intrathecal Drug Delivery (ITDD) systems for cancer pain [version 4; peer review: 2 approved, 1 approved with reservations]. F1000Res 2:96. https://doi.org/10.12688/f1000research.2-96.v4

Brogan S, Gulati A (2020) The new face of cancer pain and its treatment. Anesth Analg 130(2):286–288. https://doi.org/10.1213/ANE.0000000000004507

Bruel BM, Burton AW (2016) Intrathecal therapy for cancer-related pain. Pain Med 17(12):2404. https://link.gale.com/apps/doc/A611335392/AONE?u=hscbklyn&sid=AONE&xid=74613a8c

Deer TR, Smith HS, Cousins M et al (2010) Consensus guidelines for the selection and implantation of patients with noncancer pain for intrathecal drug delivery. Pain Physician 13:E175–E213

Deer TR, Smith HS, Burton AW et al (2011) Comprehensive consensus based guidelines on intrathecal drug delivery systems in the treatment of pain caused by cancer pain. Pain Physician 14: E283–E312

Deer TR et al (2012) Polyanalgesic consensus conference 2012: recommendations for the management of pain by intrathecal (intraspinal) drug delivery: report of an interdisciplinary expert panel. Neuromodulation 15(5):436–466. https://doi.org/10.1111/j.1525-1403.2012.00476.x

Deer TR, Pope JE, Hayek SM et al (2017) The polyanalgesic consensus conference (PACC): recommendations on intrathecal drug infusion systems best practices and guidelines. Neuromodulation 20(2):96–132. https://doi.org/10.1111/ner.12538

Gulati A, Puttanniah V, Hung J et al (2014) Considerations for evaluating the use of intrathecal drug delivery in the oncologic patient. Curr Pain Headache Rep 18(2):391

Hamza M, Doleys D, Wells M, Weisbein J, Hoff J, Martin M, Soteropoulos C, Barreto J, Deschner S, Ketchum J (2012) Prospective study of 3-year follow-up of low-dose intrathecal opioids in the management of chronic nonmalignant pain. Pain Med 13(10):1304–1313. https://doi.org/10.1111/j.1526-4637.2012.01451.x

Prager J, Deer T, Levy R, Bruel B, Buchser E, Caraway D, Cousins M, Jacobs M, McGlothlen G, Rauck R, Staats P, Stearns L (2014) Best practices for intrathecal drug delivery for pain. Neuromodulation 17(4):354–372. https://doi-org.newproxy.downstate.edu/10.1111/ner.12146

Saulino M, Kim PS, Shaw E (2014) Practical considerations and patient selection for intrathecal drug delivery in the management of chronic pain. J Pain Res 7:627–638

Sjoberg M, Nitescu P, Appelgren L et al (1994) Long-term intrathecal morphine and bupivacaine in patients with refractory cancer pain. Results from a morphine: bupivacaine dose regimen of 0.5:4.75mg/ml. Anesthesiology 80(2):284–297

Smith TJ, Staats PS, Deer T, Stearns LJ, Rauck RL, Boortz-Marx RL, Buchser E, Català E, Bryce DA, Coyne PJ, Pool GE (2002) Randomized clinical trial of an implantable drug delivery system compared with comprehensive medical management for refractory cancer pain: impact on pain, drug-related toxicity, and survival. J Clin Oncol 20(19):4040–4049. https://doi.org/10.1200/JCO.2002.02.118

Staats PS, Yearwood T, Charapata SG et al (2004) Intrathecal ziconotide in the treatment of refractory pain in patients with cancer or AIDS: a randomized controlled trial. JAMA 291(1):63–70

van den Beuken-van Everdingen MH (2016) Update on prevalence of pain in patients with cancer: systematic review and meta-analysis. J Pain Symptom Manag 51(6):1070–1090.e9. https://doi.org/10.1016/j.jpainsymman.2015.12.340

Whitehead SJ, Ali S (2010) Health outcomes in economic evaluation: the QALY and utilities. Br Med Bull 96(1):5–21. https://doi.org/10.1093/bmb/ldq033

The Components of Intrathecal Drug Delivery

Daniel A. Fung, Matthew R. Robinson, Hardik P. Parikh, and Timothy Davis

Contents

Abstract

Intrathecal drug delivery was first described by August Bier, the "father of intrathecal anesthesia," who first administered intrathecal cocaine on his colleagues in an experimental capacity and then in 1898 used this method to treat acute pain surrounding lower limb orthopedic surgery (Bier 1899). Nearly 100 years later, the FDA approved intrathecal morphine in 1984 and intrathecal baclofen in 1992 for intractable pain and intractable spasticity, respectively, followed by the approval of intrathecal ziconotide for pain (Penn et al. 1989; Duarte et al. 2016). Since the early 1980s, three pump manufacturers have achieved FDA approval for intrathecal drug delivery: Medtronic, Flowonix, and Johnson

D. A. Fung (✉) · T. Davis
Source Healthcare, Santa Monica, CA, USA
e-mail: dfung@sourcehealthcare.com

M. R. Robinson · H. P. Parikh
VA Greater Los Angeles Healthcare System, Physical Medicine and Rehabilitation Residency Program, Los Angeles, CA, USA

© The Author(s), under exclusive license to Springer Nature Switzerland AG 2022
D. P. Beall et al. (eds.), *Intrathecal Pump Drug Delivery*, Medical Radiology Diagnostic Imaging,
https://doi.org/10.1007/978-3-030-86244-2_3

& Johnson but Johnson & Johnson has ceased manufacturing their Codman pump as of 2018. Therefore, the Medtronic and Flowonix devices are the only pumps currently being implanted in an on-label manner for intrathecal drug delivery. The majority of the pumps implanted in the United States are manufactured by Medtronic (Farid 2017). This chapter will serve to discuss the components of intrathecal drug delivery systems across the two remaining manufactures that are vital in bringing the infused medication from the pump reservoir to the intrathecal space, thereby bypassing the blood-brain barrier. Medication that is infused into the intrathecal space consequently requires significantly reduced doses of all medications compared to oral bioavailability and has a far lesser tendency to cause medication tolerance (Sylvester et al. 2004). This chapter will also highlight differences in componentry which may be of value when considering the clinical appropriateness for implantation in patients with cancer or non-cancer pain as well as spasticity.

1   Intrathecal Pain Pump Models

1.1   Medtronic SynchroMed® II Intrathecal Pump

The Model 8637 SynchroMed® II is an implantable intrathecal infusion system manufactured by Medtronic, Inc. (Medtronic, Inc., Dublin, Ireland). This infusion system is comprised of a programmable pump connected to a catheter that together deliver a prescribed dose of medication from the pump's drug reservoir to the selected infusion site to help manage the patient's symptoms. The packaging contains the following sterile items: the intrathecal pump, a 22-gauge non-coring needle in a black sheath used to fill the pump, a 24-gauge non-coring needle in a purple sheath used to flush the catheter access port,

empty 20-mL syringes to empty the pump, a 0.22-μm filter, and a 10-mL syringe filled with 1–2 mL of sterile, and preservative-free saline to flush the catheter access port. The non-sterile item in the packaging is the Medtronic clinician pump programmer that is used to interrogate the pump, battery status, and pump settings prior to implantation.

The on-label indications for implantation of this infusion system in the United States include using the system for chronic intrathecal infusion of Infumorph® or Mitigo™ which are preservative-free morphine sulfate sterile solutions used for the management of chronic intractable pain. Additional indications include chronic intrathecal infusion of Prialt®, a preservative-free ziconotide sterile solution to treat chronic pain, as well as the intrathecal infusion of baclofen for the management of severe spasticity. Contraindications to implantation of the infusion system include the presence of an infection, implanting the pump at a depth greater than 2.5 cm below skin, inadequate body size to accommodate the bulk and weight of the pump, and spinal anomalies that hinder proper catheter placement or CSF flow. Additionally, the use of medications with preservatives or medication formulations with a pH of less than or equal to three is contraindicated with this drug delivery system. In regard to the management of the intrathecal drug delivery system, the delivery of an opioid pain medication via the myPTM™ Personal Therapy Manager, a self-directed intermittent bolus application, has a relative contraindication in opioid-naïve patients (SynchroMed 2020).

This model is manufactured with either a 20-mL pump reservoir (8637-20 model) or a 40-mL pump reservoir (8637-40 model). Accordingly, the approximate device specifications are unique to each model and contingent upon the volume of the pump reservoir housed within the device. The 8637-20 model has a thickness of 19.6 mL, weighs 146 g when pump is empty and 166 g when full, and contains 17.5 mL of sterile water on shipping from manufacturing. The 8637-40 model has a thickness of

26.1 mL, weighs 152 g when the pump is empty and 192 g when full, and contains 37.5 mL of sterile water on shipping from manufacturing. Both pumps have an equal diameter of 87.5 mm and residual volume of 1.4 mL ± 1.0 mL. Pump settings after manufacturing include it being set to the lowest flow rate of 0.006 mL per day. This infusion rate is called the minimum rate, and this is designed to preserve the integrity of the internal pump tubing by keeping the peristaltic pump action going. Immediately after being manufactured, the critical and noncritical alarms are disabled for shipping and storage. The decision about which pump to use is based on the dose of medication required to properly manage the underlying condition as well as implantation considerations that are unique to each patient. The goal is to maximize the time between refills as much as possible to make it convenient for the patient while keeping in mind that the maximum time that the medication is allowed to remain in the pump is 6 months.

While the device specifications vary based on the pump reservoir volume, the overall design and the components that comprise both the 8637-20 and 8637-40 models are identical. The exterior of the pump is made of titanium, and this is the part that comes into contact with human tissue on implantation. The exterior view reveals several pump features including the reservoir fill port, catheter access port, catheter port, and suture loops (Fig. 1). The reservoir fill port allows access to the interior pump reservoir by way of its silicone septum, which can withstand approximately 500 punctures. The external catheter access port also has a silicone septum with a lifetime of approximately 100 punctures that leads to the titanium catheter port to which the implanted catheter is connected. This aspect of the pump's design allows the clinician to circumvent the internal pump system to administer medication directly to the infusion site for diagnostic and therapeutic purposes and allows the indwelling medication within the catheter to be aspirated and removed. The final piece of the exterior design is the titanium suture loops through which sutures are passed to anchor the pump within the tissue pocket during the implantation process. The primary components of the internal pump mechanisms are the pump reservoir, internal pump tubing, and radiopaque identifier (Fig. 2). The titanium pump reservoir stores the drug and, as discussed in detail at the beginning of the section, is manufactured with either a volume of 20 mL or 40 mL. The reservoir leads to the internal pump tubing made of silicone rubber that serves as the conduit by which the drug

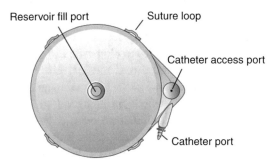

Fig. 1 Exterior view of the SynchroMed® II pump

Fig. 2 Interior view of SynchroMed® II pump components

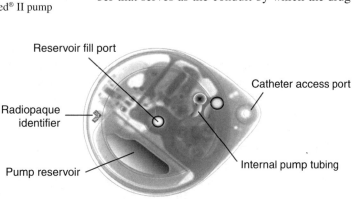

ultimately reaches the catheter attached the catheter port. In addition to the pump reservoir and tubing, a radiopaque identifier is placed inside the pump and contains the manufacturer name and model code that can be visualized by routine radiography (Fig. 2).

Given that approximately 80% of patients with spinal cord stimulators (SCS) require magnetic resonance imaging (MRI) after implantation and a similar number have a comorbid condition that is most optimally assessed by MRI, it is expected that patients with implanted programmable intrathecal drug delivery systems will likely require future MRI studies (Von Korff et al. 2005; Desai et al. 2015). The safety concerns surrounding MRI in patients with implanted medical devices stem from the interaction of the powerful magnetic field and its spatial gradients, pulsed-gradient magnetic fields, and pulsed radiofrequency fields with the device and its metallic, magnetic, and conductive components as well as some of the non-ferromagnetic and nonconductive materials. Potential complications that can result from this interaction include but are not limited to device displacement or damage, interruption of the telemetric communication between pump components, heating of the device and surrounding tissue by current induced by the magnetic field, and alteration of programmed pump parameters (Desai et al. 2015; De Andres et al. 2011). As such, these devices are not classified as "MRI safe" by the Food and Drug Administration (FDA). Rather, they are classified as "MRI conditional" because they have been deemed to be relatively safe when studied in 1.5 T and 3.0 T MRI scanners. Accordingly, the Model 8637 SynchroMed® II is MRI conditionally safe in 1.5 T and 3.0 T MRI environments. Though this model is considered to be MRI conditionally safe, there remains a concern that the pump's magnetic rotor can stall when aligned with the magnetic fields of the MRI and preclude delivery of medication with a potential delay in recovery of pump function (Desai et al. 2015). Therefore, the pump should be interrogated after an MRI scan to ensure that the hardware and software are not malfunctioning and that the pump continues to function properly.

1.2 Flowonix Prometra® II Intrathecal Pump

The Prometra® II Intrathecal Pump is also an implantable, programmable drug delivery pump manufactured by the company, Flowonix Medical Inc. (Flowonix Medical, Inc., Mt. Olive, New Jersey, USA). Similar to the SynchroMed® II device, the on-label indications for use of the Prometra® II pump include intrathecal infusion of preservative-free morphine sulfate sterile solutions (Infumorph® and Mitigo™) as well as preservative-free sterile 0.9% saline solution. The preservative-free morphine sulfate solutions are indicated for intrathecal or epidural infusion for treatment of chronic intractable pain. The FDA has also more recently approved the use of intrathecal baclofen (ITB) via the Prometra® II pump for severe refractory spasticity.

Several contraindications to Prometra® II pump implantation have been noted by Flowonix. These contraindications include the presence of infection, insufficient body habitus to accommodate the pump, a pump implantation depth more than 2.5 cm below the skin, cerebral spinal fluid flow obstruction, a spinal deformity that would preclude the acceptable placement of the intrathecal catheter, allergies to either the catheter or pump materials, and a past medical history of substance abuse. Some of the other more unusual contraindications include professional or personal exposure to high-voltage industrial equipment, high-strength magnets, radio transmitting towers, or hyperbaric exposure. Additional contraindications related to the patient's physiology include the use of anticoagulants, the presence of a bleeding disorder, and an allergy to the medication of choice.

The Prometra® II pump is MRI conditionally safe. The pump was demonstrated to be MRI safe via nonclinical testing of patients with implants located in the abdomen within a static magnetic field at 1.5 T with a maximum spatial field gradient of 1900 gauss/cm and scan duration that did not exceed 10 minutes per sequence. Additionally, for the Prometra® pump, the medication must be removed from the pump reservoir and catheter as the MRI may cause opening of inlet/outlet valves leading to inadvertent discharge of medication from the reservoir or catheter. In the event of an emergent MRI scan and the medication was not removed prior to the study, Prometra® II devices have a flow-activated valve that reduces but does not eliminate the risk of overdose and possible death. Clinicians must be mindful of alternative routes of medication administration during MRI testing to ensure no withdrawal symptoms develop from halting the patient's targeted drug delivery.

Programming of the Prometra® II pump includes four different modes: constant flow, periodic flow, multiple rates, and zero-rate technology. The possible flow rates range from 0.00 to 28.8 mL per day. The pump is capable to achieve a 0.00 mL per day flow rate owing to the constant positive pressure of the reservoir maintaining catheter patency when there is no flow. The pump's precision dosing system delivers the intrathecal medication with two microflow-controlled valves requiring less energy as compared to the peristaltic designs featured in other manufacturer's pumps. The constant flow program delivers a basal rate of intrathecal medication throughout the day without variable boluses. The multiple rate dosing can deliver up to four different flow rates throughout the day without delivering boluses. The clinician programmer is able to establish flow rates during particular specified times of day that may vary from other intervals in the day. Periodic flow schedules a basal rate throughout the day with medication boluses at fixed intervals. The programmer will establish the intervals of drug delivery as well as the dose of medication boluses in addition to the set basal rate. The zero-rate technology allows boluses to be programmed without a basal dose owing, in part, to the ability of the pump to have a zero flow. The zero flow rate may also be incorporated into one of the delivery rates of a multiple-rate programmed pump (Flowonix Medical 2020a).

The Prometra® II is only manufactured with a 20-mL reservoir (in comparison to the SynchroMed® II that also has a 40-mL variety). Its pump refill port design offers additional features made to improve efficacy of the refill procedure. The port is physically elevated slightly so as to make it more easily identified by subcutaneous palpation by the clinician prior to access. Additionally, the port is approximately 38% wider than the SynchroMed® II port, and the septum is tested to withstand around 1000 punctures by a 22-gauge non-coring Huber needle. The pump reservoir is under constant positive pressure, which potentially offers some utility in terms of safety during refills. Not only will less aspiration force be necessary to empty the pump, but increased force will be required to fill the pump. This may serve as an added failsafe during the refill procedure to ensure the medication is being delivered into the pump's reservoir. The battery life is listed as a minimum of 10 years when the flow rate is at 0.25 mL per day.

1.3 Codman® 3000 Constant Flow Pump

The manufacturing, sale, and promotion of the intrathecal pump designed by Codman® were discontinued by Johnson & Johnson in April of 2018. The company still maintains the support and ongoing care of preexisting patients who had been previously implanted with the Codman® 3000 system, and these patients remain a significant care priority with 24-h clinical and technical support services.

The Codman® 3000 intrathecal pump was used for the intrathecal delivery of analgesia, chemotherapy, and baclofen. The pump reservoir volume was available in 16, 30, and 50-mL sizes. This reservoir is also maintained under constant positive pressure via a fluorocarbon propellant and medications pumped through an antibacterial and anti-particulate filter into the intrathecal catheter. Achievable flow rates were somewhat limited ranging from 0.5 mL per day to 2.0 mL per day. The Johnson & Johnson website labels this pump as MRI conditional via nonclinical testing in both 1.5 T and 3.0 T MRI scanners. The MRI exposure time is recommended to not exceed 15 min. Any MRI studies lasting longer than 15 min requires a cooling delay of 15 min or the patient is placed at an increased risk of overdose due to increased flow rates to the intrathecal space. The Codman® MRI technical information includes a table of increased flow rates during the expected 6.5 °C rise in pump temperature after 15 min of continuous scanning. Clinicians are encouraged to completely empty the pump if the patient cannot tolerate the increased dose that the maximal listed flow rates will produce.

While Johnson & Johnson has discontinued the manufacturing of the Codman® 3000 intrathecal pump, the needed supplies for maintenance, such as refill kits, are still supplied to hospitals and healthcare providers (Medtronic 2015a).

2 Intrathecal Catheters and Catheter Insertion Kits

2.1 Medtronic Ascenda® Catheter

The catheter is the component of the infusion system that is implanted in the intrathecal space and connected to the pump to deliver the prescribed drug to the desired location. The two catheters that are compatible with the SynchroMed® II intrathecal pump are the Medtronic Model 8780 and 8781 Ascenda® Intrathecal Catheters. The catheter insertion kit contains a selection of 16-gauge stainless steel introducer needles, the pump and spinal segments of the catheter, a catheter connector with two attached collets, anchor with a dispenser tool, a non-sterile ruler, and product literature.

The basic design of these catheters is that of a pump segment that attaches to the intrathecal pump via a suture-less pump connector and a spinal segment that is advanced in the intrathecal space to the desired level under fluoroscopic guidance (Fig. 3). Both the pump and spinal segments have a polyurethane jacket. The catheter

tip has a platinum iridium radiopaque mark on the tip, interval markers of black silicone ink, a polyester braid catheter design, and an inner lumen made of radiopaque silicone. The goal of this multilayer construction is to ensure catheter integrity and provide high tensile strength capable of resisting compression and distraction. The implantable spinal segment of the catheter comes preloaded with a stainless-steel guidewire that is 0.5 mm in diameter, and it's attached to a plastic guidewire handle. Once the spinal catheter tip is positioned at the proper level, the extrathecal spinal segment of the catheter is threaded through the anchor dispenser tool that is made of polycarbonate, stainless steel, and polytetrafluoroethylene, and the anchor is attached to the lumbodorsal fascia prior to tunneling the catheter to the pump implantation site. This anchor tool holds the catheter in place, and the attachment to the fascia is done by placing sutures through its wings to secure catheter and anchor in place. The spinal segment is then tunneled from the spinal incision site to the pump pocket site, where it is trimmed to the appropriate length and attached to the pump segment via a catheter connector. The connector is made of platinum iridium and nylon with two nylon collets 4.3 mm in diameter on each end. The purpose of the non-sterile ruler is to measure the portion of the spinal catheter that is trimmed away and subtract this length from the original catheter length to calculate the final length and associated volume of the implanted catheter. The product literature is also a component of the catheter insertion kit and can be referred to as an important source of information.

Though similar in design, the approximate dimensions of the two catheters are different. The total catheter length of the Medtronic Model

Fig. 3 Pump and spinal segments of the Ascenda® Intrathecal Catheter adjoined by the catheter connector

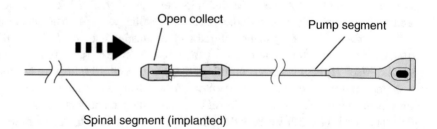

Open collect

Pump segment

Spinal segment (implanted)

8780 Ascenda® Intrathecal Catheter is approximately 114.3 cm, which is subdivided into the 86.4-cm length of the spinal segment and 27.9-cm length of the pump segment. In contrast, the Medtronic Model 8781 Ascenda® Intrathecal Catheter has a longer pump segment of 73.7 cm, which when added to the 66.0-cm spinal segment length results in a total catheter length of approximately 139.7 cm. The spinal and pump segments of both pumps have outer and inner diameters of 1.2 mm and 0.5 mm, respectively, with interval markers 1 cm apart. The tip of the spinal segment of both catheters is closed with six-side fluid-outlet holes. Both pumps have a catheter volume of 0.0022 mL per cm, and this value is multiplied by the length of the implanted catheter to calculate the final volume of the implanted catheter (Discontinuation of the Codman® Constant Flow Pump 2020; Medtronic 2015b).

2.2 Prometra® Intrathecal Catheter

The Prometra® II infusion pump attaches to a single catheter for use in the intrathecal space. The catheter is 110 cm in length and placed intrathecally via a 15-gauge Tuohy needle. It comes preloaded with an intraluminal stylet/guidewire that when in contact with saline activates a hydrophilic response that lubricates the catheter to prevent bunching when the guidewire is removed after catheter placement. Lubrication is achieved via a flushing hub on the catheter, preventing the need to lubricate the guidewire separately prior to catheter placement. The catheter is sutured to the underlying fascia via the Flowonix anchors provided in the kit. The catheter is then tunneled to the pump, and the catheter base is connected to the Prometra® II pump via the catheter connector which slides over the catheter prior to connecting to the pump stem. The catheter connector eliminates the need for suturing the catheter to the pump. Inserting the catheter connector to the pump stem will result in an audible and tactile "click." The pump stem is flexible, lessening the potential for a stress riser at the catheter-pump junction. The tip of the catheter has a tungsten tip

that is integral for identification during fluoroscopic-guided placement. This allows the physician to easily visualize the catheter tip position and to place it at a level that most appropriately delivers the medication for the desired clinical outcome via the eight staggered side holes. Measurement of catheter length is done by way of the graduated centimeter markings on the catheter (Flowonix Medical 2020b).

Similar to the Synchromed II catheter insertion kit, Flowonix also has a catheter insertion kit for the Prometra® II pump. The Prometra® II catheter insertion kit comes with a radiopaque intrathecal catheter and the preloaded hydrophilic guidewire. The kit also comes with the catheter lock for mounting to the pump stem, as well as the flushing hub. There is also an 8.9 cm, 15-gauge Tuohy needle and sterile 12-mL syringe. There is only one length of needle that comes in the kit with no longer Tuohy needle for patients who may have more soft tissue or adiposity. For anchoring, the kit comes with two angled anchors and one straight anchor.

3 Clinician Programmers and Patient Control Devices

3.1 SynchroMed® II Clinician Programmer and Patient Therapy Manager

The Medtronic Model A810 SynchroMed® II Clinician Programmer is an application designed to enable the clinician to program the settings of the Model 8637 SynchroMed® II intrathecal infusion pump following implantation. This application platform is comprised of the touchscreen clinician tablet equipped with the clinician programmer software application (app), a Universal Serial Bus (USB) connector cable, the Model 8880T2 Communicator, and the Model A902 Patient Data Service App (Fig. 4).

The clinician tablet is a portable computer device with a backlit display and touchscreen user interface, similar to those currently available to the general public, that comes loaded with the SynchroMed II clinical programmer app. When

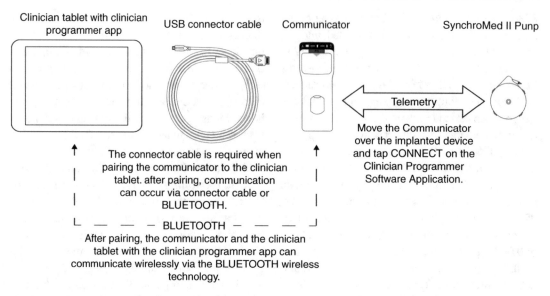

Clinician tablet with clinician programmer app   USB connector cable   Communicator   SynchroMed II Punp

The connector cable is required when pairing the communicator to the clinician tablet. after pairing, communication can occur via connector cable or BLUETOOTH.

Move the Communicator over the implanted device and tap CONNECT on the Clinician Programmer Software Application.

Telemetry

BLUETOOTH
After pairing, the communicator and the clinician tablet with the clinician programmer app can communicate wirelessly via the BLUETOOTH wireless technology.

Fig. 4 SynchroMed® II Clinician Programmer components

this app is launched, the home screen appears first, displaying the current pump settings and several workflow options from which the clinician can choose to meet their specific programming needs. These workflow options include "Refill & Adjust," "Implant/Replace Pump," "Revise Catheter," "Discontinue Therapy," and "Workflow Guide Off." Each of these options launches a separate screen containing a series of workflow tasks through which the pump parameters can be modified as indicated by the clinician for the particular task.

The Model 8880T2 Communicator enables wireless communication between the intrathecal pump and the clinician tablet and clinician programmer application via telemetry. The communicator is powered by batteries and has a LED battery level indicator on the top right of the device. This indicator flashes green for 10 seconds when the battery level is appropriate, amber when the batteries should be replaced soon, and red when the batteries should be replaced immediately. When programming the pump for the first time, the clinician tablet must be paired with the communicator using the USB connector cable. Once the clinician tablet and communicator have been paired, the USB cable can be disconnected, as the paired devices will automatically communicate wirelessly thereafter via Bluetooth tech-

nology within a 3-m range. Besides the initial pairing session, the USB cable is utilized when firmware updates must be downloaded to the communicator via the tablet as well as instances in which Bluetooth is prohibited or there is interference by other devices that preclude successful wireless communication between the devices. The communicator should be placed directly over the pump to establish a connection.

The Model A902 Patient Data Service App allows the clinician to access the various session reports, which contain information about the patient's, pump settings and programming updates, and device session history for all pumps that have been programmed on a single clinician tablet and its programmer app. These reports include the "Patient Report," "Session Short Report," "Session Long Report," and "Refill Report," and the Patient Data Service App categorizes them by patient name, date of service, or device type. This app is distinct from the aforementioned SynchroMed® II programmer app and has a separate icon by which it may be accessed from the home screen (Medtronic 2018a).

An additional software application that is compatible with the SynchroMed® II infusion system is the myPTM™ Personal Therapy Manager application. The myPTM™ app is accessible through mobile phones, and it has a

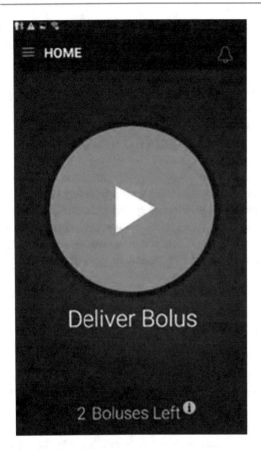

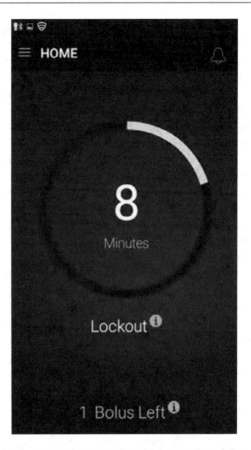

Fig. 5 myPTM™ app user interface

Fig. 6 myPTM™ app display with lockout timer following successful bolus delivery

simple, user-friendly design to facilitate ease of use for patients. This is a treatment option that is most suitable for patients who are not opioid naïve as it provides on-demand access to drug boluses prescribed to help mitigate unpredictable bouts of pain. Bolus dosing parameters that must be programmed by the treating physician include bolus dose, bolus rate, lockout period, and maximum number of daily boluses. The app displays a large blue play button at its center with "Deliver Bolus" and the number of boluses remaining captioned below the symbol when the bolus dose is to be activated (Fig. 5). Once selected, the app will notify the patient that either the bolus request was successful and the bolus is being delivered or that the request was denied because no additional bolus doses remain. If the request is successful, the app will then display a clear lockout timer that notifies patients of the time remaining until the next bolus dose can be delivered by the pump

(Fig. 6) (Medtronic 2018b). Studies have shown that this type of patient-controlled analgesia with bolus dosing options helps reduce the use of oral pain medications and increases patient satisfaction with intrathecal drug delivery systems (Bolash et al. 2018; Ilias et al. 2008).

3.2 Prometra® II Clinician Programmer and Patient Therapy Controller

The Prometra® II clinician programmer allows practitioners to set and adjust settings of the Prometra® II pump. The programmer device is a backlit, touchscreen interface to help facilitate workflow. The device incorporates a touchscreen keyboard to minimize time spent programming. The healthcare provider may adjust all dosing options available to the pump including constant flow, multiple rates, periodic flow, and zero-rate technology. The programmer communicates wirelessly with the Prometra® II pump.

The clinician programmer maintains a pump history log that is easily accessible and provides information incorporating both clinician settings and patient therapy control that shows infusion rates as well as patient-driven bolus requests and delivered boluses. Internal calculations mathematically generate a pump refill date. Clinicians can access pump flow modes and adjust as clinically appropriate. The clinician programmer also has an emergency stop function to stop all intrathecal drug delivery upon confirmation.

Patient-controlled analgesia is made possible by including patient access to the pump via the Patient Therapy Controller (PTC®). This is a stand-alone electronic device that has a touch-screen interface with a color LCD. The design is meant to be patient-friendly and is handheld (the screen is 2.7 inches when measured diagonally). The PTC has two buttons mounted for ease of operation. The two buttons are the power button and the prescription button, labeled "Rx." Pressing the Rx button when the PTC is placed over the implanted Prometra® II pump will release a pre-configured intrathecal bolus dose. The clinician configures the amount of medication bolus during a regular clinic visit via the clinician programmer as well as a total daily limit to the number of boluses and a lockout interval whereby a patient will not be allowed to initiate a subsequent bolus. This allows the patient to access a previously defined intrathecal dose of opiates without resorting to oral opiates during an unexpected pain flare (Flowonix Medical 2020c).

The PTC shows the current battery level of the PTC itself as well as the date of next Prometra® II pump refill. The PTC also keeps a record of the boluses delivered each day that can later be accessed by the Prometra® II clinician programmer. The clinician can then assess the total number boluses in a given day, which may guide treatment and further consideration of flow rate adjustments. For the PTC to be enabled, the pump must be programmed to constant flow, and a daily dose limit must be established. Clinicians can then set bolus dose amount, bolus duration, post-bolus lockout period, and the allotted number of boluses per day.

4   Flow Rate Accuracy

There are several documented complications associated with long-term implantations of intrathecal drug delivery systems. In addition to the risks associated with the surgical implantation of these devices, complications that may occur after the perioperative period in patients with long-term use of intrathecal drug delivery devices include but are not limited to infection, seroma, drug overdose, drug withdrawal, failure of pump componentry, and catheter breakage or obstruction among others. Complications rates associated with targeted drug delivery (TDD) vary widely in the literature. For instance, there has been noted an infectious complication in 8.71% of patients following a 145 patients after implant with mean follow-up of 7.24 years (Malheiro et al. 2015). Another study extrapolated that there is a risk of infection equal to 0.6% per puncture when a pump is refilled on average 57.3 days over the course of 16 years (Chan et al. 2018a). A 14-year retrospective evaluation of 430 patients noted at least one complication of some kind in 25% of implanted patients with most being attributed to failure or inaccuracy of componentry (Motta and Antonello 2014).

The accuracy of the Prometra® pump has been assessed in a clinical study evaluating the programmed drug delivery versus the actual drug delivered to the intrathecal space. Rauck et al. found that after almost 600 refill visits, 107 patients maintained a 97.1% morphine sulfate intrathecal delivery accuracy up to 6 months after implantation (Rauck et al. 2010). Only five patients fell outside of an acceptable range defined as 85–115%, and the authors hypothesized that this was due to very small flow rates that may be more susceptible to flow rate discrepancies. The same authors noted similar accuracy of 97.9% after 12 months (Rauck et al. 2013). Rosen et al. researched if there is a discrepancy between the delivery of Infumorph versus pharmacy-compounded morphine. The delivery of Infumorph in 31 patients was calculated to be 100.1%, while compound morphine was 97.4%, but this difference was not found to be statistically significant (Rosen et al. 2013).

Similarly, the SynchroMed® II pump has also been researched for accuracy of intrathecal drug delivery. Wesemann et al. evaluated 65 participants who were implanted with a SynchroMed® device and followed for 12 months (Wesemann et al. 2014). At 6 months, the calculated drug delivery was 101%. This was again demonstrated at 12 months with the same accuracy. Conversely, Farid et al. noted slight under-infusion and no infusion rates calculated to be over 100% (Farid et al. 2019). The authors hypothesize that flow rates very slightly decline over the life of the pump. This may be why calculations are different compared to the newly implanted pumps from the formerly mentioned study.

5 Pump Maintenance

A major consideration when discussing pump implantation with potential intrathecal drug delivery candidates is the longevity, or lifespan, of the pump. As the pump is powered electronically and is under constant or variable daily flow rates, the pump and/or pump components will inevitably fail if continued indefinitely. If the life expectancy of the patient is greater than the pump itself, this will dictate the timing of another surgery for the patient to continue intrathecal drug delivery. Additionally, it is important to monitor the replacement date on each pump refill as to take precautions to prevent drug withdrawal in the event the pump fails close to the time of the impending pump revision. Replacement date indicators may be accessed by the clinician at each interrogation during pump refills via the previously mentioned clinician programmers.

According to the Medtronic SynchroMed® II manual, the device longevity is listed as ranging from 4 to 7 years (SynchroMed 2020). There is variability in lifespan of the device due different flow rates and patient-requested boluses. In clinical studies of over 500 implants, the average lifespan was shown to be 5.9 years under a best-case scenario with no complications or premature revisions necessary (Bolash et al. 2015). By comparison, the Flowonix Prometra® II manual notes that when comparing flow rates and device longevity to SynchroMed® II, at 0.25 mL daily the Prometra® II device would last 10 years compared to 7 years for the SynchroMed® II pump (Flowonix 2019).

During pump refills, the reservoir is accessed via a non-coring Huber needle regardless of which intrathecal device is implanted. Per their respective manuals, the SynchroMed® II septum can withstand an average of 500 punctures, and the Prometra® II septum can withstand an average of 1000 punctures (SynchroMed 2020; Flowonix 2019). There is an obvious discrepancy between the devices, but given the number of times the pump will need to be refilled in its lifespan, there is no practical difference. In a 16-year retrospective study following infection rates with baclofen pump refills in patients with spasticity, the average refill interval was 57.3 days ± 15.4 days (Chan et al. 2018b). Even if the pump was accessed once per month over a 10-year period, the total number of punctures would be 120, well below either device's puncture threshold.

Clinicians can use various techniques to refill the pump. They can use the pump device templates that come with the refill kit, palpation only, or imaging such as ultrasound or fluoroscopy to access the reservoir port with a Huber needle. As mentioned previously, the Prometra® II reservoir has a raised edge around the reservoir port that may aid in palpating the center of the pump prior to accessing the port. There are also sonographic implications to the raised edge of the refill access port. While using ultrasound to visualize the device, the Prometra® II reservoir port appears as a dome-shaped echogenic focus which may be easier to visualize as compared to the anechoic depression that is seen with the SynchroMed® II pump (Saulino and Gofeld 2014).

6 Programming Strategies for Intrathecal Pumps

Following implantation, the pump settings must be changed from the default programmed during manufacturing to the treating physician's settings to create an infusion protocol designed to meet patients' individual treatment goals. Establishing such a protocol for drug delivery allows for a precise amount of the prescribed medication to be delivered at a preset dose and frequency that affords the patient with sufficient analgesia while mitigating the risk of adverse medication effects and drug overdose. For patients in whom the intrathecal drug delivery system is implanted for the treatment of severe spasticity, the pump may be programmed by the physician according to the following programming strategies that have been discussed above: simple continuous mode, flex dosing, and periodic bolus dosing.

The initial parameters that must be entered by the physician after implantation include the initial infusion rate and priming bolus dose. The initial infusion rate is the desired rate at which the medication is to be administered to the patient by the device. The priming bolus dose pertains to the pump and segment of the catheter that is devoid of the medication, known as the catheter's dead space, following implantation. The priming bolus dose is not delivered to the patient but serves to fill the dead space with medication. This dose in milligrams is calculated by multiplying the implanted catheter plus the fluid path volume (mL) by the drug concentration (mg/mL). The total drug volume is contingent upon the length of the implanted catheter—calculated by subtracting the trimmed catheter length from the length of the original packaged catheter in the kit—as well as the volume of the pump tubing.

For intrathecal baclofen therapy, studies recommend filling the pump and starting baclofen therapy at the time of implantation such that only the catheter is left to prime after the procedure.

This enables the medication to reach the catheter tip quickly and treatment to begin under medical supervision. Typically, the recommended dose of baclofen at the time of therapy initiation is twice the dose administered during the screening test though a starting dose equal to that of the trial may be considered for patients who had any time of unusual response to the test dose or if the clinician would like to start the dose titration more slowly. The optimal dose is contingent upon factors unique to each patient and achieved through dose titration over a period of time. The recommended daily dose increase for adults is 5–15% over 24 h for spasticity of cerebral origin and 10–30% for spasticity of spinal origin. The recommended daily dose increase over 24 h for children is 5–15%. The period over which the dose is titrated is influenced by individual factors such as the patient's response, their ambulatory status, and whether they are being titrated in a monitored setting. The titration phase is considered complete when the patient has been successfully weaned off of oral antispasmodic agents to an optimal intrathecal baclofen dose that does not result in adverse drug effects.

The dosing strategy by which an optimal dose of medication is delivered intrathecally is contingent upon the discussion between the patient and the physician regarding the goals of therapy, symptoms, timing, and patient response. A common infusion mode utilized for intrathecal baclofen delivery is the simple continuous mode in which a uniform dose of medication is administered over a 24-h cycle. A single bolus can be programmed with this mode to provide the patient with a bolus dose over a set period of time in what is called the single bolus/simple continuous mode. Flex dosing is an alternate strategy useful for optimizing functional status in patients whose symptoms fluctuate predictably over the course of a 24-h period. With this mode, a basal dose is administered with a programmed dose escalation of 10–15% in addition to their normal baseline dose when the patients' symptoms are expected to worsen or interfere with their quality of life. In most patients, the time to desired clinical effect from the dose increase or decrease is approximately 2 h. The periodic bolus dosing strategy can be employed to manage symptoms that are refractory to dose escalation. This infusion mode divides the total daily dose into a baseline dose and bolus dose. The bolus dose is calculated as a percentage of the total daily dose and divided by the number of times boluses are to be administered. In order to preserve the absolute daily dose, the basal dose is lowered when the bolus doses are administered at scheduled intervals that are typically spaced 6 h apart for a total of four boluses daily. When using this strategy, the recommendation is to trial a single bolus first to determine its effect on the patient prior to scheduling the delivery of multiple bolus doses (Boster et al. 2016).

7   Conclusion

Intrathecal drug delivery may be an appropriate treatment option for patients suffering from intractable pain or spasticity, particularly when the side effects of the systemic drug formulation cannot be tolerated. Two medical device manufacturers have developed intrathecal drug delivery devices: Medtronic manufactures the SynchroMed® II Pump and Flowonix manufactures the Prometra® II Pump. Production of a third pump—the Codman® 3000 Constant Flow Pump previously manufactured by Johnson & Johnson—has been discontinued. The FDA has approved these pumps for intrathecal delivery of baclofen, morphine, and ziconotide.

The pump componentry discussed in detail above shows several similarities as well as some differences between the pumps. These differences should always be considered in the setting of future patient care, and each patient's specific needs as the differences may impact a clinician's decision to implant a Medtronic pump versus a Flowonix pump. For instance, average battery life of the SynchroMed® II pump is approximately 7 years, while the Prometra® II pump battery will last up to 10 years so patients that have a high surgical risk or other impediments to surgical intervention may be a better candidate for a pump with a longer battery life.

Pump implant indications, implant contraindications, MRI compatibility, and flow rate accuracy are nearly indistinguishable between the pumps and may not be a factor when deciding which pump a clinician will implant. The final decision of which pump to implant may likely be more closely related to a physician's comfort or familiarity with the system or linked to the adequacy of the personnel supporting a particular pump rather than to the componentry itself.

References

Bier A (1899) Attempts over Cocainisirung of the Ruckenmarkers. Langenbecks Arch Klin Chir Ver Dtsch Z Chir 51:361–369. German

Bolash R, Udeh B, Saweris Y et al (2015) Longevity and cost of implantable intrathecal drug delivery systems for chronic pain management: a retrospective analysis of 365 patients. Neuromodulation 18(2):150–156. https://doi.org/10.1111/ner.12235

Bolash RB, Niazi T, Kumari M, Azer G, Mekhail N (2018) Efficacy of a targeted drug delivery on-demand bolus option for chronic pain. Pain Pract 18(3): 305–313

Boster AL, Adair RL, Gooch JL et al (2016) Best practices for intrathecal baclofen therapy: dosing and long-term management. Neuromodulation 19(6): 623–631

Chan DY, Chan SS, Chan EK, Ng AY, Ying AC, Li AC, Chiu CC, Cheung N, Mak WK, Sun DT, Zhu CX, Poon WS (2018a) Blessing or burden? Long-term maintenance, complications and clinical outcome of intrathecal baclofen pumps. Surg Pract 22(3):105–110

Chan DY, Chan SS, Chan EK, Ng AY, Ying AC, Li AC, Chiu CC, Cheung N, Mak WK, Sun DT, Zhu CX, Poon WS (2018b) Blessing or burden? Long-term maintenance, complications and clinical outcome of intrathecal baclofen pumps. Surg Pract 22(3):105–110

De Andres J, Villanueva V, Palmisani S, Cerda-Olmedo G, Lopez-Alarcon MD, Monsalve V, Minguez A, Martinez-Sanjuan V (2011) The safety of magnetic resonance imaging in patients with programmable implanted intrathecal drug delivery systems: a 3-year prospective study. Anesth Analg 112(5):1124–1129

Desai MJ, Hargens LM, Breitenfeldt MD et al (2015) The rate of magnetic resonance imaging in patients with spinal cord stimulation. Spine 40(9):E531–E537

Discontinuation of the Codman® Constant Flow Pump. Johnson & Johnson Medical Devices Companies. 2020. www.jnjmedicaldevices.com/en-US/codman-pumps

Duarte R, Raphael J, Eldabe S (2016) Intrathecal drug delivery for the management of pain and spasticity in adults: an executive summary of the British Pain

Society's recommendations for best clinical practice. Br J Pain 10:67–69

Farid R (2017) Problem-solving in patients with targeted drug delivery systems. Mo Med 114(1):52–56

Farid R, Binz K, Emerson JA, Murdock F (2019) Accuracy and precision of the SynchroMed II pump. Neuromodulation 22(7):805–810

Flowonix (2019) Prometra® II programmable pumps: implant manual. Flowonix, Mount Olive, NJ

Flowonix Medical (2020a) Prometra® II clinician programmer: implant manual. Flowonix, Mount Olive, NJ

Flowonix Medical (2020b) Prometra® II intrathecal catheter: implant manual. Flowonix, Mount Olive, NJ

Flowonix Medical (2020c) Prometra® II patient therapy controller guide: implant manual. Flowonix, Mount Olive, NJ

Ilias W, le Polain B, Buchser E, Demartini L (2008) Patient-controlled analgesia in chronic pain patients: experience with a new device designed to be used with implanted programmable pumps. Pain Pract 8(3):164–170

Malheiro L, Gomes A, Barbosa P, Santos L, Sarmento A (2015) Infectious complications of intrathecal drug administration systems for spasticity and chronic pain: 145 patients from a Tertiary Care Center. Neuromodulation 18(5):421–427

Medtronic (2015a) Ascenda® intrathecal catheter with an 86.4 cm spinal segment: implant manual. Medtronic, Minneapolis, MN

Medtronic (2015b) Ascenda® intrathecal catheter with a 66.0 cm spinal segment: implant manual. Medtronic, Minneapolis, MN

Medtronic (2018a) SynchroMed® II clinician programmer: clinician programming guide. Medtronic, Minneapolis, MN

Medtronic (2018b) SynchroMed® II myPTM™ personal therapy manager for patients: product guide. Medtronic, Minneapolis, MN

Motta F, Antonello CE (2014) Analysis of complications in 430 consecutive pediatric patients treated with intrathecal baclofen therapy: 14-year experience. J Neurosurg Pediatr 13(3):301–306

Penn RD, Savoy SM, Corcos D et al (1989) Intrathecal baclofen for severe spinal spasticity. N Engl J Med 320:1517–1521

Rauck R, Deer T, Rosen S, Padda G, Barsa J, Dunbar E, Dwarakanath G (2010) Accuracy and efficacy of intrathecal administration of morphine sulfate for treatment of intractable pain using the Prometra® programmable pump. Neuromodulation 13: 102–108

Rauck R, Deer T, Rosen S, Padda G, Barsa J, Dunbar E, Dwarakanath G (2013) Long-term follow-up of a novel implantable programmable infusion pump. Neuromodulation 16(2):163–167. https://doi.org/10.1111/j.1525-1403.2012.00515.x. Epub 2012 Oct 11. PMID: 23057877

Rosen SM, Bromberg TA, Padda G, Barsa J, Dunbar E, Dwarakanath G, Navalgund Y, Jaffe T, Yearwood TL, Creamer M, Deer T (2013) Intrathecal administration of Infumorph® vs compounded morphine for treatment of intractable pain using the Prometra® programmable pump. Pain Med 14(6):865–873

Saulino M, Gofeld M (2014) "Sonology" of programmable intrathecal pumps. Neuromodulation 17(7):696–698

Sylvester RK, Lindsay SM, Schauer C (2004) The conversion challenge: from intrathecal to oral morphine. Am J Hosp Palliat Care 21(2):143–147

SynchroMed® II drug infusion system brief statement. Medtronic. 2020. www.medtronic.com/us-en/healthcare-professionals/therapies-procedures/neurological/targeted-drug-delivery/indications-safety-warnings.html

Von Korff M, Crane P, Lane M et al (2005) Chronic spinal pain and physical-mental comorbidity in the United States: results from the national comorbidity survey replication. Pain 113:331–339

Wesemann K, Coffey RJ, Wallace MS, Tan Y, Broste S, Buvanendran A (2014) Clinical accuracy and safety using the SynchroMed II intrathecal drug infusion pump. Reg Anesth Pain Med 39(4):341–346. https://doi.org/10.1097/AAP.0000000000000107

Intrathecal Drug Delivery Trialing

Anjum Bux and Pooja Chopra

Contents

Abstract

Intrathecal drug delivery has been used since the 1980s to treat spasticity as well as chronic malignant and nonmalignant pain symptoms.

A. Bux (✉)
Ephraim McDowell Regional Medical Center, Harrison Memorial Hospital, Danville, KY, USA

Bux Pain Management, Danville, KY, USA

P. Chopra
Henry Ford Hospital, Detroit, MI, USA

Patients that are considered for intrathecal drug delivery systems are those with chronic pain or severe spasticity that have failed all conservative treatments including interventional and non-interventional methods. Additionally, these patients have either failed previous surgery or they are not candidates for surgical intervention. Intrathecal drug delivery systems deliver medication to the CSF to provide better relief of pain or spasticity symptoms than systemic medications with less side effects than the other more conventional routes

© The Author(s), under exclusive license to Springer Nature Switzerland AG 2022
D. P. Beall et al. (eds.), *Intrathecal Pump Drug Delivery*, Medical Radiology Diagnostic Imaging,
https://doi.org/10.1007/978-3-030-86244-2_4

of administration. In order to qualify for implantation of an intrathecal drug delivery system, patients most often will undergo a psychological evaluation and should have successful intrathecal medication trial. This chapter will focus on trialing methods along with the different medications used for spasticity and chronic pain and their side effects and complications. In addition, we will examine patient risk factors and comorbidities and their effect on trialing techniques and medication administration location.

Abbreviations

ASC	Ambulatory Surgery Center
ASRA	American Society of Regional Anesthesia
CSF	Cerebrospinal Fluid
FDA	Food and Drug Administration
MAS	Modified Ashworth Scale
ODI	Oswestry Disability Index
PACC	Polyanalgesic Consensus Committee
VAS	Visual Analog Scale

1   Intrathecal Drug Delivery Trialing

Patients that are considered good candidates for intrathecal drug delivery are those that have failed all previous conservative therapies, are not surgical candidates, or have had failed previous surgery. Once these patients are selected, they need to have undergone a successful trial before receiving an implanted drug delivery system. These trialing methods give the clinician and the patient a preview of anticipated results with an implanted intrathecal drug delivery system. The definition of a successful trial has evolved over time as have trialing methods. The purpose of an intrathecal trial is to provide information on pain relief based on objective pain scores, informa-

tion on function, the presence of side effects, adequacy of the trial dose, and the patient's response to the medication (Deer et al. 2017a). In most cases, clinicians prefer at least a 50% reduction in pain. This endpoint can vary, as in a study by Pope and Deer, where they defined an efficacy endpoint of 70% when trialing intrathecal ziconotide (Pope and Deer 2015). Using the same trial paradigm for bolus trialing of ziconotide, Mohamed et al. set the endpoint for a successful trial at 30% for reduction in VAS pain scores (Mohamed et al. 2013). Despite these substantial variances, it has been accepted that the usual criteria for success of an intrathecal trial is reduction of pain by 50% or more with acceptable side effects (Anderson et al. 2003). In addition to pain relief, many clinicians and insurance companies are looking at improvement in function as a critical endpoint of a successful trial (Deer et al. 2017a). Evaluation of function can be implemented by comparing the gait and distance the patient can walk prior to the trial to the same parameters measured after the trial dose. An alternative assessment may be performed via a formal assessment by a physical therapist prior to and after the trial dose to evaluate improvement. Finally, the use of ODI (Oswestry Disability Index) or other functional evaluation tools can be used to evaluate pre- and post-trial dose function. Regardless, it may be advisable to establish treatment goals prior to the trial to allow clinicians and patients to better evaluate responses to the dose given during the trial and their expectations of the trial prior to the intrathecal trial dose administration (Doleys and Kraus 2004). Furthermore, as part of a pretrial workup, it is recommended to obtain a psychological evaluation to document the presence of any factors that may impact the outcome of the trial and assess the suitability of the patient to undergo the trial (Deer et al. 2017a). Once a patient is selected to undergo a trial, there are various methods used to trial medications for chronic pain and spasticity. In this next section, we will review the trialing of baclofen for spasticity.

2 Intrathecal Baclofen

Baclofen is a skeletal muscle relaxant that has been commonly used since the early 1990s to treat spasticity related to various conditions including multiple sclerosis, stroke, cerebral palsy, spinal cord injury, and traumatic brain injury. Baclofen is a lipophilic derivative of the inhibitory neurotransmitter gamma-aminobutyric acid (GABA), which inhibits monosynaptic and polysynaptic reflexes at the spinal level (Penn and Kroin 1984; Krach 2001). Patients with spasticity can exhibit positive or negative symptoms. Positive symptoms are described as velocity-dependent hypertonicity, hyperreflexia, or clonus, whereas negative symptoms include weakness, discoordination, pain, and limited functional abilities (Harned et al. 2011; Ansari et al. 2008). Both types of spasticity symptoms can be difficult to control with oral baclofen, usually requiring higher doses to exert a significant clinical effect. The downside of higher baclofen doses is that they tend produce intolerable central nervous system side effects such as sedation or somnolence (Bohannon and Smith 1987). It is in these cases that intrathecal administration of baclofen has been beneficial in reducing systemic uptake and intolerable side effects prior to implantation of a pump to deliver intrathecal baclofen; it is common practice that patients must first undergo a successful trial of baclofen administered intrathecally. Baclofen trialing is most commonly done through a single bolus injection of 50–100 mcg of baclofen into the intrathecal space (Harned et al. 2011). Patients are then observed for a period of time to confirm improvement of their spasticity by utilizing the Modified Ashworth Score (MAS), one of the most commonly used criteria to measure spasticity (Table 1). The Modified Ashworth Scale measures the resistance during passive soft-tissue stretching and is graded 0–4 based on the level of tone (Ansari et al. 2008). A positive test or successful trial is indicated by a 1-point reduction in Ashworth score for spasticity of spinal origin and a 2-point reduction for spasticity of cerebral origin. Most of the time patients respond well to the single-shot bolus of intrathecal baclofen and pro-

ceed to permanent implant. There are cases, however, where patients do not have an adequate response and have to be retrialed with a higher dose of the same medication. Additionally, there have been patients that have more complex spasticity with involvement of both upper and lower limbs, where the single-shot bolus only helps lower limb spasticity with no effect on the upper limbs.

There are also patients with asymmetric disease in which one limb may have severe rigidity and spasticity while the contralateral limb has relatively well-preserved strength and no spasticity (Harned et al. 2011). A single-shot bolus trial of baclofen in these patients may provide good relaxation in the affected limb, but undesirable weakness in the non-affected extremity (Harned et al. 2011). It is for these instances that some physicians have chosen to implement an intrathecal catheter to trial baclofen. This catheter is usually placed in the lower lumbar region and advanced to the upper thoracic levels. Patients are typically given a bolus of 50 mcg of intrathecal baclofen and then assessed at 2 h and 4 h after the bolus using the Modified Ashworth Scale. After the 4-h assessment, patients are then placed on a continuous infusion to find the optimal dose for permanent implant. This is a much less common method of trialing baclofen but certainly has become more popular given the success of the technique and its versatility with the ability to

Table 1 Modified Ashworth Score (Bohannon and Smith 1987)

Ashworth Scale	Degree of muscle tone
0	No increase in tone
1	Slight increase in muscle tone, manifested by a catch and release or by minimal resistance at the end of the range of motion when the affected part(s) is moved in flexion or extension
2	Slight increase in muscle tone, manifested by a catch, followed by minimal resistance throughout the remainder (less than half) of the range of movement (ROM)
3	More marked increase in muscle tone through most of the ROM, but affect part(s) easily moved
4	Limbs rigid in flexion or extension

give multiple boluses or a continuous infusion through the intrathecal catheter. This method of trialing is dependent on the patient being in a hospital setting for several days, as opposed to the outpatient setting where one can safely perform a single-shot bolus. Furthermore, there is a higher risk of infection and development of other complications including a post-dural puncture headache with the use of a catheter. Given the increased risk of infection and the risk of headache, an extradural approach was taken by Xiulu Ruan who published a case report with a novel approach of a baclofen trial performed via an epidural catheter instead of an intrathecal catheter (Ruan et al. 2013).

Regardless of the method of trialing intrathecal baclofen, this medication remains a mainstay for the modern treatment of spasticity. We have seen baclofen used alone or in combination with other medications, but regardless of how it is utilized, it is important to understand and recognize the side effects associated with this medication. These side effects include drowsiness, lightheadedness, dizziness, nausea and vomiting, headache, seizures, and weakness. Baclofen withdrawal can also have significant clinical symptoms including agitation, confusion, seizures, psychosis, dyskinesia, hyperthermia, and increased spasticity. Baclofen withdrawal can also be severe and is a medical emergency that needs to be treated in the inpatient setting with oral baclofen as a replacement. Given the serious side effects of the medication and even more serious withdrawal effects, we must be vigilant in the care of our patients on intrathecal baclofen.

3 Pain Pump Trialing

3.1 Trialing and Type of Pain

Chronic pain can be classified into neuropathic pain, nociceptive pain, and mixed pain. Neuropathic pain is a sharp, shooting, stabbing type pain that is usually caused by nerve compression or nerve damage. Nociceptive pain is usually a mechanical, dull, aching, throbbing type pain caused by damage to tissue with result-

ing inflammation. Mixed pain is a combination of both neuropathic and nociceptive pain patterns. There is evidence that intrathecal therapy is successful in treating both neuropathic, nociceptive, and mixed type pain symptoms (Deer et al. 2012a). In the most recent PACC Guidelines, it is stated that neuropathic pain generally responds to ziconotide, opioid plus local anesthetic, opioid alone, clonidine plus opioid, and clonidine alone (Deer et al. 2017b). Nociceptive pain generally responds to an opioid, ziconotide, opioid plus local anesthetic, and local anesthetic alone (Deer et al. 2017b) (Tables 2 and 3, respectively). There is no indication of one trialing method being superior to another when treating the different types of pain. Nociceptive, neuropathic, and mixed pain are all found in malignant and nonmalignant pain types. Patients with malignant pain are often referred to interventional pain specialists late in the disease when they are suffering from poor analgesia, limited life expectancy, insufficient medical alternatives for pain relief, and even more limited interventional options and a shortened window of time for these interventions (Deer et al. 2011). Given these challenges, it has been advised that if a patient is a reasonable candidate for an implantable drug delivery device, the clinician should forego a trial and proceed directly to pump implantation to prevent delays in administering effective analgesia to the suffering patient (Deer et al. 2012a). Currently, patients with malignant pain, whether nociceptive, neuropathic or mixed, usually can forego a trial and proceed directly to implant, but patients with nonmalignant pain of any type need to undergo a trial.

3.2 Trial Dosing and Method

There are several different methods of intrathecal medication trialing, and each of these methods has site of service and dosing considerations associated with them. The trialing methods fall into four different categories, single-shot intrathecal bolus injection, multiple intrathecal bolus injections, continuous intrathecal infusion, and continuous epidural infusion. All of these trialing

Table 2 Algorithm for intrathecal medications to treat patients with neuropathic pain (Deer et al. 2012a)

Line 1	Morphine	Ziconotide		Morphine + bupivacaine
Line 2	Hydromorphone	Hydromorphone + bupivacaine or hydromorphone + clonidine		Morphine + Clonidine
Line 3	Clonidine	ziconotide + opioid	Fentanyl	Fentanyl + bupivacaine or fentanyl + clonidine
Line 4	Opioid + clonidine + bupivacaine	Bupivacaine + clonidine		
Line 5	Baclofen			

Line 1: Morphine and ziconotide are approved by the US Food and Drug Administration for IT therapy and are recommended as first-line therapy for neuropathic pain. The combination of morphine and bupivacaine is recommended for neuropathic pain on the basis of clinical use and apparent safety.

Line 2: Hydromorphone, alone or in combination with bupivacaine or clonidine, is recommended. Alternatively, the combination of morphine and clonidine may be use.

Line 3: Third-line recommendations for neuropathic pain include clonidine, ziconotide plus an opioid, and fentanyl alone or in combination with bupivacaine or clonidine.

Line 4: The combination of bupivacaine and clonidine (with or without an opioid drug) is recommended.

Line 5: Baclofen is recommended on the basis of safety, although reports of efficacy are limited.

Table 3 Algorithm for intrathecal medications to treat patients with nociceptive pain

	Morphine	Hydromorphone	Ziconotide	Fentanyl
Line 1	Morphine	Hydromorphone	Ziconotide	Fentanyl
Line 2	Morphine + Bupivacaine	Ziconotide + Opioid	Hydromorphone + Bupivacaine	Fentanyl + Bupivacaine
Line 3	Opioid (morphine, hydromorphone, or fentanyl) + clonidine			Sufentanil
Line 4	Opioid + clonidine + bupivacaine		Sufentanil + bupivacaine or clonidine	
Line 5	Sufentanil + bupivacaine + clonidine			

Line 1: Morphine and ziconotide are approved by the US Food and Drug Administration for IT therapy and are recommended as first-line therapy for nociceptive pain. Hydromorphone is recommended on the basis of widespread clinical use ad apparent safety. Fentanyl has been upgraded to first-line use by the consensus conference.

Line 2: Bupivacaine in combination with morphine, hydromorphone, or fentanyl is recommended. Alternatively, the combination of ziconotide and an opioid drug can be employed.

Line 3: Recommendations include clonidine plus an opioid (i.e., morphine, hydromorphone, or fentanyl) or sufentanil monotherapy.

Line 4: The triple combination of an opioid, clonidine, and bupivacaine is recommended. An alternative recommendation is sufentanil in combination with either bupivacaine or clonidine.

Line 5: The triple combination of sufentanil, bupivacaine, and clonidine is suggested.

methods demonstrate efficacy, and no trialing method has proven to be superior to another in regard to predicting long-term efficacy of intrathecal infusion (Deer et al. 2017a). The most recent PACC Guidelines concluded that there are equal levels of evidence for all methods of trialing; single-shot, multiple bolus injections, and continuous infusion (Deer et al. 2017a). This was demonstrated by Hamza et al., in a prospective study of 58 patients comparing the continuous method of trialing to intermittent bolus dosing method, with a 3-year follow-up after implant (Hamza et al. 2015). It was concluded that even at the 1-year follow-up time point, there was no difference in outcome regardless of trialing method (Hamza et al. 2015). The one difference that was found, however, was that patients had more frequent opioid side effects including nausea, vomiting, diaphoresis, and urinary hesitancy with the bolus dosing method compared to the continuous infusion method (Hamza et al. 2015). Research performed by Deer and colleagues also came to the same conclusion that long-term outcome was similar regardless of trial method. These authors not only compared the single-shot intrathecal bolus, multiple intrathecal boluses, or continuous infusion methods but also compared trialing via the epidural route versus an intrathecal route (Mohamed et al. 2013).

Currently, the three major insurance carriers in the United States (Medicare, United Health, and Anthem) require a catheter trial as a condition for pump implant (Deer et al. 2017a). Despite this requirement, as seen in Table 4, data from the 2015 Medtronic Product Surveillance Registry demonstrated that only 45% of the trials were performed with a continuous intrathecal infusion as compared to 44% of the trials done with a single-shot intrathecal bolus (Product Surveillance Registry (PSR) Database 2015). The remaining trials consist of 7% that were done with multiple intrathecal bolus injections, and 4% done with a continuous epidural infusion (Product Surveillance Registry (PSR) Database 2015). There are advantages and disadvantages to each trialing method, and the decision on which method to trial is often based on the patient's clinical status, diagnosis, reason for the trial, type of medication used for the trial, facility capabilities, and physician preference (Deer et al. 2017a) (Fig. 1).

The single-shot bolus method allows for a quicker trial, less risk of infection, and can be done in the office or outpatient setting (Deer et al. 2017a). However, this method increases the risk of side effects, and, if unsuccessful, the patient may need repeat injections with various doses of medication over the course of several days. The continuous infusion, whether intrathecal or epidural, allows for titration of the medication to achieve efficacy, while the patient can be directly observed for side effects over the course of several days (Deer et al. 2017a). Continuous trials must be conducted in an inpatient setting and carry a higher risk for infection, but this method also lessens the risk for side effects. Furthermore, this method allows for trialing with multiple medications and for staging a trial, especially for anticoagulated individuals and cancer patients. A staged trial involves placement of a potentially permanent intrathecal catheter and attaching it to a tunneled extension and an external pump. If the trial is successful, then the physician can proceed to implant by removing the extension and connecting to the intrathecal catheter to the implanted pump.

Table 4 Data from the Medtronic Product Surveillance Registry 2015 (Product Surveillance Registry (PSR) Database 2015)

Trialing method	Malignant pain (%)	Nonmalignant pain (%)	Spasticity (%)	Total (%)
Continuous intrathecal infusion	20	68.4	16.7	45
Single intrathecal bolus	80	26.3	50	44
Multiple intrathecal bolus infusions	0	0	29	7
Continuous epidural	0	5.3	4.2	4

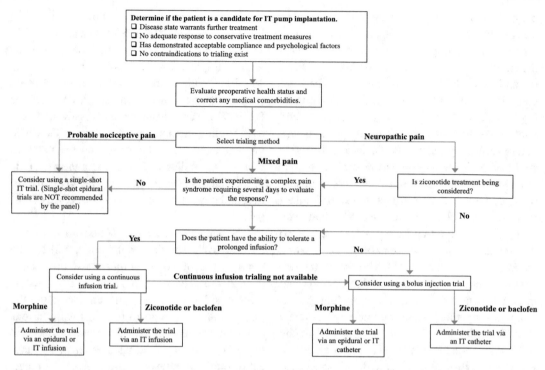

Fig. 1 Algorithm for trialing in patients who may be candidates for IT therapy for pain (Deer et al. 2012b)

Staged trials are useful in cases in which there is a small window of time from trial to implant, such as in cancer patients or those on anticoagulation with an inability to hold their anticoagulant medication for extended periods of time. Based on recent work on CSF flow by Bernards and Yaksh, bolus dosing may result in more widespread drug distribution due to the kinetic forces of the bolus overcoming the limitation of CSF flow dynamics (Bernards 2006; Yaksh et al. 2017). With evidence indicating that all trialing methods have equal efficacy and predictive value, ultimately, it is up to the physician to decide the preferred trialing method.

Morphine and ziconotide are the two FD-approved medications for intrathecal drug delivery, but many other medications have been safely used as described in the most recent PACC Trialing guidelines (Deer et al. 2017a). These medications will be discussed in greater detail later in the chapter, but their dosing for intrathecal bolus trialing is described in Table 7, and the dosing for intrathecal bolus trialing is listed in Table 8.

Table 7 Dose ranges for intrathecal bolus trialing (Deer et al. 2017a)

Medication	Recommended dose
Morphine	0.1–0.5 mg
Ziconotide	1–5 mcg
Hydromorphone	0.025–0.1 mg
Fentanyl	15–75 mcg
Sufentanil	5–20 mcg
Bupivacaine	0.5–2.5 mg
Clonidine	5–20 mcg

Taken from the 2017 PACC Guidelines Recommendations for Trialing

Table 8 Dose ranges for continuous intrathecal trialing (Deer et al. 2017a)

Medication	Recommended dose
Morphine	0.1–0.5 mg/day
Ziconotide	0.5–2.4 mcg/day
Hydromorphone	0.01–0.15 mg/day
Fentanyl	25–75 mcg/day
Sufentanil	10–20 mcg/day
Bupivacaine	0.01–4 mg/day
Clonidine	20–100 mcg/day

Taken from the 2017 PACC Guidelines Recommendations for Trialing

4 Whether or Not to Trial

Since the beginning of intrathecal drug delivery, practitioners have always performed a trial or a test to determine if the therapy will be appropriate for their patients. While this preimplantation trial has been, and continues to be, the current standard of care and is required by many insurers for approval of a permanent implant, more recently there have been questions regarding whether the success of a trial is indicative of long-term success of the therapy. There is very little evidence that shows correlation between success of an intrathecal trial and long-term success of intrathecal therapy. On the other hand, there is no evidence on success of intrathecal therapy without a trial. There are only a few reports that assess the long-term outcomes after implant and the predictive value of the intrathecal pump trial. One of these reports was a review by Dominguez et al. who evaluated 157 patients with chronic nonmalignant pain who underwent serial inpatient, single-shot intrathecal bolus trials over a 5-year period from 1996 to 2001 (Deer et al. 2017a). These patients were trialed by serial lumbar punctures starting with 0.5 mg intrathecal morphine (Deer et al. 2017a). Those patients that responded with >50% pain relief for >8 h were considered to have a successful trial (Deer et al. 2017a). Patients who had intolerable side effects from the initial dose were then trialed with 0.25 mg of intrathecal morphine (Deer et al. 2017a). Those that did not achieve adequate pain relief were trialed with 1.0 mg intrathecal morphine the next day (Deer et al. 2017a). All patients were kept in the hospital for 2–4 days during the trial period and followed for 30 months after pump implantation (Deer et al. 2017a). Of the 157 patients trialed, 134 had a successful trial and proceeded to implantation (Deer et al. 2017a). Regarding post-implant follow-up, those patients who responded to higher doses of morphine during the trial escalated their intrathecal opioid doses more quickly and required adjuvant medications and opioid substitutions, in comparison to those that responded to lower trial doses of morphine (Deer et al. 2017a).

Despite these retrospective reviews examining success of trialing, to date there has not been prospective, randomized controlled study evidence demonstrating that trialing changes long-term patient outcomes, compared to not performing a trial (Deer et al. 2017a). Although it is widely accepted that patients must undergo a successful trial to proceed to implantation of the pump, these trials have limited value in cancer patients in which it is essential to be expeditious in evaluating and implementing treatment options (Deer et al. 2011). As previously stated, cancer patients are often referred to interventional pain specialists late in the disease process, with poor analgesia, limited life expectancy, limited medical alternatives for pain relief, and even more limited interventional options and usually with a shortened window of time for implementation of these interventions (Malhotra et al. 2013). Given these challenges, it has been advised that provided these patients are reasonable candidates for an implantable drug delivery device, clinicians should forego a trial and proceed directly to pump implantation to prevent delays in administering effective analgesia to these patients (Deer et al. 2017a). Data in Table 5, from the 2015 Medtronic Product Surveillance Registry capturing trialing information on 154 patients, revealed that almost 80% of patients with malignant pain did not undergo a trial, while almost all patients with nonmalignant pain and spasticity did undergo a trial (Product Surveillance Registry (PSR) Database 2015). The success of intrathecal therapy in the cancer population without undergoing prior trialing emphasizes the need to question whether we should continue to perform trials or not and does a trial have any predictive value to long-term success of the therapy. We will continue to debate this topic for years to come, but

Table 5 Data from the Medtronic Product Surveillance Registry 2015 (Product Surveillance Registry (PSR) Database 2015)

Primary indication	Trialed before implant	
	Yes (%)	No (%)
Nonmalignant pain	88	11.9
Malignant pain	21.6	78.4
Spasticity	100	0

for now, Medicare guidelines require opioid testing via a temporary IT/epidural catheter to "substantiate adequately acceptable pain relief and degree of side effects and patient acceptance" for permanent device implantation to be covered (Medicare Coverage Issues Manual 2009). Therefore, due to current Medicare guidelines, standard practice is to implement a trial when treating nonmalignant pain, but when treating malignant pan, this remains optional, ultimately up to the clinician to decide whether a trial is warranted.

5 Dosing and Medication Selection

As previously mentioned, the FDA-approved, on-label medications for intrathecal drug delivery include morphine and ziconotide (Table 6). Morphine has been commonly used in both single-shot bolus trials and continuous catheter trials and is an opiate alkaloid that targets the mu receptors in the dorsal horn by inhibiting the release of substance P. Morphine is less lipid soluble than other opioids and has a limited volume of distribution and limited uptake into the systemic circulation (Deer et al. 2017a). Because of these properties, morphine has the highest rostral spread and highest spinal cord concentration compared to other commonly used intrathecal opioids (Deer et al. 2017a). Morphine has been used in all trialing methods, including single-shot intrathecal boluses and intrathecal or epidural continuous infusions. Morphine does have a potential for delayed respiratory depression, and, because of that, there has been some hesitancy to

Table 6 Taken from the 2017 PACC Guidelines Recommendations for Trialing (Deer et al. 2017a)

On-label medications for intrathecal use	Off-label medications for intrathecal use
Morphine Ziconotide	Hydromorphone Fentanyl Sufentanil Bupivacaine Clonidine

use this medication to trial in the outpatient setting (Deer et al. 2017a). The recommended starting dose for trialing intrathecal morphine through a continuous infusion is 0.1–0.5 mg/day and for bolus trialing is a 0.1–0.5 mg single-shot bolus (Deer et al. 2017a). Regardless of whether morphine is trialed through a single-shot bolus or continuous infusion, inpatient monitoring is advised because of the risk of delayed respiratory depression (Deer et al. 2017a). It was a recommendation from the PACC that pulse oximetry be used in the phase of recovery after trial and implant, at least once an hour for the first 12 h, every 2 h for the next 12 h, and then once every 4 h for the next 48 h (Deer et al. 2017a). It was reported by Coffey et al. that mortality risk was increased in the first 3 days after implantation if the IT dose was larger than 0.75 mg (Coffey et al. 2009). This data led to reducing the recommendations for bolus trial doses of morphine. The PACC treatment algorithms reported that bolus trial doses of morphine ranging from 0.075 to 0.15 mg were safe regarding respiratory depression (Deer et al. 2017b).

Ziconotide is a non-opioid, presynaptic N-type calcium channel blocker that acts on the dorsal horn of the spinal cord (Deer et al. 2017a). This medication is only approved for intrathecal use due to its peptide structure and pharmacodynamic effects. Ziconotide can also be trialed through a single-shot bolus or a continuous infusion. When ziconotide was first introduced, it was recommended to trial through a continuous infusion starting at 1.2 mcg/day increasing incrementally each day to 2.4 mcg/day, and then to 3.6 mcg/day while observing for efficacy and side effects. Pope and Deer reported on a trialing technique using a flex dosing algorithm that could be utilized in the outpatient setting (Deer et al. 2017a). This technique takes advantage of ziconotide's hydrophilic properties and showed equal efficacy as the continuous trialing method (Deer et al. 2017a). Initial dosing began with 2 mcg, with incremental increased in medication dose by 2 mcg each week until therapeutic efficacy was achieved (Deer et al. 2017a). Once this efficacy was attained, the patient was retrialed at that same dose to confirm analgesic efficacy and lack of side effects (Deer et al. 2017a). If side effects were observed, then the dose was reduced by 1 mcg. Hayek et al. performed this same bolus trialing technique on 15 patients with single-shot boluses starting at 2 mcg. The protocol allowed for titration increases to 4, 6, and 8 mcg as tolerated depending on efficacy and side effects (Hayek et al. 2015). Mohammed and colleagues trialed 20 patients with an initial bolus dose starting at 2.5 mcg and incrementally increasing to 3.75 mcg a week later while concurrently observing for efficacy and side effects (Mohamed et al. 2013). As a result, single-shot bolus trialing emerged as the preferred trialing method for ziconotide starting at 2 mcg with weekly increases as tolerated while simultaneously monitoring for efficacy and side effects (Pope and Deer 2015). If ziconotide is trialed in the outpatient setting, observation of the patient is recommended for any potential adverse events for up to 6–12 h prior to discharge (Deer et al. 2017a). Furthermore, it is also advised to closely monitor blood pressure as well as any potential psychotic side effects during this period (Deer et al. 2017a). Ziconotide can also be trialed in the inpatient setting with recommended doses of 0.5–2.4 mcg/day over the course of at least 3–4 days to assess efficacy and adverse events (Deer et al. 2017a).

If possible and if medically indicated, patients should first undergo a trial of one of these FDA-approved medications (Deer et al. 2017a). If that is not a possibility, one of the most common non-FDA-approved intrathecal medications trialed is hydromorphone. Hydromorphone is a hydrophilic opioid that has a mechanism of action similar to morphine, except for being more potent and utilized in lower doses and concentrations than morphine (Deer et al. 2010). The recommended trialing dose for hydromorphone in a single-shot bolus is 0.025–0.1 mg while in a continuous infusion is 0.01–0.15 mg/day (Deer et al. 2017a). Again, because of the risk of respiratory depression, it is recommended that these trials be performed in an inpatient setting where the patient can be monitored for at least 48 h.

Unlike hydromorphone and morphine, fentanyl and sufentanil are highly lipid soluble with limited rostral spread and limited uptake into the systemic circulation (Deer et al. 2017a). Many physicians have migrated toward fentanyl as the medication of choice for single-shot trialing because of its limited risk of respiratory depression (Deer et al. 2017a). It has been noted, however, that a successful trial with intrathecal fentanyl may be helpful in evaluating a response to opioids but may not predict the response to other opioids, especially with chronic use (Deer et al. 2017a). The decreased risk of respiratory depression and the lipophilicity of fentanyl have thus made it very popular in the outpatient trial setting. The recommended dose for a single-shot bolus of intrathecal fentanyl is 15–75 mcg and 25–75 mcg/day for a continuous infusion (Deer et al. 2017a). Sufentanil is more potent than fentanyl and therefore less commonly utilized in the trial setting. The recommended dose of sufentanil for a single-shot bolus is 5–20 mcg and 10–20 mcg/day for q continuous infusion (Deer et al. 2017a). When using either of these medications, it is recommended for patients to be monitored for 6–8 h after the trial for any adverse events.

Some of the more common non-narcotic medications that are used in intrathecal medication trials are bupivacaine and clonidine. Bupivacaine is an amide local anesthetic that binds to voltage-gated sodium channels and blocks the sodium influx into nerve cells thereby preventing depolarization. Bupivacaine has been safely used in the intrathecal space as a non-narcotic to provide pain relief in the acute and chronic pain setting. The recommended dosing of bupivacaine in a chronic pain trial setting is 0.5–2.5 mg for a single-shot intrathecal bolus and 0.01–4.0 mg/day for a continuous intrathecal infusion (Deer et al. 2017a). Clonidine is an apha-2 agonist that is commonly used to lower blood pressure by reducing peripheral vascular resistance and decreasing sympathetic activation. However, it has also been found to block the transmission of noxious sensory stimuli through its alpha-2 adrenoreceptor activity

(Hassenbusch et al. 2002). Clonidine has been used intrathecally alone and in combination therapy but is used less often in trialing. The recommended trialing doses of clonidine are 5–20 mcg for a single-shot intrathecal bolus and 20–100 mcg/day for a continuous intrathecal infusion (Deer et al. 2017a). Both of these non-narcotic medications can be trialed in the outpatient setting, but it is recommended that patients be monitored for 4–6 h focusing on blood pressure and heart rate to ensure that the patients return to their baseline neurological status prior to discharge (Deer et al. 2017a).

As previously said, it is recommended to trial with FDA-approved medications first and then utilize commonly used and PACC-recommended off-label medications in monotherapy, if clinically necessary. It has also become acceptable to trial combination medications within the confines of the PACC guidance for medication algorithms (Deer et al. 2017a, b). There has been some data on intrathecal trialing with combinations of medications with Rainov et al. reported on 26 patients that were trialed with an intrathecal regimen of morphine, bupivacaine, and clonidine or midazolam (Rainov et al. 2001). According to these authors, they combined morphine with clonidine, bupivacaine, and/or midazolam to achieve synergistic effects, to better treat neuropathic pain symptoms and to reduce the propensity for opioid tolerance (Rainov et al. 2001). Hayek et al. also reported on a cohort of 57 patients who were trialed with a mixture of hydromorphone and bupivacaine (Hayek et al. 2016).

When performing intrathecal trials with a combination of medications, it is recommended that the intrathecal continuous infusion method is utilized in the inpatient setting. It is also important to monitor these patients for at least 48–72 h to assess for efficacy and any adverse events that may occur including respiratory depression.

Regardless of which medication is used (Table 6), it is recommended that trialing doses (Tables 7 and 8) of intrathecal medications should be chosen conservatively, and physicians should start with the lowest reasonable dose and titrate upward slowly, based on the patient's response

and the degree of pain relief, improved function, and the presence of side effects (Deer et al. 2017a).

6 Side Effects

Side effects to intrathecal therapy are certainly dependent on which drug is being used. If adverse effects occur during trialing at the lowest reasonable dose of medication, then the trial should be considered a failure, and a different medication should be considered (Deer et al. 2017a). The most common side effects with opioid medications include pruritus, urinary retention, dizziness, nausea, vomiting, abdominal discomfort, and respiratory depression (Chaney 1995). These side effects are dose dependent and more commonly seen in the more hydrophilic opioids such as morphine or hydromorphone as compared to the more lipophilic opioids such as fentanyl or sufentanil. Most of these side effects are self-limiting and easily treated with diphenhydramine, anti-emetics, and/or low-dose naloxone, but if they persist or become intolerable, switching to a different opioid should be considered. These side effects were evident in a review done by Anderson and Burchiel in which some patients experienced intolerable morphine-related adverse events including nausea, vomiting, and pruritus during the trial and had to be retrialed with intrathecal hydromorphone (Anderson et al. 2003).

Ziconotide is a non-opioid pain medication and has its own specific set of side effects. These side effects include nausea, abdominal pain, anxiety, forgetfulness, change in speech, confusion, delusions, hallucinations, unsteadiness, nystagmus, and paranoia (Mayo clinic drugs and supplements 2020). Interestingly, side effects of intrathecal ziconotide are mostly related to bolus dosing or a rapid rate of increase of the medication in a continuous infusion rather than a final dose. In other words, if a patient with intrathecal ziconotide experiences side effects, then it is recommended to decrease the rate of infusion of the medication or to slow or stop the rate of dose titration (Rauck et al.

2006). These strategies typically result in the resolution of adverse effects (Rauck et al. 2006). In a previous study of bolus trialing of intrathecal ziconotide, Hayek et al. had six patients that experienced cognitive side effects and syncope that were severe enough to result in their removal from the study (Hayek et al. 2015). Deer and Pope also experienced the same scenario in their study of bolus trialing of intrathecal ziconotide with three patients experiencing urinary retention and one patient with psychotic effects (Pope and Deer 2015).

Side effects of other non-opioid medications, such as bupivacaine, include hypotension, syncope, extreme motor and sensory neurological changes, urinary retention, and bradycardia. Again, these adverse effects are dose dependent and usually more profound with bolus intrathecal delivery rather than a continuous infusion. The side effects associated with intrathecal clonidine include hypotension, bradycardia, headache, drowsiness, fatigue, dizziness, and constipation (WebMD n.d.). These adverse effects, much like the other medications, are dose dependent and more profound with bolus dosing of the medication.

In comparing a single-shot bolus injection to continuous infusion trialing Anderson et al. found more frequent opioid side effects including nausea, vomiting, diaphoresis, and urinary hesitancy in patients who underwent single-shot bolus of intrathecal morphine versus those who had undergone a continuous infusion (Anderson et al. 2003). Overall, side effects vary according to the particular drug that is trialed and whether it is given in a bolus fashion or by continuous infusion. These medication side effects and methods of trialing dictate the setting in which the trial can be performed.

7 Trial Environment

There are basically three settings in which a trial can be done, the office setting, the outpatient ambulatory surgery center (ASC) setting, or in the hospital (Table 9). There are many factors which determine the setting in which a trial is conducted. These factors include method of trialing, patient characteristics and comorbidities, medication used, and insurance considerations. As previously stated, there are four methods of trialing: single-shot intrathecal bolus injection, multiple intrathecal bolus injections, continuous intrathecal infusion, and continuous epidural infusion. The single-shot bolus injection and multiple intrathecal bolus injections can be performed safely in the outpatient setting, either the office or the ASC and usually without a catheter. Given the fact that the three major players in the United States (Medicare, Anthem, and United Health) require a catheter trial as a condition for pump implant, most of these bolus trials are done with temporary catheter placement (Deer et al. 2017a). For infusion trials including continuous intrathecal infusion or continuous epidural infusion, PACC guidelines recommend inpatient trialing in the hospital setting for these patients (Deer et al. 2017a). More importantly, patient risk factors and patient comorbidities will dictate the setting in which the trial can be done. Patients with significant risk factors including obesity, sleep apnea, elderly, significant pulmonary or cardiac disease, concurrent use of sedative medications including benzodiazepines, and opioid naïve patients may need to be trialed in an inpatient setting where adequate monitoring can be done for 48–72 h (Deer et al. 2017a). Also, inpatient trialing should be considered for those patients in whom accessing the intrathecal space may prove to be difficult or those patients that may have increased anesthesia requirement for the trial procedure.

Patients that are opioid tolerant and have little or no risk factors may be safely trialed in the outpatient setting with adequate monitoring for

Table 9 Settings in which trial can be performed (Deer et al. 2017a)

Trial setting	Method of trialing
Office-outpatient	Single-shot bolus or multiple bolus injection
ASC-outpatient	Single-shot bolus or multiple bolus injection
Hospital-inpatient	Continuous intrathecal or epidural trial

4–8 h depending on which medication is trialed (Deer et al. 2017a). According to the most recent PACC guidelines, the only medications that should be considered for trialing in the outpatient setting include intrathecal fentanyl, ziconotide, bupivacaine, and possibly clonidine (Deer et al. 2017a). The decision to use these medications in the outpatient setting, however, needs to take into consideration the patient risk factors, comorbidities, and the ability to adequately monitor the patient after the trial. The one exception to this recommendation is for those cancer patients nearing end of life where a trial can be performed in a home setting in the presence of a healthcare infusion nurse to adequately monitor the patient (Deer et al. 2017a).

Ultimately, the decision on which setting to trial the patient is up to the physician based on his or her comfort level with the patient's risk factors, method of trialing, medication being used, and the facility.

8 Comorbidities and Medication Interactions

As previously stated, patients with significant comorbidities or risk factors need to be trialed in an inpatient setting. Also, there are certain medications that need to be adjusted and possibly held before a trial. Patients that are being trialed with an opioid may benefit from a pretrial opioid taper especially those patients that are opioid tolerant or have opioid induced hyperalgesia. The PACC guidelines recommend that systemic opioid therapy be markedly reduced or eliminated prior to initiating intrathecal therapy, especially for those patients that may be at high risk for opioid-induced respiratory depression (Deer et al. 2017a). In these patients, it was discovered that opioid reduction or cessation coupled with very small doses of morphine given during intrathecal trialing resulted in improved outcomes for patients after the implantation of their intrathecal drug delivery systems (Deer et al. 2017a). The opioid reduction protocol was demonstrated by

Hamza et al., who weaned the patients from their baseline systemic opioid medications to half of their original dose then conducted an intrathecal medication trial using morphine given as a bolus (Hamza et al. 2012). Those patients that underwent a successful trial were weaned off of the other half of their systemic opioids over 3–5 weeks on an outpatient basis. After 7–10 days of being off opioids, these patients were implanted with an intrathecal drug delivery system (Hamza et al. 2012). It was found that these patients did well shortly after the surgical implantation, and their dose stabilized out at 1.5 mg/day of intrathecal morphine without the concurrent use of oral opioids (Hamza et al. 2012). Grider et al. also weaned patients off oral opioids prior to performing an intrathecal trial. In his retrospective case review, Grider followed patients that were weaned completely off systemic opioids 6 weeks prior to their intrathecal trial (Grider et al. 2011). These patients also did very well after implantation with their dose stabilizing at 0.36 mg/day of intrathecal morphine 12 months after implant without concomitant use of oral opioids (Grider et al. 2011). As these studies demonstrated, patients that weaned down or off their oral opioids prior to intrathecal trial showed good long-term success with their intrathecal drug delivery systems at lower doses.

In addition to oral opioids, patients need to wean down or off all benzodiazepines and any other sedating medications. Benzodiazepines and other sedating medications may compound the opioid side effects including respiratory depression that is known to be seen with intrathecal opioids. In addition, concurrent antidepressant or anticonvulsant treatment may increase the risk of adverse events when given in conjunction with intrathecal ziconotide (Deer et al. 2017a).

Finally, as with other interventional procedures, anticoagulants need to be temporarily discontinued for the appropriate time prior to the intrathecal trial. It is best to follow the guidelines from the American Society of Regional Anesthesia (ASRA) for guidance on the duration of holding anticoagulants.

9 Complications of Trialing

Some of the most common complications from intrathecal medication trialing include bleeding, infection, overmedication, cerebrospinal fluid leakage, spinal cord injury, and nerve injury. As previously stated, patients on anticoagulants should be off of them for the appropriate amount of time based on ASRA guidelines. There is no evidence that antibiotic prophylaxis is needed prior to an intrathecal pump trial. The decision to give antibiotic prophylaxis prior to pump trial depends on patient risk factors for infection, the method of trialing, and the duration of trial. Given the paucity of evidence for antibiotic prophylaxis in the trial period, it can be assumed that most physicians do not give prophylactic antibiotics for single-shot intrathecal bolus trialing but may give antibiotics for continuous intrathecal catheter trials. If patient risk factors are present such as diabetes, history of previous infections, or the presence of an indwelling catheter, consideration should be made for prophylactic antibiotic administration. It is rare to develop an infection during the trial period, but it is certainly possible, as shown in a slow-titration study of continuous intrathecal ziconotide by Ver Donck and colleagues, in which 4 of the first 40 patients enrolled developed meningitis after the third week of trialing (Ver Donck et al. 2008). In addition, 14% of patients developed a CSF leak with concomitant post-dural puncture headache (Ver Donck et al. 2008). Given the risk of CSF leakage and post-dural puncture headache, it is recommended to advise patients on what to look for after an intrathecal trial and on the appropriate conservative measures to take if they develop a post-dural puncture headache. The clinician should also remain vigilant for the possibility of the patient developing a spinal headache, and a lumbar epidural blood patch should be performed if the patient is unresponsive to noninvasive treatments. It should also be noted that although rare, clinicians should also remain vigilant for any signs of meningitis in the posttrial period.

In order to lessen the risk of overmedication, it is recommended that trialing doses of intrathecal medications should be chosen conservatively, and physicians should start with the lowest reasonable dose and gradually titrate up based on the patient's response in regards to pain relief, improved function, and the occurrence of side effects (Deer et al. 2017a). The complication of spinal cord injury or nerve injury is rare but is mentioned due to the possibility of occurring and the potential severity of these complications. To limit the potential for any nerve injuries, including that of the spinal cord, general anesthesia should be avoided when possible and the use of fluoroscopy and intrathecal contrast helps minimize the abovementioned risk.

10 Catheter Dislodgement

Catheter complications comprise a majority of the device-related complications that occur with intrathecal drug delivery systems. In a report from Sterns and colleagues, the annual rate for device-related complications was approximately 10.5%, with the majority being catheter-related (65%) versus pump-related (35%) (Grider et al. 2011). Complications occur in permanently implanted pumps, but catheter dislodgement can also occur during continuous catheter trials. Since we are also evaluating patient function during the trial and patients are usually in the hospital for several days, it is important to secure the catheter to the skin to prevent it from being pulled out of the intrathecal space. Some practitioners suture the catheter to the skin at the entry site, while others may use Steri strips or another type of adhesive device to secure the catheter. Either method is acceptable as long as care is taken to adequately secure the catheter to the skin at the entry point. If the catheter is pulled out of the intrathecal space, the trial can either be terminated or the patient can be retrialed. Another site where the catheter commonly disconnects is at the connection to the pump. Usually if the catheter becomes dislodged at this site, it can be swabbed with alcohol and reconnected. The longer the trial and the more active or mobile the patient, the higher the risk for catheter dislodgement. With proper technique in securing the intrathecal catheter and vigilance in care of the catheter, we can significantly reduce the risk of dislodgement.

11 Conclusion

Trialing is important, especially in patients with nonmalignant pain, as it provides the clinician and the patient a preview of the anticipated response to a permanent intrathecal drug delivery system. As we said at the beginning of this chapter, most patients that are candidates for intrathecal drug delivery systems have failed all conservative treatments for their chronic pain symptoms. Regardless of the trialing method or medication used, physicians must be familiar with side effects, complications, and their management. Knowledge of patient comorbidities, pain type, and risk factors may determine the setting in which the trial is conducted. Ultimately, it is up to the physician, based on their knowledge, experience, and comfort level, to decide the medication, trialing method, and setting for the intrathecal trial. Success of the intrathecal trial relies on selecting the right patient that has had an appropriate pretrial psychological evaluation and who has participated in a thorough discussion of the intrathecal medication delivery process and their expectations. The more familiar we are with the different medications, trial settings, trialing methods, side effects, and complications, the better chances we have for a successful outcome.

References

Anderson VC, Burchiel KJ, Cooke B (2003) A prospective, randomized trial of intrathecal injection vs epidural infusion in the selection of patients for continuous intrathecal opioid therapy. Neuromodulation 6:142–152

Ansari NN, Naghdi S, Arab TK, Jalaie S (2008) The interrater reliability of the modified Ashworth scale in the assessment of muscle spasticity: limb and muscle group effect. Neurorehabilitation 23(3):231–237

Bernards CM (2006) Cerebrospinal fluid and spinal cord distribution of baclofen and bupivacaine during slow intrathecal infusion in pigs. Anesthesiology 105:169–178

Bohannon RW, Smith MB (1987) Phys Ther 67(2):206–207

Chaney MA (1995) Side effects of intrathecal and epidural opioids. Can J Anaesth 42(10):891–903

Coffey R, Owens M, Broste S et al (2009) Mortality associated with implantation and management of intrathecal opioid drug infusion systems to treat noncancer pain. Anesthesiology 111:881–891

Deer TR, Smith HS, Cousins M et al (2010) Consensus guidelines for the selection and implantation of patients with noncancer pain for intrathecal drug delivery. Pain Physician 13:E175–E213

Deer TR, Smith HS et al (2011) Comprehensive consensus based guidelines on intrathecal drug delivery systems in the treatment of pain caused by cancer pain. Pain Physician 14:E283–E312

Deer TR, Prager J, Levy R et al (2012a) Polyanalgesic consensus conference 2012: recommendations for the management of pain by intrathecal (intraspinal) drug delivery: report of an interdisciplinary expert panel. Neuromodulation 15:436–464

Deer TR, Prager J, Levy R, Burton A, Buchser E, Caraway D et al (2012b) 2012 polyanalgesic consensus conference-2012: recommendations on trialing for intrathecal (intraspinal) drug delivery: report of an interdisciplinary expert panel. Neuromodulation 1(Suppl):420–435

Deer TR, Hayek S, Pope JE et al (2017a) The polyanalgesic consensus conference (PACC) recommendations for trialing of intrathecal drug delivery infusion therapy. Neuromodulation 20(2):133–154. https://doi.org/10.1111/ner.12543

Deer TR, Pope J et al (2017b) The polyanalgesic consensus conference (PACC) recommendations on intrathecal drug infusion systems best practices and guidelines. Neuromodulation 20(2):96–132

Doleys DM, Kraus JK (2004) Psychological and addiction issues in intraspinal therapy. Semin Pain Med 2:46–52

Grider JS, Harned ME, Etscheidt MA (2011) Patient selection and outcomes using a low-dose intrathecal trialing method for chronic nonmalignant pain. Pain Physician 14:343–361

Hamza M, Doleys D, Wells M et al (2012) Prospective study of 3 year follow up of low dose intrathecal opioids in the management of chronic nonmalignant pain. Pain Med 13:1304–1313

Hamza M, Doleys DM, Saleh IA, Medvedovsky A, Verdolin MH, Hamza MA (2015) Prospective, randomized, single-blinded, head-to-head long-term outcome study comparing intrathecal boluses with continuous infusion trialing techniques prior to implantation of drug delivery systems for the treatment of severe intractable chronic nonmalignant pain. Neuromodulation 18:636–649

Harned ME, Salles SS, Grider JS (2011) An introduction to trialing intrathecal baclofen in patients with hemiparetic spasticity: a description of 3 cases. Pain Physician 14:483–489

Hassenbusch SJ, Gunes S, Wachsman S, Willis KD (2002) Intrathecal clonidine in the treatment of intractable pain: a phase I/II study. Pain Med 3:85–91

Hayek SM, Hanes MC, Wang C, Veizi IE (2015) Ziconotide combination intrathecal therapy for non-cancer pain is limited secondary to delayed adverse effects: a case series with a 24 month follow up. Neuromodulation 18:397–403

Hayek SM, Veizi E, Hanes M (2016) Intrathecal hydromorphone and bupivacaine combination therapy for post laminectomy syndrome optimized with patient-activated bolus device. Pain Med 17(3):561–571. Epub ahead of print

Krach LE (2001) Pharmacotherapy of spasticity: oral medications and intrathecal baclofen. J Child Neurol 16:31–36

Malhotra VT, Root J et al (2013) Intrathecal pain pump infusions for intractable cancer pain: an algorithm for dosing without a neuraxial trial. Anesth Analg 116(6):1364–1370

Mayo clinic drugs and supplements. Ziconotide (intrathecal route). 2020

Medicare Coverage Issues Manual (2009) Coverage issues—durable medical equipment. www.cms.hhs.gov/manuals/downloads/Pub06_PART_60.pdf. Accessed 19 Aug 2009

Mohamed SI, Eldabe S, Simpson KH et al (2013) Bolus intrathecal injection of Ziconotide to evaluate the option of continuous administration via implanted intrathecal drug delivery system: a pilot study. Neurostimulation 16:576; discussion 582

Penn RD, Kroin JS (1984) Intrathecal baclofen alleviates spinal cord spasticity. Lancet 1:1078

Pope JE, Deer TR (2015) Intrathecal pharmacology update: novel dosing strategy for intrathecal monotherapy ziconotide on efficacy and sustainability. Neuromodulation 18:414–420

Product Surveillance Registry (PSR) Database (2015) Medtronic plc, Minneapolis

Rainov NG, Heidecke V, Burkert W (2001) Long term intrathecal infusion of drug combinations for chronic back and leg pain. J Pain Symptom Manag 22:862–871

Rauck RL, Wallace MS, Leong MS et al (2006) A randomized, double-blind, placebo controlled study of intrathecal ziconotide in adults with severe chronic pain. J Pain Symptom Manag 31:393–406

Ruan X, Chen T, Bungardner GW, Hamilton J, Peavy A et al (2013) Novel epidural baclofen infusion trial for intractable spasticity with long-term follow-up observation and a focused review of the literature. J Pain Relief 2:121

Ver Donck A, Collins R, Rauck RL, Nitescu P (2008) An open-label, multicenter study of the safety and efficacy of intrathecal ziconotide for severe chronic pain when delivered via an external pump. Neuromodulation 11:103–111

WebMD (n.d.) Clonidine side effects by likelihood and severity

Yaksh TL, Fisher C, Hockman T, Wiese A (2017) Current and future issues in the development of spinal agents for the management of pain. Curr Neuropharmacol 15(2):232–259. Epub ahead of print

Targeted Drug Delivery Perioperative Planning Considerations

Lissa Hewan-Lowe and Corey W. Hunter

Contents

L. Hewan-Lowe (✉)
Department of Rehabilitation and Human
Performance, Icahn School of Medicine at Mount
Sinai Hospital, New York, NY, USA
e-mail: lissa.hewan-lowe@mssm.edu

C. W. Hunter
Ainsworth Institute of Pain Management,
New York, NY, USA
e-mail: chunter@ainpain.com

© The Author(s), under exclusive license to Springer Nature Switzerland AG 2022
D. P. Beall et al. (eds.), *Intrathecal Pump Drug Delivery*, Medical Radiology Diagnostic Imaging,
https://doi.org/10.1007/978-3-030-86244-2_5

Abstract

Intrathecal drug delivery systems (IDDS) have been utilized successfully in the treatment of a wide variety of chronic issues providing effective relief from pain and spasticity for almost 40 years (Onofrio et al. 1981; Prager et al. 2014). Indications for placement of these systems are categorized as treatment for conditions that are either diffuse or focal. Intrathecal drug delivery is a proven therapy that is valuable in the treatment of both cancer and noncancer pain as it has been demonstrated to reduce or eliminate the need for systemic opioid medications and has been shown to dramatically decrease the adverse side effects associated with systemic opioid delivery (Candido et al. 2017; Mitchell et al. 2015). Morphine, ziconotide, and baclofen are approved by the Food and Drug Administration (FDA) for use in IDDS, but off-label medications also show efficacy and are widely used intrathecally. Generally, implanted IDDSs work by infusing medication from a subcutaneously implanted pump directly into the intrathecal space via a catheter. The target of the infused medication is the dorsal horn of the spinal cord, and the intrathecal delivery targets this area directly and avoids the harsh side effects of many of the oral alternatives. Baricity refers to the medication's density relative to CSF and is an important variable of IDDS, as the baricity of the medication has to be taken into consideration when determining an optimal catheter tip placement location. When placing an IDDS, the proximal end of the catheter is tunneled and connected to the pump, which has been implanted and secured to the anterior abdominal wall (Lynch 2014). The pump contains a reservoir that pumps medication through the catheter into the intrathecal space. The medication stored in the implanted reservoir is retrieved and refilled percutaneously through a central access port. It is generally agreed that a trial should be conducted prior to implantation to determine the initial medication dose and patient response to the medication. The implanted pumps will need replacement when they near the end of their battery life or if there is a pump malfunction. The catheter may also need replacement or revision if there is disruption of the integrity or a blockage of the catheter. This chapter will feature the appropriate indications for IDDS, discuss on-label and novel medications, and will review important considerations in candidate selection, catheter tip placement, preoperative/intraoperative/postoperative planning, dealing with complications, and in the clinical management of patients undergoing intrathecal drug delivery therapy.

Abbreviations

ASA	Aspirin
ASRA	American Society of Regional Anesthesia and Pain Medicine
BMI	Body mass index
CBC	Complete blood count
CDC	Centers for disease control and prevention
CK	Creatinine kinase
CMP	Comprehensive metabolic panel
CRP	C-reactive protein
CRPS	Chronic regional pain syndrome
CSF	Cerebral spinal fluid
CT	Computed tomography
ERI	Elective replacement indicator
FDA	Food and Drug Administration
IDDS	Intrathecal drug delivery systems
INR	International normalized ratio
IT/ITT	Intrathecal/intrathecal therapy
ITB	Intrathecal baclofen
LMWH	Low molecular weight heparin
MR	Magnetic resonance
MRI	Magnetic resonance imaging
NICE	National Institute for Health and Care Excellence
NSAIDs	Nonsteroidal anti-inflammatory drugs
PACC	Polyanalgesic Consensus Conference
PMP	Prescription monitoring program
SSI	Surgical site infection
WBC	White blood cell count

1 Intrathecal Drug Delivery

Since the first reservoir implantation in 1981, intrathecal drug delivery systems (IDDS) have provided effective relief from pain and spasticity to patients with a wide variety of chronic issues (Onofrio et al. 1981; Prager et al. 2014). Its success has been demonstrated as a valuable in treatment of spasticity and intractable pain from cancer that aids in the reduction or elimination of oral opioid medications (Candido et al. 2017; Mitchell et al. 2015). Intrathecal (IT) drug delivery systems are comprised of a catheter and a pump that delivers medication either through an external or an internal drug delivery system. In the case of an external pump, the catheter is implanted and connected percutaneously to an external medication source. Generally, the percutaneous system is reserved for the treatment of acute and temporary pain (Xing et al. 2018). In implanted systems, a catheter is placed into the intrathecal space at the level of the lumbar spine and threading it cranially to target the dorsal horn of the spinal cord. The external end of the catheter is then tunneled to the location of the pocket that has been created for the pump, attached to an electronic pump, and then secured to the anterior abdominal wall (Lynch 2014). Regardless of the type of pump, the reservoir pumps medication through the catheter into the intrathecal space. Medication stored in the implanted reservoir is percutaneously accessed through a silicon access port, with a non-coring needle. This technique of accessing the pump is a more durable option than a percutaneous catheter, and it also has less risk of infection and/or catheter migration (Xing et al. 2018). For the purposes of this chapter, only intrathecal implanted drug delivery systems will be discussed. A discussion of external pumps can be found in chapter "The Components of Intrathecal Drug Delivery".

1.1 Indications

Intrathecal therapy has been used successfully for cancer and chronic nonmalignant pain (Shah and Padalia 2020a). In the past, IDDSs were only indicated for patients suffering from chronic pain who failed all other treatments as evidenced by poor pain control or intolerable side effects from oral medications (Shah and Padalia 2020a). However, IT therapy for chronic pain is increasingly becoming utilized as part of a multimodal pain control strategy, not just reserved for failed treatments (Xing et al. 2018). Analgesic response to intrathecal drug delivery (IDD) has been seen in patients with neuropathic, visceral, deafferentation, and mixed pain. Anecdotal evidence suggests IT therapy may also be used to treat focal extremity pain (Deer et al. 2017a). Intrathecal baclofen therapy is used to treat muscle spasticity from a variety of conditions such as spinal cord injury, stroke, multiple sclerosis, and cerebral palsy and is discussed further in chapters "Introduction and Background for Intrathecal Pumps Used for Pain and Spasticity", "Intrathecal Drug Delivery Trialing", and "Pump Management: Intrathecal Baclofen Pumps".

Cancer pain: Because cancer pain is often difficult to control and treated with high-dose opioids, IDD (which does not interfere with oncologic care) is often employed as studies have shown better efficacy improved toxicity and more optimal cost-effectiveness as compared to systemic opioids (Xing et al. 2018). Indications include single or multiple pain generators from primary or metastatic tumors, chronic postsurgical pain, and nerve injury or neuropathy after chemotherapy and/or radiation (Xing et al. 2018). In the case of end-of-life care, palliation with optimal pain control is the main objective (Deer et al. 2017a).

Noncancer pain: Indications include chronic pain from spinal pathology where the patient is not a surgical candidate, truncal pain, refractory axial back pain, abdominal pain, failed back surgery syndrome, peripheral neuropathy, complex regional pain syndrome (CRPS), arachnoiditis, and connective tissue disorders.

In both cancer and noncancer-related pain, there should be consideration for other interventional pain therapies such as thermal ablation techniques, chemo-embolization, vertebral augmentation, neurostimulation, and many other techniques. In the most recent recommendations from Polyanalgesic Consensus Conferences (PACC), IT therapies are recommended at the same level of as neurostimulation (Fig. 1) in neuropathic pain with stable disease course, but it is generally recommended that if the patient's pain can be effectively treated with neuromodulation, then that should be the first treatment that is offered (Deer et al. 2017a). However, it was also noted that neurostimulation therapies may lose efficacy and require revisions or explantation which should be incorporated into the decision-making process (Deer et al. 2017a). An algorithmic approach to intrathecal pump implantation should be part of a stepwise treatment plan and that includes a discussion of risks and benefits

with both patients and caregivers (Shah and Padalia 2020a).

Spasticity: Patients may be evaluated in a multidisciplinary rehabilitation setting and those that fail to achieve adequate functionality or spasticity management with oral medication, botulinum toxin injections, or both may be considered for intrathecal baclofen (ITB) (Lake and Shah 2019). Children with spasticity, limb deformity, joint dislocation, poor motor function, muscle tightness, and progressive neurologic diseases are typical candidates for ITB plus rehabilitation, and this can be initiated after an appropriately conducted IT baclofen trial (Saulino et al. 2016).

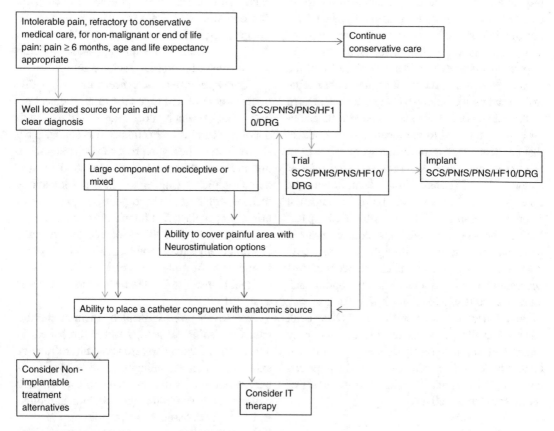

Fig. 1 Algorithm for device placement within the pain care algorithm for non-cancer patients or patients with pain not at the end of life. *DRG* dorsal root ganglion, *HF10* high frequency stimulation, *PNfS* peripheral nerve field stimulation, *PNS* peripheral nerve stimulation, *SCS* spinal cord stimulation). Blue arrows indicate an affirmation or positive response; red arrows signify a negative response. (Adapted from: Deer TR, Pope JE, Hayek SM, Bux A, Buchser E, Eldabe S et al. The Polyanalgesic Consensus Conference (PACC): Recommendations on Intrathecal Drug Infusion Systems Best Practices and Guidelines. Neuromodulation. 2017;20(2):96–132. https://doi.org/10.1111/ner.12538)

1.2 Medications

Choosing medication for intrathecal therapy should take into consideration the diagnosis, the patient life expectancy, potential duration of therapy, the pain type and location, drug properties of the chosen medication, the type of catheter and placement target, and the type of dosing. For example, IT pain management works better with multiple bolus doses as compared to continuous infusion, whereas spasticity management dosing strategies may differ depending on severity, anatomic location, and the time of day that the spasticity is at its worst (Deer et al. 2017a). Additionally, changing medications to influence the physicochemical properties, solubility, permeability, kinetics, and metabolism of medication can affect cerebrospinal fluid (CSF) spread and help to guide medication selection (Deer et al. 2017a).

Morphine sulfate, ziconotide, and baclofen are the only medications approved by the US Food and Drug Administration (FDA) for intrathecal use (Xing et al. 2018; Deer et al. 2017a; Grider et al. 2008). Intrathecal opioid therapy is safer and has less risk of diversion as compared to oral therapy. Higher concentrations of opioids, however, come with increased risk of granuloma formation (Deer et al. 2017a). Off-label agents such as clonidine and bupivacaine have proven efficacy and will be discussed in more detail below (Candido et al. 2017).

Neuropathic pain typically responds to single agents such as ziconotide, local anesthetic, or clonidine but is also known to respond to clonidine combined with an opioid or an opioid combined with a local anesthetic. Medication combinations are sometimes required to produce the necessary treatment effect and should be considered after failure or inadequate response to a single on-label medication. *Nociceptive pain* generally responds to opioids, ziconotide, or a local anesthetic but is also known to respond to a combination of medications, most commonly an opioid combined with bupivacaine.

Cancer pain: When treating patients with neoplastic pain, the clinician should consider combination therapy as a first-line treatment choice. If the patient responds to morphine or ziconotide, however, the initial use of a single on-label medication is recommended (Deer et al. 2017a).

1.2.1 Morphine

Morphine is a mu-opioid receptor agonist that if injected into the CSF effects the neural elements by binding to receptors in the substantia gelatinosa located in the dorsal column. Pre- and post-synaptic receptor activation with morphine controls ascending pain-related neural activity. The first randomized controlled study for cancer pain showed an advantage to its use in pain control with reduced toxic side effects, and a subsequent study showed no difference in pain relief but consistently reduced toxicity (Xing et al. 2018).

1.2.2 Ziconotide

Ziconotide is a potent non-opioid drug derivative of neurotoxic venom from the cone snail that has demonstrated strong clinical evidence for its efficacy. Ziconotide works in nociceptive neurons in the dorsal horn as a reversible antagonist to presynaptic N-type voltage-gated calcium channels. It is non-granulomagenic and does not have the same association with cardiopulmonary depression fatalities that opioids do. Effective dosing starts at a low dose and is increased slowly as studies have shown it to have an improved safety profile and better tolerability with a slow titration (Xing et al. 2018; Padfield 2012).

1.2.3 Baclofen

By bypassing the blood-brain barrier, ITB offers spasticity reduction with less cognitive side effects than oral medications that is particularly helpful for spastic patients with cognitive deficits (Saulino et al. 2016). Baclofen can help to reduce pain but has limited utility as a primary medication to treat chronic pain (Deer et al. 2017a). The baricity of baclofen allows it to effectively float in the CSF, whereas morphine at higher concentrations will sink. So, if a patient is supine with a posteriorly placed IT catheter, it is likely that the hyperbaric morphine will sink down toward the arachnoid matter and be absorbed, losing its effect on the cord.

1.2.4 Off-Label Therapies and Medication Combinations

Off-label therapy for pain management is recommended for consideration if FDA-approved medications are contraindicated or a patient fails their therapy with one of the on-label medication (Deer et al. 2017a). Although there is limited research support for their intrathecal use, the following medications have been used in an off-label manner intrathecally and could be considered for use: octreotide, neostigmine, baclofen, clonidine, bupivacaine, fentanyl, sufentanil, hydromorphone, midazolam, and ketamine (Xing et al. 2018). In patients with cancer-related pain, there is widespread acceptance for using fentanyl as a primary IT medication, as well as hydromorphone or morphine or fentanyl combined with bupivacaine, ziconotide, or clonidine for failed relief with first-line agents (Table 1) (Xing et al. 2018; Deer et al. 2017a).

In addition to giving a single medication intrathecally, there is also evidence that supports combining medications can produce better pain control. Combining ziconotide and morphine as well as morphine with bupivacaine, levobupivacaine, ropivacaine, baclofen, clonidine, and dexmedetomidine have been shown to improve pain levels in patients' refractory cancer pain (Candido et al. 2017; Xing et al. 2018)

1.2.5 Novel Agents

There are currently novel agents under investigation for their potential role in intrathecal pain management including transcription factor inhibitors, conopeptides, a capsaicin analog that acts on a heat sensor receptor involved in pain signaling, and a destruction agent for c-fiber neurons (Xing et al. 2018).

1.3 Baricity

Baricity is the density of a substance relative to CSF. As hyperbaric solutions are denser than CSF, they will follow gravity, and hypobaric solutions will rise to the top of the space containing the CSF. The medication's baricity helps to predict its behavior within the intrathecal space.

In a vertical patient, for example, as the drug or drug mixture is infused through the intrathecal catheter, a hyperbaric solution will fall caudally, and a hypobaric solution will rise cephalad. Catheter tip placement should therefore take into account both the baricity of an infused solution and the typical patient position in order to achieve optimal treatment effects (Boster et al. 2016b).

The relationship between the concentration and density of both morphine and bupivacaine is linear and so at higher concentrations they are hyperbaric and may sink posteriorly in a supine patient (Boster et al. 2016b). Conversely, the relationship between the concentration and density of both clonidine and baclofen is logarithmic and thus hypobaric (Boster et al. 2016b). The intrathecal formulation of ziconotide is highly diluted with normal saline, which is hypobaric, and so the formulation as delivered is hypobaric (Boster et al. 2016b). Hydromorphone has a baricity that varies with the concentration from similar to CSF at lower concentrations to hyperbaric with higher concentrations.

2 Preoperative Management

2.1 Patient Selection

Identification of appropriate candidates is critical to achieving an optimal clinical benefit of IT therapy, and patients should meet acceptable selection criteria in addition to the appropriate physical indications prior to intrathecal pump placement (Shah and Padalia 2020a). Patients appropriate for intrathecal therapy should have a clear, accurate diagnosis that is derived via a thorough history and physical examination and a condition that is likely to respond to IT medications (Prager et al. 2014; Deer et al. 2017a). A comprehensive evaluation incorporates any necessary specialists and care team members in an effort to identify patients who are likely to have positive outcomes of IT therapy (Xing et al. 2018). This will help to refine the preoperative identification of appropriate patients and will facilitate the optimization of the patient's health, physical status, and family support prior to pump

Table 1 Recommendations for first-, second-, and third-line intrathecal pain medications in patients with noncancer-related nociceptive or neuropathic pain and in patients with cancer-related pain

	First line	Second line	Third line
Noncancer-localized pain	*Strong evidence:* ziconotide or morphine *Moderate evidence:* fentanyl alone or fentanyl + bupivacaine	Fentanyl + clonidine ± bupivacaine Hydromorphone or morphine + bupivacaine Bupivacaine	Fentanyl ziconotide + bupivacaine Morphine or hydromorphone + clonidine Ziconotide + clonidine or bupivacaine or both Bupivacaine + clonidine
Noncancer diffuse pain	*Strong evidence:* Ziconotide or morphine Moderate evidence: hydromorphone Morphine or Hydromorphone + bupivacaine		Morphine or hydromorphone + clonidine or ziconotide Fentanyl + bupivacaine
Cancer-related localized pain	Strong evidence: Ziconotide or morphine *Moderate evidence:* fentanyl morphine or fentanyl + bupivacaine	Hydromorphone + bupivacaine Hydromorphone or fentanyl or morphine + clonidine or ziconotide	Hydromorphone or fentanyl or morphine + bupivacaine + clonidine or ziconotide Ziconotide + bupivacaine or clonidine Sufentanil
Cancer-related diffuse pain	*Strong evidence:* Ziconotide or morphine *Moderate evidence:* Hydromorphone Morphine or hydromorphone + bupivacaine	Hydromorphone or morphine + ziconotide or clonidine	Hydromorphone or morphine or fentanyl + bupivacaine + clonidine or ziconotide Ziconotide + bupivacaine or clonidine Sufentanil

Adapted from: Deer TR, Pope JE, Hayek SM, Bux A, Buchser E, Eldabe S et al. The Polyanalgesic Consensus Conference (PACC): Recommendations on Intrathecal Drug Infusion Systems Best Practices and Guidelines. Neuromodulation. 2017;20(2):96–132. https://doi.org/10.1111/ner.12538

implantation (Xing et al. 2018). In addition to the issues listed above, environmental as well as psychosocial factors should also be evaluated (Prager et al. 2014). Clinicians should make every effort to obtain prior medical records and conduct a chart review in the process to optimally determine candidacy and to accurately stratify risk (Prager et al. 2014). Appropriate patients include those individuals with at least 3 months predicted survival, more than 50% pain relief during the preimplantation trial, and anatomy that allows for optimal catheter placement. Although IT therapy is indicated for a very wide variety of conditions, some diagnoses such as headache, fibromyalgia, atypical facial pain, and nonmalignant head-neck pain have failed to show good outcomes (Prager et al. 2014). Any chronic pain condition may also be complicated by untoward psychological issues which can make painful conditions much less responsive to any form of treatment including IT drug delivery. It is recommended that all patients undergo psychological evaluation in addition to physical evaluation prior to the IT medication trial. The psychological evaluation aims to assess a patient's understanding of IDD and its purpose and its limitations as well as their ability to cope with pain. The evaluation also is designed to rule out underlying mental disorders that may interfere with IDD. Psychological screening may be performed by trained mid-level providers in the absence of a fully trained psychological professional.

Patients may also develop new psychological symptoms after pump implantation that can often require follow-up and ongoing treatment by a mental health professional (Prager et al. 2014; Lynch 2014; Shah and Padalia 2020a; Deer et al. 2017a). In patients with cancer pain, the psychological assessment may be optional prior to an IT medication trial or pump implantation, but ongoing psychological treatment of pain may be a necessary adjunct (Deer et al. 2017a). *Cancer-related pain*: In patients with cancer pain, the decision to place a pump is more straightforward and increasingly considered earlier in the patient's course of treatment (Xing et al. 2018; Lynch 2014). *Spasticity*: Patients with severe

chronic spasticity of spinal or cerebral origin that have failed oral medication management are optimal for consideration of ITB. During the process of evaluating the patient in regard to their diagnosis, condition, and treatment options, the treatment plan should include a pain treatment algorithm that outlines the course of treatment starting with the least invasive options and ending with the least invasive treatment option that provides sufficient relief of pain and adequate functional improvement (Deer et al. 2016).

2.2 Preoperative Patient Workup and Considerations

General Assessment: During the preoperative workup, the patient's general medical condition should be assessed. Practitioners should look for straightforward causes of pain that can be treated or reversed. Other considerations prior to surgery are assessing the patient for any type of ongoing infection, to ensure the hemoglobin A1c is 7.5 or less and to assess their nutritional status as a poor status can contribute to slow healing and compromised pocket integrity (Prager et al. 2014).

2.3 Comorbidities and High-Risk Patients

Many patients that are optimal candidates for intrathecal therapies are considered high risk and have significant comorbidities and are often prominently debilitated. In general, comorbidities that increase the risk of complications during IT therapy include obstructive sleep apnea, chronic cardiopulmonary issues, smoking, venous insufficiency, metabolic syndrome, hypertension, diabetes mellitus, and immunosuppression (Xing et al. 2018). Opioid therapy should be accompanied by hypervigilance in patients with cardiopulmonary dysfunction and in those with reduced medication clearance such as geriatric patients or those with kidney or liver dysfunction as opioid therapy can depress respiratory drive (Deer et al. 2017a). As there is a potential for interactions between IT-delivered medications and CNS-active medications, guidelines suggest that benzodiazepines, antidepressants, anticonvulsants, muscle relaxants, and alcohol consumption be monitored for their effects and any potential adverse interaction (Deer et al. 2017a). Additionally, before starting intrathecal ziconotide, a creatinine kinase (CK) level should be established at baseline because ziconotide is known to elevate CK levels two or three times the upper limit of normal, but the causation mechanism of this increase and the significance of the high CK levels are unclear (Deer et al. 2017a).

Pain management considerations: In an effort to minimize adverse outcomes including death and to optimize the benefit of intrathecal therapies, it is recommended that systemic opioids be eliminated when possible (Deer et al. 2017a). Respiratory depression is a common concern in systemic opioid therapy and encompasses a range of severity from mild rate changes to respiratory arrest. In order to reduce risk, physicians should attempt to coordinate care, insist patients disclose all current prescriptions, and conduct regular prescription monitoring program (PMP) surveillance checks. It may also be prudent to conduct a drug screen prior to trial to establish a baseline or if illicit medication use is suspected (Prager et al. 2014; Deer et al. 2017a). Long-term opioid therapy is known to have potential adverse effects on hypothalamic-pituitary adrenal and gonadal axes and may affect neuroendocrine function (Prager et al. 2014). Therefore it is suggested that candidates undergo endocrine evaluation prior to the initiation of IT opioid therapy, with as needed intermittent ongoing surveillance for suppression (Prager et al. 2014; Deer et al. 2017a).

2.4 Medical Conditions that Prohibit Intrathecal Drug Delivery

Absolute contraindications to IDD include ongoing systemic or localized infection, bleeding diathesis, allergy to intrathecal medications or materials of the IT system, septicemia, localized infection near the pump implant site, obstructed (CSF) flow, the presence of an unstable mental health disorder, active substance abuse, and anticoagulation at time of implantation (Lynch 2014; Lake and Shah 2019; Awaad et al. 2012; Smyth et al. 2015).

Relative contraindications include a failed IT trial, immunosuppression, mental health disorders, epidural metastases, poor patient adherence, difficult spinal anatomy, unrealistic goals, psychosocial factors affecting compliance, and financial burdens caused by either the implantation surgery or the ongoing pump refills (Lynch 2014; Smyth et al. 2015). Ventriculoperitoneal shunting for hydrocephalus may affect cerebrospinal fluid flow, and this should be considered prior to initiating IDD therapy. A history of seizures, prior abdominal, or pelvic surgery is important and should be assessed, and the patient determined to be an eligible candidate for pump implantation prior to even conducting an IT trial (Saulino et al. 2016). Also before any type of surgical procedure to implant, the pump smoking cessation should be encouraged and anticoagulation stopped (Prager et al. 2014). There are special considerations for patients with cancer prior to placing an intrathecal pump. It is recommended to understand the primary cancer diagnosis, the degree of metastatic spread, and the patient's prognosis and to review all of the recent imaging to determine the exact location of tumor and the likelihood of pain to spread to other locations. All of these assessments should take place prior to scheduling the patient for an intrathecal medication trial (Deer et al. 2017a).

2.5 Other Considerations in Cancer Patients

The literature suggests IT therapy is a reasonable therapeutic option for patients undergoing chemotherapy and/or radiation. The initiation or continuation of IT therapy would not interfere with chemotherapy or radiation, and the pump implantation should be timed to take place between cancer treatments (Deer et al. 2011b). For patients undergoing radiation therapy, the radiation field may drain the battery or cause electrical failure of the device, and so caution should be taken to adequately shield the pump with lead to minimize the device's radiation exposure. If this is not possible, relocation of the pump may be considered (Deer et al. 2011b).

Contraindications for IT therapy include a white blood cell count (WBC) of $\leq 2 \times 10^9/L$ and/or an absolute neutrophil count (ANC) of $\leq 1000/\mu L$, but patients receiving colony-stimulating factors (CFS) or other growth factor treatments may still be candidates for IT therapy. Additionally, platelet counts in these patients should exceed 50,000/μL, and ideally they should have the ability to keep their platelet counts between 70,000 and 100,000/μL as these patients will need to have continued interventions including pump refills and, potentially, catheter and rotor checks. The pump implantation can occur between treatments when the patient's white blood cell counts are higher. This should be carefully coordinated with the treating oncologist and the other clinicians involved in the patient's care (Deer et al. 2011b).

2.6   Trialing

Intrathecal medication trials consist of either medication titration, lasting days to weeks, or bolus trialing with a single injection of medication, and the patient kept overnight. Regardless of the method of trialing, they are both conducted as an inpatient so the patient's vital signs and respirations can be monitored. An intrathecal trial conducted prior to permanent implantation demonstrates an individual's response to IDD. In cases of terminal illness or if the patient is in extreme intractable pain, the trial may be skipped (Prager et al. 2014; Deer et al. 2017a). As mentioned, the trial options include either a single injection or an infusion trial infusion. Both of these trialing methods are an option, and the intrathecal trialing of medications will

be discussed further in chapter "Intrathecal Drug Delivery Trialing". Each of the trialing methods has their advantages and disadvantages, and the specific method should be chosen on a case-by-case basis (Lynch 2014). In theory, an intrathecal trial should involve the proposed medication and mimic the dosing, the infusion rate, and the catheter placement level (Prager et al. 2014). Opioid trials must be monitored overnight, and patients who use positive pressure respiration devices for their sleep apnea should continue their use throughout the trial (Prager et al. 2014). Pain relief during the trial is only one indicator of success for IDD, and additional diagnostic evaluations may be needed. In patients who are appropriate candidates for an IT trial and if there are no contraindications for the trial, an IT trial is highly recommended to determine the effectiveness of the medication and to assess the ability of the patient to tolerate the medication.

A baclofen trial to assess for the patient's response to ITB is typically conducted prior to pump placement and is important for identifying candidates, determining the optimal starting dose and for refining the patient treatment goals. The contraindications to trialing are the same as the contraindications to intrathecal trialing for pain (Boster et al. 2016a). Patients who have partial ambulatory capability may be considered for an intrathecal trial so they can evaluate how a lowered lower extremity muscular tone effects their ambulation. Typically, during a lower dose ITB trial, a bolus of 50 mcg of medication is given. In special circumstances including very small children and patients that utilize their spasticity for mobility, bolus trial dosing may be reduced to 25 mcg (Boster et al. 2016a). Conversely, some patients may require a larger dose of 75–100 mcg. Regardless of the intrathecal dose given, 24 h must pass between bolus doses to allow clearance of the medication and normalization of the patient's spasticity. During the first portion of an ITB trial, the patient's cardiopulmonary function should be monitored while measuring the patients modified Ashworth Scores and monitoring for the point when the patient's spasticity returns

(Boster et al. 2016a). Additionally, patient observation should include watching for adverse events such as headaches, nausea, vomiting, urinary retention, hypotension, seizures, sedation, respiratory depression, and even coma (Boster et al. 2016a).

2.7 Preimplantation Planning Considerations

Prior to implantation, some of the important issues to consider are the starting dose and drug concentration, the medication delivery mode, the pump size and location, and the target level for catheter tip placement (Boster et al. 2016a).

Timing of implantation: Neurostimulation can be considered for the treatment of noncancer pain if the pain is well localized and not likely to spread. If the pain is multifocal, cancer related, or likely to spread, IT therapy should be considered as a primary treatment rather than neurostimulation. The PACC guidelines cite literature suggesting IT therapy may provide greater flexibility than neurostimulation when pain is likely to spread or increase in severity (Deer et al. 2017a). In cancer-related pain, the timing of pump implantation depends on the stage of the disease and the patient's life expectancy (Deer et al. 2017a).

Catheter tip placement: The patient's response to the IT medication response depends on a number of different elements including catheter tip location, the medications hydrophilicity and baricity and the dermatomal, sclerotomal, or viscerotomal level of the pain generator (Table 2). In

Table 2 Catheter tip placement level as determined by the primary location of the patient's pain

Pain generator site	Level
Head, neck, and arm	T3–T6[a]
Back and leg	T8–T10
Abdomen	T8–T11
Rectal/pelvic	T11–L2

[a]Some literature suggests cervical placement to cover head and neck pain generators; however, this should be done with caution as more cephalad placement will give more spread of medication and may produce more CNS side effects (Deer et al. 2016) (Chan et al. n.d.).

regards to the catheter tip location, some of the medication flow analyses have shown that the medication infused through the catheter has limited spread beyond the tip and that it produces slightly improved segmental pain relief in the focal area around the catheter tip (Xing et al. 2018; Deer et al. 2017a). Recent PACC guidelines highlight that there is limited data to inform optimal tip placement (Deer et al. 2017c). Ideally, the catheter tip should be aimed at the center of the spinal dermatome in the dermatomal area correlated with the area producing pain (Table 2) (Shah and Padalia 2020a; Deer et al. 2017a). In some cases, such as children with CP, the catheter tip can be placed into the pre-brainstem area to combat both dystonia and spasticity (Saenz et al. 2021) *(s)*. (Deer et al. 2017d).

The preoperative assessment of the intrathecal space and the degree of patency can facilitate appropriate anatomic insertion and for placement of the intrathecal catheter. Catheter insertion and accurate tip placement may be technically difficult in patients with severe spasticity that may have neuromuscular derived scoliosis and spinal torsion and previous spinal fusion surgeries (Robinson et al. 2017). The presence of the spinal deformities can complicate not only the lumbar catheter insertion but can make getting the catheter tip placed in the correct position difficult (Robinson et al. 2017). The intrathecal compartment containing the CSF delivers the medication to the spinal cord, and this space can have barriers or can form compartments due to spinal deformity or prior surgery and therefore sometimes needs to be assessed for resistance or limitation of CSF circulation (Deer et al. 2017a). This can be done by way of magnetic resonance (MR) imaging CSF flow studies or through computed tomography (CT) myelography. Additionally, certain unusual anatomic variants may inhibit the use of intrathecal catheters. Therefore the investigation of spinal deformities, assessment of previous spinal or abdominal surgeries, and consideration of other relevant comorbidities should take place during the initial assessment of the patient under consideration for IDD (Prager et al. 2014).

Table 3 Catheter insertion level as determined by different pathology locations (Chan et al. n.d.)

Insertion	
Cervical	Head and neck cancers with refractory pain in upper cervical dermatomes C1–5
Thoracic	Breast, lung mediastinal tumors with referred intercostal pain in thoracic dermatomes
Lumbar	Abdominal tumors (i.e., esophageal, pancreatic, gastric, and colorectal cancers) for upper thoracic and lumbar pain

Alternative placement techniques include surgical placement through a laminotomy created by drilling through fusion masses and/or the lumbar lamina with a high-speed bur down to the level of the dura creating a channel for inserting the catheter. The catheter can also be inserted at other levels of the spine including at the thoracic spine, cervical spine, or foramen magnum (Table 3) (Robinson et al. 2017). Alternate imaging modalities may also be used to guide the catheter placement including the use of conventional CT or cone beam CT that is widely available on many C-arm fluoroscopy units (Robinson et al. 2017). One of the primary considerations when placing the catheter is the presence and severity of spinal stenosis. Patients with spinal stenosis can be implanted if the catheter is placed above the location of the stenosis including above the level of the conus medullaris provided the patient is neurologically stable and the imaging guidance is optimal (Lake and Shah 2019; Albright et al. 2006).

Some literature suggests a cervical catheter tip placement to cover pain generators located in the head and neck (Deer et al. 2016; Chan et al. n.d.). This should be done with caution; however, as more cephalad placement will give more spread of the medication and may produce more CNS side effects (Deer et al. 2016; Chan et al. n.d.).

Pump placement: Selecting pump size and planning for placement. Preoperatively, the integrity of possible pump placement sites should be assessed, and the planned pocket location should be determined and discussed with the patient (Awaad et al. 2012). Pump manufacturers typically recommend anterior abdominal place-

ment and attachment to Scarpa's fascia, and the vast majority of the pumps are implanted subcutaneously in either the right or left lower quadrants (Prager et al. 2014; Deer et al. 2017a; Teodorczyk et al. 2013). Despite this convention, there is no significant evidence showing one pump implantation method is superior to another so we suggest the decision be guided by the patient's body habitus, condition of the typical sites of implantation, the therapy goals, and the patient's personal preference. In abdominal placement, the patient's abdominal and flank anatomy will need to be able to withstand device placement onto the anterior abdominal wall and have enough subcutaneous tissue and integrity of the overlying skin to withstand the tunneling across the flank (Knight et al. 2007b). During the assessment, the clinician may find that an abdominal wall implantation may not be appropriate for implantation due to an unusual body habitus, anatomic impediments, lack of sufficient subcutaneous fat, scar tissue from previous surgeries, prior radiation therapy, poor skin quality because of infection or inflammation, or increased skin tension on the overlying abdomen. In these cases, an alternative placement site may be necessary.

In patients with very low body mass index (BMI), a subfascial or submuscular placement is well vascularized, stable, and minimizes the dangers of pump infection and movement. In the abdomen, this approach places the pump into a pocket in the subfascial plane or within the rectus sheath (Deer et al. 2016; Bogue et al. 2020; Fiaschi et al. 2018; Follett et al. 2004). A benefit to placing the pump into a deeper layer is possible prevention of wound dehiscence and skin erosion over the surface of the pump, but a deeper device placement makes refills more painful and more challenging (Follett et al. 2004). In morbidly obese patients, it may not be practical to place the pump against the abdominal fascia as this placement may be too deep. Options include placing the pump farther lateral than the mid-clavicular line in a region that tends to have less adipose tissue or placing the pump into the mid-fat plane of the lower quadrant of the abdomen (Knight et al. 2007a, b). Placing the pump in adipose tissue should be avoided if at all possible as the device cannot be securely anchored and there will be an increased risk of the device flipping resulting in kinking or twisting of the catheter. Pumps may be placed posteriorly in the flank in the location of the superior lumbar (Grynfeltt-Lesshaft) triangle or superior to the hip in the gluteal region. Alternate locations include overlying the pectus major, on the anterior portion of the upper thigh and in the mid-abdomen (Narang et al. 2016; Devine et al. 2016). These alternative regions can be applied to the patient treatment plan as their body habitus and the needs of the therapy dictate. In patients who cannot tolerate traditional lateral decubitus surgical positioning and who require prone positioning instead, a posterior placement should be considered. Currently, available implantable pumps come with either a 20 mL or 40 mL reservoir. Small reservoirs should be implanted in patients who have a smaller body habitus, in patients who have a lower IT dose requirement, or in patients who would like a smaller profile device. The pump, when placed in the lumbar triangle location, should reside approximately 10 cm above the iliac crest for optimal comfort and to minimize the possibility of erosion (Padfield 2012; Deer et al. 2016). *Anticoagulation Guidelines: when to stop and when to restart.* According to recent PACC guidelines, anticoagulation medications should be held anywhere between 24 h and 14 days prior to trial depending on the type of medication, the indication, and the comorbidities of the patient. Additionally, herbal supplements that may cause anticoagulation, such as ginkgo biloba or ginger, are also encouraged to be held prior to performing a trial. All anticoagulants should be held for the duration of the trial and in general can be restarted 24 h after catheter removal. In the case of permanent implantation, anticoagulation may resume 24 h after surgery (Deer et al. 2017a). The PACC guidelines note that subcutaneous and IV heparin recommendations are on a case-by-case basis.

As per the most recent guidelines for anticoagulation put forth by the American Society of Regional Anesthesia and Pain Medicine (ASRA), when performing neuraxial procedures, subcutaneous heparin may be stopped 6 h prior to procedure. Table 4 shows the most recent guidelines that were published in 2019. They emphasize the importance of identifying risk prior to the procedure, maintaining accurate medication lists, and stratify risks in consultation with other physicians treating the patient (American Society of Regional Anesthesia and Pain Medicine 2010).

Risk Assessment: Medications that may contribute to respiratory depression should be identified and potentially stopped prior to trial and implantation (Deer et al. 2017a). Many patients being considered for intrathecal opioid therapy are already opioid tolerant and have a relatively low risk for respiratory depression form these medications (Deer et al. 2017a). Additionally, occult high intracranial pressure can increase the risk of a CSF leak, and thus patients at risk of high intracranial pressures may need to be screened with imaging and measurement of the intrathecal pressure prior to pump and catheter implantation.

Pre-op labs: Preoperative labs assess for infection, coagulation dysfunction, endocrine function, ability to properly heal the surgical wound, and for an overall laboratory evaluation of medical stability. It is recommended to acquire a complete blood count (CBC), comprehensive metabolic panel (CMP), coagulation studies, and an endocrine evaluation. As mentioned before, a hemoglobin A1c value may be checked if uncontrolled diabetes is suspected.

Imaging: Preoperative imaging should focus on assessing the patient's anatomy and on determining the best approach for the intrathecal medication trial and pump and catheter implantation procedure. Imaging evaluations include MR imaging of the thoracic and lumbar spine or CT myelography if the patient is unable to undergo an MRI (Deer et al. 2017a). In addition to the cross-sectional imaging, X-rays of the spine may be useful to assess the anatomy and any postsurgical changes that may be present (Deer et al. 2017a).

Table 4 Anticoagulation recommendations based on the 2019 American Society of Regional Anesthesia and Pain Medicine guidelines (American Society of Regional Anesthesia and Pain Medicine 2010)

Medication	When to discontinue prior to procedure			
	High risk	Medium risk	Low risk	
Warfarin	5 days	5 days	a	INR should be checked prior to procedure and be within normal range during procedure. Warfarin and acenocoumarol may be restarted at 6 and 24 h post procedure, respectively
Acenocoumarol	3 days	3 days	a	
P2Y12 inhibitors				Clopidogrel can be restarted 12–24 h and Prasugrel, Ticlopidine, Cangrelor restarted 24 h post procedure
Clopidogrel	7 days	7 days	a	
Prasugrel	7–10 days	7–10 days	a	
Ticlopidine	5 days	5 days	a	
Cangrelor	3 days	3 days	a	
GP IIb/IIIa inhibitors				
Abciximab	2–5 days	2–5 days	2–5 days	
Tirofiban/eptifibatide	8–24 h	8–24 h	8–24 h	Restart 8–12 h post procedure
LMWH				Restart 4 h post low-risk procedure. For medium-/high-risk restart 12–24 h post procedure
Prophylaxis	12 h	12 h	12 h	
Treatment dose	24 h	24 h	24 h	
Unfractionated heparin				
Subcutaneous	24 h	6 h	6 h	Can restart subcutaneous heparin 2 h post low-risk procedures and 6–8 h post intermediate and high-risk procedures
IV	6 h	6 h	6 h	Restart IV heparin 2 h post procedure
Fibrinolytics: Fondaparinux	4 days	4 days	a	Restart 6 h after low-risk procedures, otherwise restart after 24 h
Dabigatran	4 days	4 days	a	Restart 24 h post procedure
Rivaroxaban/Apixaban/Edoxaban	3 days	3 days	a	
ASA and ASA combinations				Restart 24 h post procedure
Primary prevention	6 days	a	a	
Secondary prevention	a	a	a	
NSAIDs	5 half-lives	a	a	Restart 24 h post procedure

NSAIDs can be continued for medium- and low-risk procedures.
Consider discontinuing ASA and NSAIDs in some medium-risk procedures.
aRecommend shared assessment and risk stratification; refer to the ASRA guidelines for specific recommendations regarding continuation

3 Intraoperative Management

3.1 Sedation Versus General Anesthesia

Placement under general anesthesia warrants careful needle placement and catheter advancement to avoid spinal cord trauma, as patients cannot provide feedback as monitoring as they can with moderate sedation (Prager et al. 2014). It is suggested by some that general anesthesia be avoided for "percutaneous placement of an intrathecal catheter, except under special circumstances such as a patient's inability to be still during placement despite moderate sedation (i.e., due to spasticity or tremor associated conditions (Prager et al. 2014). General anesthesia is preferred in pediatric patients and in patients where the clinician is confident of the catheter placement (Awaad et al. 2012). Clinical experience indicates that an awake but sedated patient is an acceptable scenario for the individual undergoing the procedure as the clinician can use the patient's complaints of pain or paresthesia as an indicator of an adverse neurological event, but the degree of invasiveness of an intrathecal pump placement and the length of time necessary to place the pump and catheter may make it preferable to have the patient anesthetized with either spinal or general anesthesia. It has been recommended by the Polyanalgesic Consensus Conferences (PACC) that the choice of anesthetic should be left to the managing clinician and tailored to the patient's best interest (Deer et al. 2017c).

3.2 Prophylactic Medications

Preoperative antibiotics are recommended for prevention of surgical site infection, prior to trial and 1 h before the system implantation (Awaad et al. 2012). In the case of immunosuppressed patients, additional preoperative measures may be warranted to prevent injection (Saulino et al. 2016). In regards to infection prophylaxis, recent PACC guidelines recommend:

- *Pre-op*: Antibiotic should be given 1 h prior to implantation with the dose depending on the weight of the patient; after entering the operating room, shave or remove the hair in the locations of the planned incisions; the patient should receive prophylactic preoperative antibiotic with weight-based dosing prior to trials; a preoperative nasal culture should be obtained and nasal bacitracin given if positive for staphylococcus.
- *Intra-op*: The patients skin should be prepped with chlorhexidine gluconate; the clinician performing the surgery should double glove.
- *Post-op*: An occlusive dressing should be applied after the trial if a catheter is used; the clinician should be aware of the increased possibility of a deep surgical site infection that may occur up to 1 year after implantation; post-op antibiotics should be given after 24 h in both catheter trial patients and after pump and catheter implantation.

3.3 Appropriate Patient Positioning

The patient is anesthetized and then positioned in the lateral decubitus position on the operating room table with the side of the pump placement upward and the patient placed on a surgical beanbag immobilizer or something similar to hold their position (Fig. 2). In some cases, off-label pump placement positions will dictate alternate patient positioning such as placing the patient prone or supine. The patient is then sterilely prepped and draped, and a C-arm is put into place to guide needle access to an intrathecal location and for the positioning of the catheter tip (Fig. 2).

3.4 Location and Placement of the Intrathecal Needle and Catheter

Catheter complications are the most common cause of failure in long-term intrathecal medication delivery. Thus the needle and catheter placement are critical steps in the implantation process.

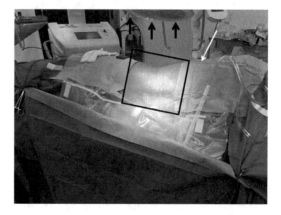

Fig. 2 Typical patient positioning on the operating room table should be in a lateral decubitus position with the pump implantation side up (white arrow) and the surgical site prepped (area within the black rectangle). The surgical beanbag immobilizer is placed beneath the patient and cannot be seen as it is blocked by the overlying blue surgical drapes. The C-arm is seen to be in place over the patient (black arrows)

3.5 Needle Placement

Under fluoroscopic guidance, the needle should be positioned for entry at L2–3 or L3–4 (one to two levels below dural puncture site) to avoid injury to the conus medullaris and using a para-median approach with an oblique shallow angle on the side ipsilateral to the pump placement site. This approach aims to prevent the catheter from crossing midline, which reduces the risk of breakage or dislodgement (Prager et al. 2014; Padfield 2012). A cut down may be required in order to reduce the entry angle of the needle, and longer needles should be used either in place of a cut down or for patients with larger body habitus (Padfield 2012).

3.6 Selecting Catheter Length

Catheter length depends on the chosen pump implantation site. The conventional catheter lengths are sufficient for all but the most extreme cases, and typically there is excess catheter that should be trimmed to the appropriate size. The excess catheter should be cut, but adequate catheter length should be left in order to create a relief loop in the midline and behind the pump to reduce unnecessary tension on the catheter. Care must be taken not to leave too much catheter redundancy as too much length may increase the risk of the catheter kinking (Shah and Padalia 2020a).

3.7 Techniques and Considerations for Tunneling Catheters

The pathway of tunneling should be decided upon prior to surgery, and the pathway for the tunnel should be marked for the purpose of identifying the location for placement of the local anesthetic. This pathway should consider the patient's bony structures including the rib margin and the iliac crests along with other factors such as the amount of subcutaneous soft tissue, previous abdominal and spine surgeries, and truncal deformities. Once the catheter is placed with the tip at the appropriate location and the catheter secured with the anchor, local anesthesia is injected along the marked tunneling path (Padfield 2012). A tunneling rod is used and placed through the subcutaneous soft tissue from the point where the catheter is anchored to the pump pocket or vice versa. Confirmation of correct tunneling rod placement in the subcutaneous tissue is done with palpation, but imaging guidance can be used if necessary. After the catheter has been successfully tunneled, the excess portion is trimmed, the connector is added to the proximal end of the catheter, and then the catheter is attached to the pump.

3.8 Anchoring

The pump should be anchored by using permanent sutures to attach the pump to Scarpa's abdominal fascia in the location of the pocket (Knight et al. 2007b). When anchoring the pump into place, we recommend the device be sutured with strong non-dissolvable sutures such as a 2-0 fiber wire sutures or 2-0 silk. The use of a Dacron pouch and that would scar it into place in lieu of sutures has fallen out of favor as the soft tissue's reaction to this pouch produces extensive scar tissue, and any revisions are made more difficult and typically require a prolonged dissection time in order to take out the patch.

3.9 Wound Closure

Prior to closure, adequate hemostasis should be already been achieved, and the wound should be closed in a layered approach to stabilize the implanted pump and to prevent the risk of postoperative infections (Knight et al. 2007b; Follett et al. 2004). In regards to wound closure technique, study results are mixed. Although some evidence suggests the use of staples for wound closure as it has been shown to significantly reduce risk of wound dehiscence and infection, recent literature reviews show no difference in closure methods overall regarding these rates

(Kim et al. 2017; Newman et al. 2011; Mitigation of Infection Risk n.d.; Cochetti et al. 2020; Krishnan et al. 2019). One study notes that infection rates and complications of closure methods may be due to varying techniques among clinicians and variance between institutions regarding post-op care (Luo et al. 2020). Additionally, staples may be added to suture closures to reinforce and reduce tension (Shah and Padalia 2020b). Overall, given the wide variability in wound closure techniques and with the improvement in suture quality and wound dressings, we believe that the closure method should be the surgeon's choice.

3.10 Wound Dressing

A non-bulky sterile occlusive dressing that fully covers the incision should be applied intraoperatively immediately after wound closure to reduce the risk of infection. This will also serve as protective barrier for device programming, which involves non-sterile equipment and begins shortly after placement by placing the communicator over the pump. The first postoperative dressing change will vary according to the surgeon's preference, but both the Centers for Disease Control (CDC) and NICE recommend using sterile occlusive dressings for 24–48 h (Follett et al. 2004; Deer et al. 2017b). Existing evidence, however, does not definitively support the use of these dressings past 24 h (Follett et al. 2004; Deer et al. 2017b).

4 Postoperative Management

4.1 Postoperative Considerations

An abdominal binder should be used postoperatively to reduce the risk of hematoma formation and facilitate healing of the intrathecal pump to the anterior abdominal wall. This will not only facilitate the patient's postoperative discomfort but will keep the pump from coming detached from the abdominal wall and flipping in the pocket. Postoperatively, the patient should be monitored for signs of complications such as fever and swelling indicating a hematoma or a CSF leak. Titration of the patient's intrathecal pain medication may begin 24 h after procedure and for baclofen it can start immediately (Deer et al. 2011a). Operative documentation should include the specific anatomic location of the pump so the practitioners who will be performing future refills can reference this. Any anticoagulation that the patient is on can be started 24 h after surgery.

4.1.1 Postoperative Wound Care and Restrictions

Topical antimicrobial agents are not recommended for use on surgical wounds that heal by primary intention (Deer et al. 2017c). Recommendations for postoperative antibiotics typically suggest their stopping the antibiotics 1 day after surgery. In fact, most of the evidence shows the use of antibiotics past 48 h increases hospital stays and may slow healing (Deer et al. 2017b). Exceptions for this include patients that are immunocompromised, institutionalized patients, or patients undergoing revision implantation where the antibiotics may be continued for up to 2 weeks following implantation for maximum prophylaxis against infection. Postoperative follow-up should first occur 10–14 days after the procedure to ensure proper wound healing, to make sure the patients are recovering normally from the procedure and to adjust the IT medication if necessary (Deer et al. 2017b). An additional follow-up should be done at 6 weeks postoperatively to check for signs of surgical site infection (SSI), to check the patients healing and to make additional dosing changes to the medication of needed. If infection is suspected, the C-reactive protein (CRP) may be checked as this will be persistently or increasingly elevated with an infection. After any procedure, the CRP will rise due to stress but will subsequently decrease over normal course of the follow-up, and failure to normalize or if an unexpected spike in the level is detected, these indicators are highly sensitive for infection (Deer et al. 2017b).

Postoperative instructions should be given to patients and should include advice against lifting more than 10 pounds, strenuous activity, bending, twisting, or exposure to extreme heat or cold for 6–8 weeks (About Your Intrathecal Pump 2010).

4.1.2 Complications and Their Management

Complications may include respiratory depression or issues associated with medication infusion, pocket infection, seroma, hematoma, CSF leak, spinal headache, meningitis, pump or catheter malfunction, and catheter tip granuloma (Xing et al. 2018).

- *Under or over infusion of medication*: In evaluating for this, consider the mechanism of action of the medication, the symptoms of over or under dose, previous resistance or tolerance to the medication being infused, the likelihood of pump or catheter system failure, the current catheter location, or the possibility of catheter tip granuloma formation (Teodorczyk et al. 2013). If withdrawal is suspected, inpatient admission should be strongly considered. The workup for a medication or ITT system complication should include laboratory testing for the blood and/or urinary levels of the IT medication, pump interrogation, catheter aspiration via the catheter access port, test bolus through the pump, and reservoir aspiration to verify amount of medication in the pump (Lake and Shah 2019). An MRI or a CT myelogram scanned along the course of the catheter may help to diagnose difficult causes such as catheter granuloma formation that has been reported with the use of most drugs except fentanyl, sufentanil, and ziconotide (Lynch 2014).
- *Positional headache*: This may be due to intracranial hypotension that develops due to a CSF leak around the catheter, catheter displacement out of the CSF, or rupture or disconnection of the catheter or connectors. The treatment for this requires the repair or correction of whatever is causing the CSF leak and can involve such treatments as putting the patient in an 0 abdominal binder, requiring bed rest, providing intravenous hydration or

medications for a spinal headache, placing an epidural blood patch, or revising or replacing the catheter.
- *Suspected CSF leak*: As mentioned previously, if a CSF leak is suspected, it should be diagnosed with a combination of physical examination, imaging studies, and catheter aspiration/injection. After the leak is appropriately identified, the treatment can be rendered. If the leak is present around the catheter, an epidural blood patch is an appropriate treatment of this issue. If a single epidural blood patch is not effective, it can be repeated twice more and if the leak persists, one can perform an exploration of the lumbar wound and over sewing the dura in the location of the leak or patching it using a dural sealant such as Duraseal® Spine Sealant (Integra LifeSciences Corporation, Princeton, NJ, USA). If this is still not effective to abate the flow of CSF, the system can be removed or the cerebrospinal fluid can be diverted via a ventriculostomy.
- *Infection*: Infection following placement of an IDD system can include superficial skin infection, catheter implantation site infection, a pump pocket infection, or meningitis. Any infection of the components of the IDD system warrants the removal of all components of the system, culturing the existing infection and treatment with intravenous or the appropriate antibiotics (Lake and Shah 2019). In the pediatric population, one study showed that the overall infection rate was 9.8% and identified the risk factors for infection were a younger patient age, shorter height, lower weight, the presence of a wound dehiscence or a CSF leak, and previous wound or pump revisions within 6 months of the incident pump placement (Spader et al. 2016). Infection certainly is not rare or unusual as another study demonstrated infection rates as high as 16% (Bolash et al. 2015).
- *Catheter migration*: There are various things that can lead to catheter migration including improper anchoring or suturing, not placing enough catheter length into the intrathecal space and flipping of the pump that causes kinking or retraction of the catheter. Although

the incidence of catheter malfunction is low, it can cause loss of drug efficacy, medication withdrawals, and CSF leakage, which can lead to hygromas and the need for a catheter revision (Padfield 2012). Proper anchoring starts with a good needle entry site, a steep needle entry angle, and optimal catheter placement within the CSF which can help mitigate risk of migration. Once the catheter is inserted, a purse string suturing technique can be used in the location of the catheter entry site to try reinforce against a CSF leak in the short term and to facilitate the tissue fibrosis around the catheter in the longer term (Padfield 2012). As mentioned previously, a small redundant loop of catheter called a strain loop or a relief loop is left in the midline and around the pump to allow movement during healing and to prevent tension on the catheter (Padfield 2012).

- *ITB complications*: Similar to that of complications related to intrathecal pain medication delivery, ITB complications are usually related to either infection or failure of the pump or catheter to deliver the medication due to the variety of different scenarios previously mentioned. Surgical site infections (SSIs) are usually seen at and beyond 4 weeks after implantation, typically approximately 6 weeks following placement of the pump (Woolf and Baum 2017). Complications related to the catheter are typically seen later than SSIs and usually present at about 3–6 months postimplantation (Woolf and Baum 2017).

4.2   Replacements and Revisions

Intrathecal pain pumps sound alarms to indicate a malfunction, a low reservoir, or a low battery. As mentioned in chapter "The Components of Intrathecal Drug Delivery", the life of the intrathecal pump battery is variable and partially depends on usage and varies between the two manufacturers. One manufacturer claims that the pump life is 10 years, and the other manufacturer states that the pump battery life generally lasts from 4 to 7 years (Bolash et al. 2015; Prometra®Pump 2020). In regards to the need for

revision of intrathecal pumps, one study showed infection rates of 16%, lack of therapeutic efficacy at 11%, surgical complications at 3%, and granuloma formation at 1% (Bolash et al. 2015). The elective replacement indicator (ERI) specifies the battery life left on the pump and can be seen when the pump is interrogated. Baclofen pumps should be scheduled for surgical replacement 3–6 months prior to the ERI to ensure that the pump will be replaced in time (Boster et al. 2016b). If the need for a catheter revision arises, it is prudent to admit and monitor patients prior to revision. In the case of a suspected but unverified baclofen catheter malfunction, the ITB dosing should be weaned prior to surgery, and the patient should be observed for side effects. If there is the presence of baclofen withdrawal symptoms and/or increase spasticity, a malfunction of the drug delivery system is likely (Boster et al. 2016b). As the actual ITB dose that the patient is receiving through a malfunctioning pump or catheter is unknown, a reduced postoperative dose or initial starting trial dose is recommended. This should be started intraoperatively, and inpatient admission is recommended to monitor for signs of over- or underdosing (Boster et al. 2016b).

5   Conclusion

Since its inception, IDDS has emerged as a widely used and effective treatment option for a broad range of indications in the treatment of chronic conditions associated with various types of pain and spasticity. This chapter has provided an overview of current IT therapeutic agents and their properties and indications in treating neuropathic pain, nociceptive pain, and spasticity. Research and development in intrathecal drug delivery continue to produce new medications, devices, and treatment recommendations. The authors of this chapter recommend that practitioners seek guidance on IDDS therapy from current PACC guidelines to help guide the optimal application of intrathecal drug therapy in patients. Prior to implantation, we recommend practitioners focus on comprehensive patient assessment and planning by establishing an accurate diagnosis, performing proper patient selection, refining the timing of the implantation, selecting the appropriate medication, and ensuring correct catheter tip placement. Optimizing these factors is essential to produce the greatest degree efficacy and maximal duration of therapy. We also discussed the use of IDDS trialing and pretrial management to determine the appropriate patient candidates for device implantation and to ensure the medication selected is effective and can be tolerated by the patient. This chapter also presents surgical implantation considerations of the IDDS including anesthesia, sedation, medication prophylaxis, appropriate pump size selection, pocket placement, and patient positioning. We suggest using most recent anticoagulation guidelines set forth in Table 4 and performing a proper patient risk assessment. The risk assessment should be accompanied by preoperative lab work and cross-sectional imaging in order to adequately plan for device implantation and long-term intrathecal therapy. Additionally, we discuss tips for intrathecal needle placement, catheter tunneling, catheter length and tip location, pump anchoring, wound closure, sterile dressing application, and tips for reducing surgical site infections. We suggest that the ideal catheter placement location is in part based on the location of the identified pain generator as well as the intrathecal medication choice and the baricity of that medication. This chapter also discusses postoperative management, which includes wound care, patient restrictions, management of postoperative complications, and the indications for pump and/or catheter revisions. Proficient patient assessment and operative planning are required for optimal outcomes in intrathecal medication therapy. We have provided objective evidence-based information, medical literature, and expert recommendations in an effort to assist the interested practitioner in optimizing their targeted drug delivery practice. Our hope is this chapter will contribute substantially to the appropriate identification, treatment, and management of chronic pain and spasticity for those patients without an alternative treatment option.

References

About Your Intrathecal Pump. Memorial Sloan Kettering. https://www.mskcc.org/cancer-care/patient-education/intrathecal-pump-treatment-pain. Accessed 10 Sept 2010

Albright AL, Turner M, Pattisapu JV (2006) Best-practice surgical techniques for intrathecal baclofen therapy. J Neurosurg 104(4 Suppl):233–239. https://doi.org/10.3171/ped.2006.104.4.233

American Society of Regional Anesthesia and Pain Medicine. https://www.asra.com/asra-news/article/199/updates-to-the-asra-guidelines-for-inter. Accessed 10 Sept 2010

Awaad Y, Rizk T, Siddiqui I, Roosen N, McIntosh K, Waines GM (2012) Complications of intrathecal baclofen pump: prevention and cure. ISRN Neurol 2012:575168. https://doi.org/10.5402/2012/575168

Bogue JT, Wald G, Iosim S, Greenfield JP, Otterburn DM (2020) Submuscular placement of baclofen infusion pumps: case series and technique. Ann Plast Surg 85(S1 Suppl 1):S8–S11. https://doi.org/10.1097/SAP.0000000000002347

Bolash R, Udeh B, Saweris Y et al (2015) Longevity and cost of implantable intrathecal drug delivery systems for chronic pain management: a retrospective analysis of 365 patients. Neuromodulation 18(2):150–156. https://doi.org/10.1111/ner.12235

Boster AL, Bennett SE, Bilsky GS et al (2016a) Best practices for intrathecal baclofen therapy: screening test. Neuromodulation 19(6):616–622. https://doi.org/10.1111/ner.12437

Boster AL, Adair RL, Gooch JL et al (2016b) Best practices for intrathecal baclofen therapy: dosing and long-term management. Neuromodulation 19(6):623–631. https://doi.org/10.1111/ner.12388

Candido KD, Kusper TM, Knezevic NN (2017) New cancer pain treatment options. Curr Pain Headache Rep 21(2):12. https://doi.org/10.1007/s11916-017-0613-0

Chan XH, Li L, Tan KH Intrathecal catheter insertion and analgesia is a safe and effective method of pain control in patients with advanced and intractable cancer pain. J Pain Relief 6:289

Cochetti G, Abraha I, Randolph J et al (2020) Surgical wound closure by staples or sutures?: systematic review. Medicine (Baltimore) 99(25):e20573. https://doi.org/10.1097/MD.0000000000020573

Deer T, Buvanendran A, Diwan S (2011a) Intrathecal drug delivery for pain and spasticity, vol 2. Saunders

Deer TR, Smith HS, Burton AW et al (2011b) Comprehensive consensus based guidelines on intrathecal drug delivery systems in the treatment of pain caused by cancer pain. Pain Physician 14(3):E283–E312

Deer TR, Verdolin MH, Pope JE (2016) Placement of intrathecal needle and catheter for chronic infusion. In: Deer T, Pope J (eds) Atlas of implantable therapies for pain management. Springer, New York. https://doi.org/10.1007/978-1-4939-2110-2_37

Deer TR, Pope JE, Hayek SM et al (2017a) The poly-analgesic consensus conference (PACC): recommendations on intrathecal drug infusion systems best practices and guidelines [published correction appears in neuromodulation. 2017 Jun;20(4):405–406]. Neuromodulation 20(2):96–132. https://doi.org/10.1111/ner.12538

Deer TR, Provenzano DA, Hanes M et al (2017b) The neurostimulation appropriateness consensus committee (NACC) recommendations for infection prevention and management [published correction appears in neuromodulation. 2017 Jul;20(5):516]. Neuromodulation 20(1):31–50. https://doi.org/10.1111/ner.12565

Deer TR, Pope JE, Hayek SM et al (2017c) The polyanalgesic consensus conference (PACC): recommendations for intrathecal drug delivery: guidance for improving safety and mitigating risks. Neuromodulation 20(2):155–176. https://doi.org/10.1111/ner.12579

Deer TR, Pope JE, Hayek SM et al (2017d) The polyanalgesic consensus conference (PACC): recommendations on intrathecal drug infusion systems best practices and guidelines [published correction appears in neuromodulation. 2017 Jun;20(4):405-406]. Neuromodulation 20(2):96–132. https://doi.org/10.1111/ner.12538

Devine O, Harborne A, Lo WB, Weinberg D, Ciras M, Price R (2016) Unusual placement of intrathecal baclofen pumps: report of two cases. Acta Neurochir 158(1):167–170. https://doi.org/10.1007/s00701-015-2636-9

Fiaschi P, Cama A, Piatelli G, Moretti P, Pavanello M (2018) A novel skin and fascia opening for subfascial inserting of intrathecal baclofen pump. World Neurosurg 110:244–248. https://doi.org/10.1016/j.wneu.2017.11.086

Follett KA, Boortz-Marx RL, Drake JM et al (2004) Prevention and management of intrathecal drug delivery and spinal cord stimulation system infections. Anesthesiology 100(6):1582–1594. https://doi.org/10.1097/00000542-200406000-00034

Grider JS, Brown RE, Colclough GW (2008) Perioperative management of patients with an intrathecal drug delivery system for chronic pain. Anesth Analg 107(4):1393–1396. https://doi.org/10.1213/ane.0b013e318181b818

Kim KY, Anoushiravani AA, Long WJ, Vigdorchik JM, Fernandez-Madrid I, Schwarzkopf R (2017) A meta-analysis and systematic review evaluating skin closure after total knee arthroplasty—what is the best method? J Arthroplast 32(9):2920–2927. https://doi.org/10.1016/j.arth.2017.04.004

Knight KH, Brand FM, Mchaourab AS, Veneziano G (2007a) Implantable intrathecal pumps for chronic pain: highlights and updates. Croat Med J 48(1):22–34

Knight KH, Brand FM, Mchaourab AS, Veneziano G (2007b) Implantable intrathecal pumps for chronic pain: highlights and updates. Croat Med J 48(1):22–34

Krishnan RJ, Crawford EJ, Syed I, Kim P, Rampersaud YR, Martin J (2019) Is the risk of infection lower with sutures than with staples for skin closure after ortho-

paedic surgery? A meta-analysis of randomized trials. Clin Orthop Relat Res 477(5):922–937. https://doi.org/10.1097/CORR.0000000000000690

Lake W, Shah H (2019) Intrathecal baclofen infusion for the treatment of movement disorders. Neurosurg Clin N Am 30(2):203–209. https://doi.org/10.1016/j.nec.2018.12.002

Luo X, Zhang W, Yan P et al (2020) Skin closure tape and surgical staples in primary total knee arthroplasty: a systematic review and meta-analysis. Biomed Res Int 2020:4827617. Published 2020 Jan 10. https://doi.org/10.1155/2020/4827617

Lynch L (2014) Intrathecal drug delivery systems. Contin Educ Anaesth Crit Care Pain 14(1):27–31

Mitchell A, McGhie J, Owen M, McGinn G (2015) Audit of intrathecal drug delivery for patients with difficult-to-control cancer pain shows a sustained reduction in pain severity scores over a 6-month period. Palliat Med 29(6):554–563. https://doi.org/10.1177/0269216315570514

Mitigation of Infection Risk. American Society of Regional Anesthesia and Pain Medicine (n.d.)

Narang S, Srinivasan SK, Zinboonyahgoon N, Sampson CE (2016) Upper antero-medial thigh as an alternative site for implantation of intrathecal pumps: a case series. Neuromodulation 19(6):655–663. https://doi.org/10.1111/ner.12469

Newman JT, Morgan SJ, Resende GV, Williams AE, Hammerberg EM, Dayton MR (2011) Modality of wound closure after total knee replacement: are staples as safe as sutures? A retrospective study of 181 patients. Patient Saf Surg 5(1):26. Published 2011 Oct 19. https://doi.org/10.1186/1754-9493-5-26

Onofrio BM, Yaksh TL, Arnold PG (1981) Continuous low-dose intrathecal morphine administration in the treatment of chronic pain of malignant origin. Mayo Clin Proc 56(8):516–520

Padfield N (2012) Atlas of implantable therapies for pain management. Br J Clin Pharmacol 73(2):311. https://doi.org/10.1111/j.1365-2125.2011.04057.x

Prager J, Deer T, Levy R et al (2014) Best practices for intrathecal drug delivery for pain. Neuromodulation 17(4):354–372. https://doi.org/10.1111/ner.12146

Prometra®Pump (2020) Flowonix Medical Inc. website. https://flowonix.com/healthcare-provider/products/prometra-pump. Accessed 15 Aug 2020

Robinson S, Robertson FC, Dasenbrock HH, O'Brien CP, Berde C, Padua H (2017) Image-guided intrathecal baclofen pump catheter implantation: a technical note and case series. J Neurosurg Spine 26(5):621–627. https://doi.org/10.3171/2016.8.SPINE16263

Saenz A, Grijalba M, Mengide JP, Argañaraz R, Ford F, Mantese B (2021) Baclofen pump with pre-brainstem catheter tip placement: technical note and case series. Childs Nerv Syst 37(1):203–210. https://doi.org/10.1007/s00381-020-04679-3

Saulino M, Ivanhoe CB, McGuire JR, Ridley B, Shilt JS, Boster AL (2016) Best practices for intrathecal baclofen therapy: patient selection. Neuromodulation 19(6):607–615. https://doi.org/10.1111/ner.12447

Shah N, Padalia D (2020a) Intrathecal delivery system. [Updated 2020 Apr 27]. In: StatPearls [Internet]. StatPearls Publishing, Treasure Island. https://www.ncbi.nlm.nih.gov/books/NBK538237/

Shah N, Padalia D (2020b) Intrathecal delivery system. [Updated 2020 Apr 27]. In: StatPearls [Internet]. StatPearls Publishing, Treasure Island. https://www.ncbi.nlm.nih.gov/books/NBK538237/

Smyth C, Ahmadzai N, Wentzell J et al (2015) Intrathecal analgesia for chronic refractory pain: current and future prospects. Drugs 75(17):1957–1980. https://doi.org/10.1007/s40265-015-0471-1

Spader HS, Bollo RJ, Bowers CA, Riva-Cambrin J (2016) Risk factors for baclofen pump infection in children: a multivariate analysis. J Neurosurg Pediatr 17(6): 756–762. https://doi.org/10.3171/2015.11.PEDS15421

Teodorczyk J, Szmuda T, Siemiński M, Lass P, Słoniewski P (2013) Evaluation of usefulness of scintigraphic imaging in diagnosis of intrathecal drug delivery system malfunction—a preliminary report. Pol J Radiol 78(3):21–27. https://doi.org/10.12659/PJR.889130

Woolf SM, Baum CR (2017) Baclofen pumps: uses and complications. Pediatr Emerg Care 33(4):271–275. https://doi.org/10.1097/PEC.0000000000001090

Xing F, Yong RJ, Kaye AD, Urman RD (2018) Intrathecal drug delivery and spinal cord stimulation for the treatment of cancer pain. Curr Pain Headache Rep 22(2):11. Published 2018 Feb 5. https://doi.org/10.1007/s11916-018-0662-z

Key Steps in the Intrathecal Pain Pump Procedure

Annie Layno-Moses, Terry Nguyen, Afrida Sara, and Timothy Davis

Contents

Abstract

Intrathecal drug delivery has expanded since the inception of this technology in the 1980s and is utilized for several different conditions including pain control and management of spasticity. The use of intrathecal pumps is less common than most other techniques for interventional pain management but is essential in such conditions as refractory pain, cancer pain, multifocal pain, severe spasticity, and in patients who are not candidates for surgical correction of their underlying condition. This chapter highlights the key necessary steps for the implantation of a pain pump including patient positioning, needle and catheter placement, pump pocket creation, catheter tunneling, and catheter to pump connection. Methods for minimizing infection and optimizing cosure are also discussed as well as potential alternative pump locations in the event, and abdominal placement is an undesirable location.

A. Layno-Moses · T. Nguyen · A. Śara · T. Davis (✉)
Source Healthcare, Santa Monica, CA, USA
e-mail: amoses@sourcehealthcare.com;
tnguyen@sourcehealthcare.com;
asara@sourcehealthcare.com

Abbreviations

BMI   Body mass index
CSF   Cerebral spinal fluid
IDDS   Intrathecal drug delivery system

Intrathecal drug delivery directly into the cerebral spinal fluid (CSF) is highly effective at lowering the overall required systemic drug dose and is especially useful for cases in which delivery of medications via less-invasive routes, such as oral or transdermal, is either ineffective or associated with detrimental adverse effects.

Candidates for intrathecal drug delivery system (IDDS) pump implantation should be properly screened for contraindications to the placement of a system, undergo a thorough preoperative history assessment, have an appropriate physical exam, understand the risks and benefits of such implantation, and in most cases undergo an intrathecal medication trial prior to selecting that pump location and proceeding with implantation. At the time of implantation, the IDDS includes the insertion of an intrathecal catheter that is tunneled to the pump that is typically attached to the sheath of the external oblique muscle which lies just subjacent to the plane containing the fascia of Scarpa. This surgical technique requires some additional tools and materials not typically seen with many interventional techniques, and it is helpful to have a list of supplies necessary for pump implantation (Table 1).

1   Positioning

The pump is most commonly placed in the right or left lower quadrant of the abdomen. For this type of pump placement, securing the patient in a lateral decubitus position is recommended to allow access to both the lower spine and the abdomen (Jones 2011). This also prevents the need to reposition the patient during the surgery, thus lowering the risk of surgical site infection. All pressure points should be properly padded to ensure patient comfort and to prevent potential nerve compression injuries during surgery (Furnish and Wallace 2014). Prior to surgery, the site of implantation should be marked, while the patient is in a sitting position rather than the lateral position. If the patient is marked in the lateral position, this could result in incorrect final placement of the pump and possibly postoperative discomfort associated with the pump being located against the ribs or pelvis or in another unintended location due to shifting of the soft tissue when the patient moves from the lateral position to standing or sitting (Furnish and Wallace 2014). This is especially problematic in patients who are morbidly obese or in patients with unusual anatomy (Furnish and Wallace 2014).

An intrathecal pain pump placement necessitates a paraspinal lower lumbar incision for the catheter placement and a lower abdominal incision for the pump implantation. These areas should be prepped and draped accordingly after positioning the patient in a lateral decubitus position. The C-arm should also be positioned at the desired lumbar level for imaging guidance throughout the procedure. The catheter tip will need to be visualized during insertion of the catheter so the C-arm should be set up to optimally visualize all areas of the lumbar and thoracic spines. Both an anteroposterior and lateral view will be used to guide the needle and to determine proper needle depth within the intrathecal space, and a lateral view is sufficient to determine the final catheter tip position (Jones 2011).

2   Needle/Catheter Placement

The desired interspace for needle/catheter placement is located by palpating the spinous processes approximately one vertebral body level below the preferred lumbar entry point. The entry is a paramedian entry into the interlaminar space that avoids transgressing the tenacious supraspinous ligament. To avoid risks of spinal cord injury, the ideal point of needle entry will be below the level of the conus medullaris which is typically located from T12 to L2 and most commonly at the L1–2 level. Depending on the patient's anatomy, the dural entry point is typically between L2 and L5.

Table 1 Supply list for intrathecal drug delivery system implantation

1.	Synchromed II intrathecal pump, Ascenda catheter, SynchroMed II clinician programmer, and catheter insertion kit
2.	Electrocautery
	(a) The PEAK® Surgery System includes PEAK PlasmaBlade® soft tissue dissection devices and the PULSAR® II Generator.—Medtronic
3.	Medtronic Tyrx absorbable antibiotic pouch
	(b) http://www.tyrx.com/index.htm
4.	Amniovo amniotic membrane allograft
	(c) 3.0 cm × 3.0 cm size
5.	Suture:
	(d) 2-0 vicryl (2 sutures)
	• Deep tissue and subcutaneous skin closure of catheter incision

Suture construction	Suture color	Available sizes	Suture BSR* profile		Absorption completed by:
Braided	Violet/white (undyed)	5/0 through 2	2 weeks	75%	56–70 days
			3 weeks	50%	
			4 weeks	25%	

	(e) 2-0 Ethibond (1 suture)
	• Securing catheter anchor

Size	2-0
Brand	ETHIBOND
Color	Green
Length	45 cm/18″
Arms	Single armed
Material	Polyester
Construction	Braided
Absorbability	Nonabsorbable
Absorption rate	NA
Breaking strength retention (BSR)	Indefinite
Directionality	Unidirectional
Control release	N

	(f) 0 FiberWire suture (two sutures)
	• Attaching the pump to the abdominal fascia −0 FiberWire, 38″ (blue) with tapered needle, 22.2 mm 1/2 Circle—AR-7250
	(g) Stratafix suture (1 suture)
	• Subcuticular Closure with 2-0 MONOCRYL® Plus Antibacterial (poliglecaprone 25) suture
6.	Surgical instruments
	(h) Scalpel and #11 blade
	(i) Self-retaining retractors
	• Blunt Weitlaner—5.5 to 6.5 in
	• Spread Gelpi—5.5 to 7.0 in
	(j) Surgical scissors
7.	Sterile saline irrigation
8.	Vancomycin powder (3.0 g)
9.	Dermabond Prineo wound closure system
	(k) This is a two-part system with an applicator and liquid adhesive two-octylcyanoacrylate topical skin adhesive (Dermabond) that sets in approximately 60 s when applied to mesh tape
	(l) Patient can shower after Prineo application
10.	Abdominal binder
	(m) Patient wears binder during the day for 4 weeks

Published guidelines recommend that patients are not put under heavy sedation or anesthesia during and the placement of the intrathecal catheter to reduce the chance of neurological complications (Deer et al. 2017). If deep sedation or general anesthesia is not used during the initial catheter placement, copious amounts of local anesthetic should be injected into to the skin and subcutaneous tissue to facilitate patient comfort (Belverud et al. 2008).

In practice, the needle can be placed prior to making the incision or the incision can be made before placement of the needle. If the incision is made first, this requires that the approach to the spine and the level of entry be adequately planned to accurately predict where the needle will pierce interlaminar dura and to make sure the superior angulation of the needle is sufficient enough to allow a smooth insertion of the catheter to the desire intrathecal level. The paramedian approach is used while monitoring the needle depth on the lateral view, and the needle tip is guided into the intrathecal space while taking care to identify CSF prior to placing the catheter and to make sure the catheter feeds into the needle and advances easily. Keeping all of these factors in mind, the incision is first made one vertebral body lower than the planned needle dural entry point just paramedian to the spinous process (Fig. 1). The distance of the incision inferior to where the needle would pierce the dura will vary based on body mass index (BMI), and a more inferior needle starting point may be necessary in patients with large amounts of subcutaneous fat in order to keep an adequate amount of inferosuperior angulation. An incision at this location allows for thorough dissection of tissue down to the lumbodorsal fascia which has a whitish color and is an optimal anchoring point for the catheter anchor sutures. The superficial tissue can then be easily mobilized to accommodate for the needle trajectory (Fig. 2). An anteroposterior fluoroscopic view is used to predict the trajectory from the paramedian skin entry point to the chosen interlaminar space where the needle will pass through the dura.

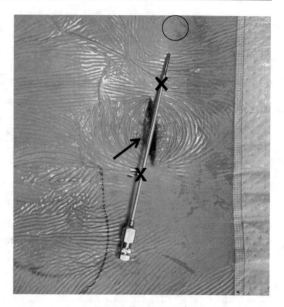

Fig. 1 Photograph showing a left paraspinal needle placement with the appropriate needle trajectory (indicated by the black X's) directed toward the midline and the dura insertion point (black circle). The incision for the catheter insertion (black arrow) is placed approximately one vertebral body height inferior to the planned dural entry point

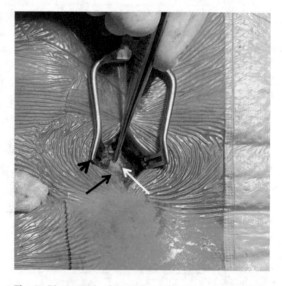

Fig. 2 Photograph of the catheter insertion site shows the incision (black arrow) that is held open by a Weitlaner retractor (black arrowhead) demonstrating the lumbodorsal fascial layer (white arrow). Electrocautery (not shown) and other retractor tools can be used to create the appropriate access for catheter insertion and anchoring

Once the fascia is noted and an anchoring site identified, a 16-gauge Tuohy introducer needle can be inserted directly through the fascia using the paramedian approach. From the anteroposterior view, the needle is angled 10°–15° lateral to medial toward the midline and advanced with a cephalad angulation (Fig. 3). If the needle contacts the lamina, it is repositioned with the tip directed toward the correct interlaminar location using a "walk-off" technique to advance the needle more cephalad until it reaches the epidural space. Compared to the midline approach, this technique more directly penetrates the ligamentum flavum rather than the supraspinous and interspinous ligaments.

The needle will then be advanced, and a loss of resistance either to air or fluid (depending on the technique used) may be noted when the needle passes through the epidural space (Furnish and Wallace 2014). The bevel of the needle should then be rotated 90° toward the midline until it is parallel to the dura fibers. This is done in order to reduce the likelihood of post-dural puncture headaches (Furnish and Wallace 2014).

Using lateral imaging to visualize depth, the needle can be advanced into the intrathecal space (Jones 2011). Brief removal of the stylet from the needle will demonstrate CSF flow, indicative of appropriate needle placement in the intrathecal space. If there is no CSF return, the needle should be periodically rotated and only advanced with the bevel parallel to the dura fibers. If there is negligible CSF return or there is still uncertainty as to the needle tip position, one or two cc's of noninionic contrast can be injected through the needle. If it is present in the CSF, it will outline the cauda equina and opacity of the intrathecal space. It is imperative to avoid significant loss of CSF during initial placement as this can affect correct the certainty of appropriate intrathecal placement. Once the catheter tip advances beyond the distal portion of the needle, caution should be taken to not withdraw the catheter against resistance as this would likely lead to shearing of the catheter itself (Furnish and Wallace 2014). In the event that catheter advancement is met with a lot of resistance, care should be taken when withdrawing and repositioning the catheter. If there is

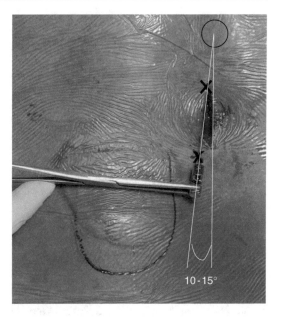

Fig. 3 Photograph showing the introducer needle will be inserted at an angle 10°–15° (white angle and measurement) lateral to medial and advanced with a cephalad angulation to a midline target where the needle should transgress the dura (black circle). The appropriate needle trajectory is indicated by the black X's

still substantial resistance to catheter movement, the introducer and catheter should be removed together before attempting to reinsert the introducer needle (Jones 2011).

As soon as correct placement of the introducer needle is confirmed by fluoroscopy, the catheter and the catheter guidewire should be inserted through the needle to the desired spinal level (Fig. 4) (Jones 2011). This target level is determined preoperatively based on a thorough review of patient history, physical exam findings, condition being treated, anatomic location of the primary pathology, and the medication being used. When using intrathecal baclofen, there is evidence demonstrating that placing the catheter more cephalad can improve upper extremity spasticity scores (Belverud et al. 2008). Additionally, placement of the catheter at the level of pain may be important when using lipophilic analgesic agents (i.e., fentanyl) (Belverud et al. 2008). Additional evidence is needed to more completely define the relationship between catheter location and clinical response in patients

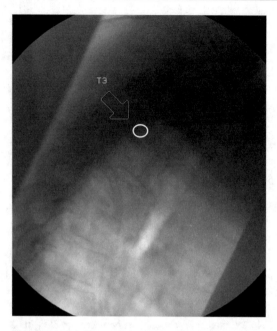

Fig. 4 Lateral fluoroscopic view of the upper thoracic spine shows an intrathecal catheter and its radiopaque catheter tip (white circle) just posterior to the T2–3 intervertebral disc. The catheter tip was designated to be at the superior margin of T3 as indicated by the fluoroscopic labeling

after intrathecal drug delivery systems for a variety of different medications.

Although some authors create the incision prior to needle insertion, an alternative technique is to identify an optimal access to the intrathecal space under fluoroscopy, place the needle intrathecally, advance the catheter to the appropriate position, and then make the incision from the point of needle entry into the skin and extend that incision inferiorly (Figs. 5a and b). The following alterative techniques can be used to make the incision following the needle insertion:

(a) The incision can be made superior and inferior to the site of the needle entry, but it is best made inferior to the needle as this lead to an anchor insertion point inferior to the needle entry point which lessens the chance of catheter kinking at the anchor point. Soft tissue dissection is carried out down to the level where the needle pierces the lumbodorsal fascia (Jones 2011). During tissue dissection, care must be taken to avoid damage to

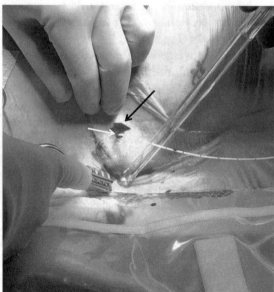

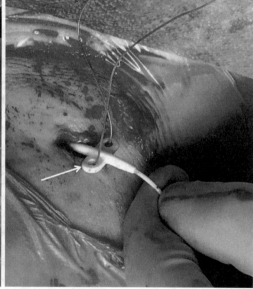

Fig. 5 (**a** and **b**) An incision (black arrow in **a**) is made around the catheter (white arrow in **a**) and the catheter anchor (white arrow in **b**) is placed over the catheter and anchored to the lumbodorsal fascia. (Adapted from: Beall

D.P. et al. (2021) Intrathecal Pain Pumps: Placement and Management. In: Munk P.L., Babu S.B. (eds) Interventional Radiology in Palliative Care. Medical Radiology. Springer, Cham)

the catheter. For this reason, some physicians prefer to leave the Tuohy needle in place while dissecting, but this technique has the possibility of needle heating when using electrocautery for tissue dissection. The length of soft tissue dissection depends on the BMI of the patient, and care must be taken when dissecting from lateral to medial and inferior to superior to not create too much potential space. An extensive amount of potential space can have a greater amount of healing time when compared to smaller dissections and can create a space for fluid collections including seromas or CSFomas.

(b) The incision can be made at the midline over the spinous processes just medial to the needle insertion point, and the dissection is then extended down to the supraspinous ligament (Furnish and Wallace 2014). Unlike the previous method, the incision is made medial to the needle entry site and not directly adjacent to the needle itself. Dissection should aim for exposure of the traversing needle down to the level of the fascia (Jones 2011). This technique requires the catheter to be pulled through the original insertion site either through the needle or after the needle has been removed. The authors recommend that, if this technique is used, the needle should be left in place as pulling the catheter through the skin where the needle originally entered exposes the catheter to the epidermis and dermis increases the risk of bacterial introduction.

Prior to the anchoring step, a nonabsorbable suture can be placed in the muscular fascia around the Tuohy needle prior to its removal, and a purse string suture can be placed. This is done in addition to the anchoring of the catheter to help secure the catheter and to prevent CSF leakage into subcutaneous tissue (Brand et al. 2007). Following suture placement, the needle is then removed, and the guidewire is withdrawn from the catheter.

A hemostat can then be placed on the end of the catheter end to prevent CSF loss while anchoring and tunneling, and the end of the catheter is best kept clipped at the upper end of the surgical field to avoid the possibility of contamination. After removal of the Tuohy needle, the purse-string suture surrounding the catheter should be tightened, and care should be taken to ensure that there is no kinking or obstruction of the catheter. A catheter anchor can then be slid onto the catheter and sutured to the fascia layer (Fig. 5b) (Jones 2011). Larger gauge permanent suture such as 0 or 2-0 silk or Ethibond can be used to close the anchor wings together or to attach the wings to the lumbodorsal fascia. A second suture may be placed to secure the anchor neck to the underlying fascia. It is important that the catheter is properly anchored in order to prevent catheter migration or pistoning that can loosen the anchor points and lead to catheter migration. Once the catheter is secure, the incision can be draped with sterile gauze before directing attention to the site of the pump implantation. The CSF flow from the catheter should be checked after placement of the pump and catheter to identify occlusion or disruption that can occur during anchoring and placement of the IDDS and to ensure patency of the catheter prior to wound closure (Brand et al. 2007).

3 Pump Pocket Creation

The next steps involve creating the subcutaneous pocket in the preferred location for pump placement. Anesthesia for this segment of the procedure can be augmented by injecting preservative free lidocaine directly into the intrathecal catheter after ensuring that the catheter is at the appropriate level to provide the anesthesia at the correct level or by using ample amounts of local anesthetic at the site of pocket creation (Furnish and Wallace 2014). The pump is typically placed in the right or left lower quadrant of the abdomen at the midclavicular line and halfway between the iliac crest and the lower costal margin. At this point, a 7-cm skin incision is made, and traction is applied as the incision is extended through the subcutaneous fat typically using electrocautery (Fig. 6). The pocket is extended down to Scarpa's fascia which lies just superficial to the myofascial

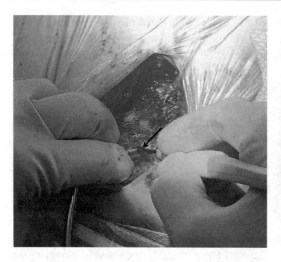

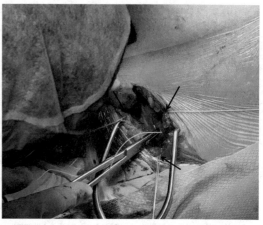

Fig. 6 The lower quadrant abdominal incision is make through the skin and down through the subcutaneous fat usually using electrocautery (black arrow). (Adapted from: Beall D.P. et al. (2021) Intrathecal Pain Pumps: Placement and Management. In: Munk P.L., Babu S.B. (eds) Interventional Radiology in Palliative Care. Medical Radiology. Springer, Cham)

Fig. 7 Permanent sutures are placed through the anterior portion of the abdominal wall (black arrows) which will later be used to secure the pump to the anterior abdominal wall. (Adapted from: Beall D.P. et al. (2021) Intrathecal Pain Pumps: Placement and Management. In: Munk P.L., Babu S.B. (eds) Interventional Radiology in Palliative Care. Medical Radiology. Springer, Cham)

covering of the external oblique muscle. The fascia of Scarpa is membranous and pulls off of the myofascial plane easily with retraction of the subcutaneous fat. In very thin patients, care must be taken to avoid penetration through the oblique abdominal musculature and, if violated, repaired with primary closure to avoid postsurgical hernia formation. The pocket is created in this location by dissecting a space is just large enough for the pump and also of sufficient size to allow closure of the soft tissue over the pump without undue tension. Undermining the pocket cephalad or caudal to the incision will prevent the final incision from lying directly on top of the pump refill port thereby allowing for a more comfortable access to the port for future pump refills (Furnish and Wallace 2014). The depth of the pocket is also important as depths more than 2.5 cm can make refilling the pump much more difficult, and too much soft tissue overlying the pump can interfere with communication with the pump. In patients with large amounts of abdominal fat, the deep fascia layer may not be a practical location for pump anchoring, and the pump may also be placed within the subcutaneous fat layer superfi-

cial to Scarpa's fascia. This should be avoided if possible as pumps that are placed within the fat layer may not heal in place adequately and may cause complications associated with movement of the pump including problems with pump movement or difficulties in pump refilling and programming (Jones 2011).

Hemostasis is important to maintain at both incision sites, but this is especially imperative at the abdominal incision, as this wound tends to have more blood vessels and is more prone to hemorrhage. Wound hemostasis is typically easily achieved using either monopolar or bipolar electrocautery. After pocket creation, four permanent sutures (0 or 2-0 silk, Ethibond or FiberWire) are placed in the myofascial tissue covering the external oblique muscle that function as the anchor points of the pump (Fig. 7). The sutures are placed through the fibrous covering of the external oblique muscle with a horizontally oriented pass through the tissue so as not to penetrate into the peritoneum and potentially injure the underlying bowel (Fig. 7). Placing the sutures prior to placing the pump in the pocket will make the pump insertion and suture anchoring easier.

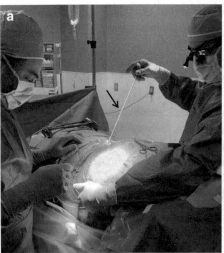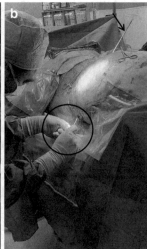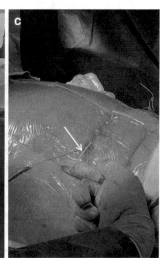

Fig. 8 (**a–c**) The malleable tunneling device (black arrows in **a** and **b**) is passed from the pump pocket superiorly to the more inferiorly located paramedian spine incision where the catheter placement has been performed. The catheter is then placed into the distal end of the tunneling device (indicated by black circle in **b**) and external portion of the catheter is advanced completely into the tunneling device. The tunneling device is then removed leaving only the catheter extending out of the pump pocket (white arrow in **c**). The flow of CSF out of the end of the catheter can be checked at this time to ensure patency. (Adapted from: Beall DP, Wagoner DD, Yoon E, Koenig BM, Witherby J, Flamm ME, Knoll AS, Farve A. Intrathecal Pain Pumps: Placement and Management. In: Munk PL, Babu S, editors. Interventional Radiology in Palliative Care. New York, NY: Springer, 2020)

4   Catheter Tunneling

Once the pump pocket has been created, a malleable tunneling device will be used to tunnel from the lumbar catheter insertion site to the pump or vice versa (Fig. 8). The tunneling device can be curved or modified to aid in tunneling through the subcutaneous soft tissue.

The type of intrathecal catheter used will dictate the tunneling strategy and catheter connection. When using a one-piece catheter, the tunneling device is typically inserted at the pump pocket site and passed subcutaneously through to the lumbar incision. The catheter can then be fed through the lumen of the tunneling device which is subsequently withdrawn leaving the catheter that has been tunneled to the pump site (Jones 2011). After this the catheter can be trimmed leaving an excess of approximately 5–10 cm proximal to the point where the catheter enters into the pump pocket.

The two-piece catheter has two separate segments, a spinal segment and a pump segment. When placing the two piece catheter, the tunneling is done just the opposite of the one-piece catheter with the tunneling device typically inserted into the lumbar incision and tunneled through to the pump pocket. The pump segment of the catheter will then be pulled through the lumen of the tunneling device from the pump pocket to the lumbar incision (Jones 2011). Similarly to the one-piece placement, excess catheter will be needed at the pump pocket incision.

Given the substantial variability of patient size, anatomy, and body mass index, there may be a large degree of variation in tunneling strategies and locations. The primary goals are to tunnel the catheter in an anatomic location that protects the catheter from kinking, connect an optimally placed pump and catheter with the least amount of tunneling possible, and leave enough length of catheter to connect the catheter together and to the pump. The tunneling may be done from the pocket site to the catheter insertion site and vice versa depending on the situation. The tunneling handle may be removed so the tunneling device may be removed bi-directionally.

5   Catheter Pump Connection and Pump Placement

After the successful tunneling of the catheter, flow of CSF from the spinal catheter should be observed to confirm there is no obstruction or kinks in the catheter (Furnish and Wallace 2014). For the one-piece catheter, the proximal portion of the catheter is secured to the connector (Fig. 9) via a collet, and the proximal portion of the connector is attached to the pump (Furnish and Wallace 2014). The attachment hub should snap on to the pump and rotate without resistance and should be thoroughly checked to ensure it is securely connected. The excess catheter is then loosely coiled and placed behind the pump (Jones 2011). The amount of catheter present in the abdominal pump pocket will of course be lengthened by the proximal catheter connector.

For a two-piece catheter, the spinal and pump segments can be connected using a titanium pin, and a strain-relief sleeves is placed over the connector. Connection of the two segments is done at the site of the lumbar incision, and the strain-

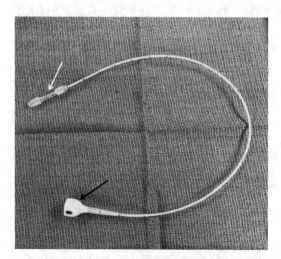

Fig. 9 Proximal catheter attachment that includes the collet (white arrow) that attaches to the remainder of the intrathecal catheter and the catheter attachment mechanism that attaches to the intrathecal pump (black arrow). (Adapted from: Beall DP, Wagoner DD, Yoon E, Koenig BM, Witherby J, Flamm ME, Knoll AS, Farve A. Intrathecal Pain Pumps: Placement and Management. In: Munk PL, Babu S, editors. Interventional Radiology in Palliative Care. New York, NY: Springer, 2020.)

relief sleeve is then anchored to the lumbodorsal fascia via the lumbar incision (Belverud et al. 2008).

Regardless of whether a one-piece or a two-piece catheter is used, it is important to coil the excess catheter and place it behind the pain pump. Measuring the entire length of the catheter is critically important for accurate pump programming, as it affects the rate of drug delivery so all components of the catheter that are trimmed off should be measured, recorded, and taken into consideration regarding the calculation of the final catheter length.

The pump is then placed in the pocket with the refill port facing outward and the catheter access port directed medially, and the pump is then anchored to the anterior abdomen using the permanent sutures placed during the pump pocket creation (Furnish and Wallace 2014). The sutures are placed through the loops on the side of the pump and tied to avoid any pump rotation or movement. When coiling the excess catheter to place behind the pump and during the process of placing the pump in the pocket, care should be taken to ensure the catheter does not kink and the sutures do not surround and construct the catheter (Jones 2011). The catheter should not be present along the anterior portion of the pump so as to avoid possible damage during pump medication refills. The catheter access port is typically directed medially as the soft tissue is usually thicker in this direction which will help to mitigate against skin erosion over the pump, especially in very thin patients. Both the lumbar and the pump incisions should then be irrigated with sterile saline and Betadine and/or antibiotic solution prior to wound closure.

6   Minimizing Infection

Additional measures can be taken to limit the chances of injection including preoperative washing with Hibiclens® daily for 3 days prior to surgery. An absorbable antibiotic pouch such as the Tyrx™ antibacterial envelope can be added to the wound in addition to a powdered antibiotic such as vancomycin. The Tyrx™ pouch was originally designed for implantable cardiac devices, and the material is made from a surgical mesh with two antibiotics (rifampin and minocycline) that resorbs over time (Kolek et al. 2013). Infection reduction has been shown for implantable cardiac devices (Kolek et al. 2013; Krahn et al. 2011a), but objective information has not yet been produced demonstrating a decreased infection rate in patients after intrathecal pump placement. Regardless this can be used at the discretion of the implanting physician in an attempt to keep the infection rate as low as possible.

One to 2 g of vancomycin powder can also be added to the wound and has been shown to be effective against gram-positive bacteria for patients undergoing surgery for intrathecal pump placement (Ghobrial et al. 2014). Vancomycin powder has also demonstrated safety and improved efficacy for reducing surgical site infections when used in addition to the standard antibiotic prophylaxis (Abdullah et al. 2016). Routine use of vancomycin powder is supporting by existing surgical literature, and there is little evidence that the routine use of topical vancomycin powder leads to antibiotic resistance.

The use of perioperative antibiotics is similar to other procedures with a non-insignificant risk of infection. Intravenous access is established, and the patient is given intravenous antibiotics just before the implantation of the IDDS. Recommended antibiotics include 1–2 g of cefazolin (Ancef) and 80–160 mg of Gentamycin with the Gentamycin dose depending on the patient's age and renal function. Patients that have an allergy to penicillin should be given 600–900 mg of clindamycin instead of the cefazolin with a higher dose of clindamycin used for patients weighing 90 kg or more.

7 Closure

After the irrigation and the above described antimicrobial measures have been utilized, the catheter insertion site is ready to be closed. Both incisions are typically close using a layered technique starting with a resorbable suture such as a 0 or a 2-0 vicryl suture placed in the deeper soft

tissues. Vicryl sutures typically resorb completely in 56–70 days and may be used for closing both the deep subcutaneous tissue and the skin using interrupted subcuticular sutures. The incision for the catheter insertion site is usually small enough to be closed using vicryl suture alone. One deep vicryl suture is used to close the deep fascia, and then the skin is closed using interrupted vicryl sutures with a subcuticular suturing technique. The abdominal wound is larger, and interrupted vicryl sutures can be used to close the deeper layer of soft tissue (known as Campers fascia), and then the skin closure can be performed with either interrupted vicryl sutures or a unidirectional barbed resorbable suture such as Stratafix™ or V-loc™. These unidirectional barbed sutures hold the tissue against the back side of the unidirectional barb after passing through it and are designed to be placed using a running suture technique rather than as an interrupted suture which should allow for a more rapid wound closure. If the skin tension exceeds what is optimal or if the edges of the skin are not tightly approximated, surgical staples may be used to reinforce the skin sutures. A topical adhesive such as 2-octylcyanoacrylate (Dermabond) can be added to the skin. This sets in rapidly (in approximately 60 s) and provides a physical barrier to superficial bacteria. An additional physical barrier such a Prineo mesh tape may also be used. The combination of Dermabond and Prineo will allow the patient to shower immediately after they return home.

8 Alternative Pump Location Selection

The location of the pump implantation is determined after a detailed review of the patient's anatomy, prior surgeries, comorbidities, and preference. The most common site of pump implantation is typically the right or left lower abdominal quadrant due to both its proximity to the lumbar catheter insertion site and the layer of fat that protects the pump from pressure erosions and/or external trauma. The pump is usually very well tolerated when placed in this location, and the patients usually report little interference with their normal activities of daily life. However, in patients that have extensive abdominal scarring from previous surgeries, aggregated metastatic abdominal masses, or if the adipose tissue around the mid-section is too thick, the abdomen may no longer be an acceptable location for pump implantation. Other factors including pelvic pathology, hip contracture, and cachexia may also preclude the possibility of placing the pump in the abdomen. In these cases, the physician implanting the pump may choose to select an alternative site such as the axilla, infraclavicular space, anteromedial thigh, or iliac fossa.

According to a case series done by Narang et al., the anteromedial thigh may be a good alternative site despite having less vascularity of the subcutaneous adipose tissue (Narang et al. 2016). All nine of the thigh implantation procedures outlined in this case series were deemed successful with only one wound dehiscence complication due to the patient's lack of muscle mass. After this patient underwent a revision surgery and had the pump placed in the alternate thigh, no further complications were noted. While this alternative site implantation is somewhat similar to the conventional procedure, care should be taken to stay within the subcutaneous layer and to avoid injuring any of underlying or adjacent neu-

rovascular structures including the femoral nerve, artery or vein, or the superficial femoral artery (Narang et al. 2016).

Another potential alternative site for pump implantation is the infraclavicular fossa (Fig. 10). This site is located substantially farther from a lumbar catheter insertion site and carries with it other potential complications including the possibility of damaging breast tissue, axillary vascular puncture, or injury to the brachial plexus (Narang et al. 2016). Another challenge for implanting in this location is that it may be difficult to create a pocket large enough pocket to fit a 40 mL pump, but if this situation is encountered, a 20 mL pump may be an acceptable alternative option (Rocque and Leland Albright 2010). Prepping the pocket adjacent to the pectoral fascia is similar that of the traditional abdominal wall where the soft tissue is dissected down to the pectoral fascia via electrocautery and the pocket is formed just over the fascia (Rocque and Leland Albright 2010). The pump is then secured to the pectoralis myofascial tissue by looping four 0 or 2-0 permanent sutures through the loops on the side of the pump (Rocque and Leland Albright 2010). The pump should be placed to maximize comfort and should be placed so it doesn't impact the adjacent clavicle with normal arm and shoulder girdle movement (Rocque and Leland Albright 2010).

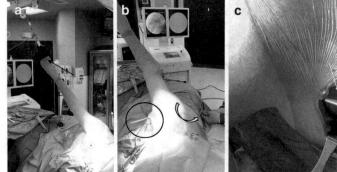
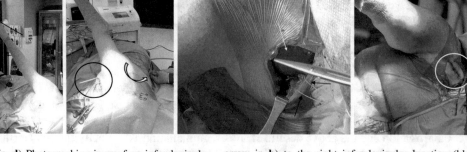

Fig. 10 (**a–d**) Photographic views of an infraclavicular (pectoral) placement of an intrathecal drug delivery pump shows the patient in a lateral decubitus position with their right arm elevated and held by an arm trap (black arrow in **a**). A long tunnelling device is used to tunnel the catheter from the lumbar catheter insertion site (white curved arrow in **b**) to the right infraclavicular location (black circle in **b**). The pump (white arrow in **c**) is placed adjacent to the pectoral fascia and tied down using permanent suture (black arrows in **c**). The incision is then closed using deep and subcuticular sutures and covered with Dermabond and Prineo (white circle in **d**)

A case series that followed four patients after their infraclavicular pump implantation procedure reported good patient tolerance to the procedure and to the pump location and no immediate intraoperative nor perioperative complications (Rocque and Leland Albright 2010). There was one death reported, although investigation of this mortality attributed the death to respiratory failure which was unrelated both the pump implantation procedure and the choice of pump location (Rocque and Leland Albright 2010).

In patients with very little subcutaneous fat, the pump can be placed in a subfascial plane. The upside of placing the pump deep in the subfascial layer below the myofascial covering of the rectus abdominus, oblique muscles, and the tranversus abdominus rather than between Scarpa's and the external oblique muscle fascia is the reduced risk of pump movement post procedure (Rocque and Leland Albright 2010). The disadvantages of pump placement in the intrafascial plane are that it is more invasive to place, is more prone to muscular damage during placement, and usually causes the patient more discomfort during pump refills.

9 Conclusion

Intrathecal drug delivery has proven to be dramatically effective in treating refractory pain and generalized spasticity refractory to systemic medications delivered via alternative routes (Deer et al. 2017). This chapter outlines the key steps and goes into extensive detail on the surgical implantation of the intrathecal pump including the optimal location of the pump and the appropriate patient positioning and clarifies some of the important steps in the pump implantation procedure. The significant steps in the surgical implantation of an IDDS such as the catheter placement, the pump pocket preparation, connecting the pump catheter, and closing the incisions are also discussed in detail, and important tips are provided to optimize the outcomes of implantation and to make the system stable over time. These recommendations can be combined with other consensus guidelines to help guide the

appropriate patient selection and medication choice when initiating intrathecal drug delivery.

In addition to the evidence-based information provided and the objective medical literature used in the preparation of this chapter, we have also provided subjective expert analysis and recommendations in order to help the reader of this text enhance their practice as much as possible.

References

Abdullah KG, Chen HI, Lucas TH (2016) Safety of topical vancomycin powder in neurosurgery. Surg Neurol Int 7(Suppl 39):S919–S926

Belverud S, Mogilner A, Schulder M (2008) Intrathecal pumps. Neurotherapeutics 5(1):114–122

Brand FM, Mchaourabiano AS, Veneziano G (2007) Implantable intrathecal pumps for chronic pain: highlights and updates. Croat Med J 48(1):22–34

Deer TR et al (2017) The polyanalgesic consensus conference (PACC): recommendations for intrathecal drug delivery: guidance for improving safety and mitigating risks. Neuromodulation 20(2):155–176

Furnish T, Wallace MS (2014) Intrathecal drug delivery: patient selection, trialing, and implantation. In: Practical management of pain. Mosby, Maryland Heights, pp 953–965

Ghobrial GM, Thakkar V, Singhal S, Oppenlander ME, Maulucci CM, Harrop JS et al (2014) Efficacy of intraoperative vancomycin powder use in intrathecal baclofen pump implantation procedures: single institutional series in a high risk population. J Clin Neurosci 21:1786–1789

Jones R (2011) Spinal cord stimulation and implanted intrathecal drug infusion. In: Pain procedures in clinical practice. Hanley & Belfus, Philadelphia, pp 483–506

Kolek MJ, Dresen WF, Wells QS, Ellis CR (2013) Use of an antibacterial envelope is associated with reduced cardiac implantable electronic device infections in high-risk patients. Pacing Clin Electrophysiol 36(3):354–361. https://doi.org/10.1111/pace.12063. Epub 2012 Dec 17

Krahn AD, Lee DS, Birnie D et al (2011a) Predictors of short-term complications after implantable cardioverter-defibrillator replacement: results from the Ontario ICD database. Circ Arrhythm Electrophysiol 4(2):136–142. https://doi.org/10.1161/CIRCEP.110.959791. Epub 2011 Feb 15

Narang S et al (2016) Upper antero-medial thigh as an alternative site for implantation of intrathecal pumps: a case series. Neuromodulation 19(6):655–663

Rocque BG, Leland Albright A (2010) Infraclavicular fossa as an alternate site for placement of intrathecal infusion pumps. Neurosurgery 66(2):E402–E403

Intrathecal Pump Management

Daniel R. Kloster

Contents

Abstract

Intrathecal therapy was introduced in the 1980s. Since that time, it has evolved into a very beneficial therapy for chronic pain, cancer pain, and spasticity. Patients are considered optimal candidates for intrathecal therapy when conservative treatments have been ineffective or when patients have intolerable side effects from systemic medications. By delivering medication directly to the intrathecal space, profound analgesia can be achieved with far fewer side effects. This also applies to patients suffering from spasticity that respond poorly to oral medications. This chapter will highlight proper patient selection, intrathecal dosing, medication compounding, and training requirements for implanting and managing physicians and will provide strategies to optimize the sustainability of intrathecal opioid therapy.

Abbreviations

CT   Computed tomography
CYP   Cytochrome P450
FDA   Food and Drug Administration
IDDS   Intrathecal drug delivery system
ITB   Intrathecal baclofen
MRI   Magnetic resonance imaging
OIH   Opioid-induced hyperalgesia
PTC   Patient therapy controller
PTM   Patient therapy manager
TDD   Targeted drug delivery

D. R. Kloster (✉)
Crimson Pain Management, Overland Park, KS, USA

© The Author(s), under exclusive license to Springer Nature Switzerland AG 2022
D. P. Beall et al. (eds.), *Intrathecal Pump Drug Delivery*, Medical Radiology Diagnostic Imaging,
https://doi.org/10.1007/978-3-030-86244-2_7

1   Patient Selection

Patient selection regarding intrathecal therapy is arguably the most important aspect of this treatment. Providers and patients alike desire an optimal outcome, and it is imperative to select an appropriate patient for this treatment modality (Przybyl et al. 2003; Wallace et al. 2015; Mekhail 2014). The Food and Drug Administration (FDA) states that intrathecal therapy is indicated for moderate to severe trunk and limb pain and intractable pain where more conservative therapies have failed. In accordance with this, providers typically choose patients who have a painful pathologic process and have responded suboptimally to more conservative therapies (Befverud et al. 2008). These typical painful problems usually encompass several areas. For example, intrathecal therapy can be helpful for nonsurgical axial neck or back pain, painful degenerative scoliosis, spinal degenerative processes associated with pain and muscle spasm, and failed back surgery syndrome (Hagedorn and Atallah 2017). It also can be useful for complex regional pain syndrome, arachnoiditis, and trunk pain consistent with post herpetic neuralgia or post thoracotomy syndrome (Demartini et al. 2010; van der Plas et al. 2011). Other axial pain such as visceral and pelvic pain may fall into this category as well as appendicular pain either from a radicular origin or from prominent degenerative joint disease. In essence, intrathecal medication therapy may be effective for pain from any somatic location when more conservative treatments have been tried and have been met with a suboptimal response (Deer et al. 2017).

Even when a patient appropriately meets the clinical indications for targeted drug delivery (TDD) indications and is a good candidate from a painful pathology standpoint, the clinicians must also determine if a patient is a good candidate for the surgical procedure itself. The patient's general state of health should be adequate to tolerate the intrathecal medication therapy and to provide proper wound healing. A provider must also consider if a patient has bleeding tendencies and if a patient needs to or has the ability to stop their anticoagulant therapy. If a patient does not meet these conditions, they will not qualify for surgical procedure necessary to initiate the intrathecal therapy. The consideration of the patient's wound healing capability and their blood clotting proficiency are necessary components to assess prior to even the consideration of IT therapy as the patient will need to be healthy enough to heal the surgical wounds after placement of a subcutaneous titanium implant (Wang et al. 2018; Brown and Phillips 2010; Serrano et al. 2014; Horlocker 2011). Additional considerations are that the patient has an adequate body habitus to support placement of a pump, has sufficient insurance or financial means, and has the family support necessary to make it to future appointments to manage and refill the pump. If the patient is malnourished, for example, they may not either be able to heal the incisional sites or they may be too cachectic to have a suitable anatomic option for placement of the pump. An additional requirement that is especially pertinent to patients with cancer-related pain is that they should have a life expectancy greater than 3 months (Hassenbusch et al. 1997). If these conditions cannot be met, the patient will usually not qualify for intrathecal therapy.

Patients suffering with late stage or metastatic cancer are very often good candidates for intrathecal therapy, especially those patients with neoplasms that can be especially painful such as pancreatic carcinoma or osseous metastases (Bruel and Burton 2016; Hayek et al. 2011a). The literature supports using TDD as it not only helps with improved pain control but can also prolong the patient's life expectancy (Smith et al. 2002). The patients are correspondingly more likely to desire additional treatments of their underlying cancer if their pain is well managed. In all patients but especially in the patients with cancer pain on numerous other medications, their systemic pain medications may have numerous intolerable side effects (Moryl et al. 2010; Gulati et al. 2014). Nausea is common with oral opioids, and the inevitable constipation that is associated with these medications can be severe and very debilitating in these patients whose health is already significantly compromised. These side effects caused by systemic opioids will be dramatically decreased or eliminated with intrathecal therapy. Sedation and short-term memory loss are also often present in patients who take systemic opiate medications. Replacing systemic opioid therapy with intrathecal therapy eliminates or greatly reduces these sedating side effects. Patients on systemic opioid therapy are also subject to waxing and waning doses of their medications due to normal medication metabolism and intermittent dosing. This has continued to be an issue despite long-acting opioids and can result in intermittent exacerbations of the patient's pain that may be difficult to control with systemic therapy. These peaks, and troughs seen with the use of systemic medications are absent with intrathecal therapy. In addition to the constant rate intrathecal drug delivery, both the Medtronic pump and the Flowonix pump have the ability to provide intermittent bolus dosing that can be useful in treating intermittent surges of pain. The Medtronic system has a controller that is designated as the patient therapy manager (PTM), and the Flowonix system's controller is called the patient therapy controller (PTC). Both of these systems allow patients to safely give themselves intermittent boluses of medication above their baseline dosing. Generally, the patients will feel a response in 15 to 30 minutes after an intrathecal bolus. Patients with cancer-related pain will often have a combination of both neuropathic and nociceptive pain, and TDD allows for combinations of medications to be used that are beneficial for treating both types of pain (Stearns et al. 2005). By using multiple medications in combination in the intrathecal pump, the managing clinician may be able to provide the patients with better pain relief and fewer side effects compared to treatment with systemic medications (Deer et al. 2017). In addition to medications used for pain control, it is also possible to use intrathecal droperidol in patients with significant biliousness as a treatment to help control their nausea (Gulati et al. 2014). Although droperidol is usually effective in controlling symptoms of nausea and vomiting in most circumstances, it may

have little effect in patients with chemotherapy-induced nausea (Gulati et al. 2014).

In addition to the previously discussed patients, another group of patients that will typically have a very good outcome with TDD is the elderly population. Elderly patients will often have nociceptive pain that is responsive to low-dose systemic opioids but may not be able to tolerate these medications due to their side effect, especially the constipation and short-term memory loss (Chau et al. 2008). These side effects, if significant enough, may lead to a decrease in patient function or may cause the patient to refuse to take the medication (Saunders et al. 2010). At this point, an intrathecal medication trial may be effective in determining the degree of pain relief and for showing the patient that very effective pain relief may be accomplished without life-altering side effects. The subsequent placement of an intrathecal pump will allow the patient to resume an active lifestyle without the substantial discomfort caused by the pain and/or medication side effects.

Patients with diffuse pathology such as multi-site pain or multi-pathology pain may also benefit greatly from TDD (Wallace et al. 2015; Mekhail 2014). An example would be somebody who has had previous neck surgery and low back surgery that now has recurrent pain from adjacent segment degenerative disease. If just one of these two sites is painful, other treatments such as spinal cord stimulation can be a good option, but for patients with multiple locations affected by pain, the anatomic coverage from one stimulator would not be sufficient. Additionally, patients that have undergone previous spine surgery may also be affected by other pain producing pathologies such as arachnoiditis. Once patients have diffuse symptomatology and/or are affected by more than one pain producing pathologic process, choosing a therapy for only one region in the body is unwise and will ultimately lead to treatment failure.

The most common group of patients typically identified as candidates for TDD is patients that have failed all other treatments. Although these patients are good candidates for intrathecal therapy, they are the most difficult patient population to treat as they have proven to not be responsive to any of the other treatments attempted thus far. Often these patients have been on high doses of systemic narcotics and will require correspondingly high doses of intrathecal narcotics to overcome their opioid tolerance built up over time (Chau et al. 2008). This patient population can certainly be treated with higher than typical doses of intrathecal opioids but is helpful to wean the patients down off of their systemic narcotics prior to starting TDD (this is discussed in further detail in chapter "Intrathecal Drug Delivery Trialing"). It is important to understand the most likely outcome for this patient population and to discuss their expected outcomes prior to even performing an intrathecal medication trial. Sometimes patients that have been through different surgical procedures who have failed back surgery syndrome and are on high doses of opioids with multiple intolerances to medications or expectations that are difficult to meet can be nearly impossible to treat successfully without setting realistic expectations and a having a viable treatment strategy. Psychological testing in this subgroup of patients may also be beneficial (Deer et al. 2017; Doleys 2003; Doleys and Brown 2001). Patients need to understand the goals of TDD and that this treatment, like any other, is about improving functionality and quality of life, and although it is expected that the pain scores will be improved, this is a subjective measurement and cannot be guaranteed.

An intrathecal pump does have the advantage of utilizing medications that are not available orally such as bupivacaine, ziconotide, and fentanyl (Deer et al. 2017; Hassenbusch et al. 2002; Deer et al. 2002). By utilizing medications that work via different delivery routes and at different receptors (i.e., the inhibition of the N-type voltage-sensitive calcium channel by ziconotide), there is a better opportunity to achieve an adequate analgesic response. In addition to the improved efficacy, intrathecal medications have been shown to be safer from a mortality and morbidity standpoint and have less risk of diversion (Centers for Disease control (CDC) 2011). Intrathecal medication delivery can be especially useful for patients that

have difficult pain control due simply to their particular underlying condition. Patients with systemic diseases such as lupus erythematosus, Crohn's disease, and rheumatoid arthritis can benefit from this treatment similar to other patients with nonsystemic disease-related pain. In patients with systemic disease, it's always best to control the underlying disease process in a way that optimizes systemic therapy, but if this is not sufficiently effective to control the pain, TDD can be initiated. Although these patients are good candidates for intrathecal medication therapy, there are additional issues in this patient population that must be taken into consideration prior to considering TDD. Patients with systemic diseases often have compromised immune systems which increase the already not insubstantial risk of infection associated with placement of an intrathecal drug delivery system (IDDS). The increased risk of infection may be compounded by the patient's medications as many of these medications used to treat autoimmune diseases are immunosuppressive and may potentiate the risk of infection. This is similarly true for cancer patients on immunosuppressive therapy and chemotherapeutic agents.

In addition to chronic pain and cancer pain patients, patients with severe spasticity that are not effectively managed with systemic medications are also good candidates for intrathecal therapy (Schiess et al. 2020; Saulino et al. 2016). The US Food and Drug Administration (FDA) approves and indicates intrathecal baclofen therapy (ITB) for the management of severe spasticity of spinal and cerebral origins in children between the ages of 4 and 18 suffering from severe chronic spasticity that is unresponsive to oral antispasmodics. There is no clear definition of spasticity or severe spasticity, but it should be implied that if spasticity causes significant discomfort or interferes with activities of daily living, mobility, positioning, or caregiver aid, this will qualify as severe. If these patients' spasticity is suboptimally controlled, they can have significant persistent systemic issues and discomfort. Children with developmental deformities are a good population to consider for ITB. They can have spasticity and muscle tightness that is exacerbated by the continued growth of their musculoskeletal system. Effective spasticity management will allow these individuals to be more functional. Additionally, patients who already have impaired cognition can experience worsening in their mentation with many systemic medications used to treat spasticity. Intrathecal therapy can allow relief from spasticity without the detrimental effect on cognition at a dose that is much smaller than that taken orally. Given the high degree of efficacy and very low side effect profile associated with ITB, it should optimally be considered early in the treatment of patients with severe spasticity rather than as a last resort. In conjunction with rehabilitation, ITB can be immensely beneficial in helping to preserve function and maximize comfort. If a patient suffers from contractures, it can be very difficult for them or their caregiver to clean those areas and those areas which are also much more prone to skin breakdown. Baclofen dosed in small amounts into the intrathecal space can significantly decrease muscle tone which can lead to an improvement in the patient's contractures. The improvement in muscle tone can also improve and facilitate activities of daily life such as ambulation or wheelchair transfers. There is evidence to show that patients treated with intrathecal baclofen are very satisfied with the results and that this benefit is long lasting with literature documenting the efficacy of this therapy up to 24 years after the initial pump implantation (Mathur et al. 2014). The timing of when to initiate intrathecal Baclofen therapy is somewhat controversial in some situations. The typical post-injury delay prior to initiating ITB is 1 year after injury, but it has been shown that the use of ITB can decrease the severity of spasticity produced by TBI, and several studies suggest that earlier intervention would be more beneficial (Saulino et al. 2016). The historical strategy to delay therapy was based on the assumption that patients would be too sick to receive benefit and that they should maximize their neural healing prior to intervening with ITB therapy. Delaying therapy, however, can contribute to additional adverse sequelae such as flexion contractures, skin breakdown, and joint ankylosis. Earlier initiation of ITB has been shown mitigate these processes (Saulino et al. 2016).

2   Compounded Medications

The use of compounded intrathecal medications is common (Deer et al. 2017). When using medications that have been combined together to create a compound designed to meet the individual needs of a patient, it is important to understand the role of the compounding pharmacy that produces these medications (Kienle 2020). Pharmacy compounding is defined as combining, mixing, or altering of ingredients to create a customized medication for an individual patient in response to a licensed practitioner's prescription. These pharmacies are not regulated by the FDA but rather by individual state pharmacy boards. There are approximately 4000 compounding pharmacies in the United States, but only about a third of these have undertaken the currently voluntary national accreditation process through either of the two leading accreditation organizations: the Accreditation Commission for Healthcare's Pharmacy Compounding Accreditation Board (ACHC/PCAB) and the National Association of Board of Pharmacy Accreditation (NABP). Both of these organizations hold any licensed compounding pharmacy accountable to United States Pharmacopeia chapters (USP) sterile compounding standards and the FD&C act 503A compounding pharmacy requirements to compound patient-specific medications pursuant to a legally written prescription order. A great resource to find such an accredited pharmacy is to either directly contact the ACHC/PCAB or the NABP or go to their websites:

Accreditation Commission for Health Care, Cary, NC, USA. http://www.achc.org
National Association of Boards of Pharmacy, Mount Prospect, IL, USA. http://nabp.pharmacy/programs/accreditations-inspections/compounding-pharmacy/

Though using compounded medications is an off-label use, the vast majority of practitioners are utilizing intrathecal compounded medications in their practice (FDA 2018). The use of devices or medication in an off-label manner is very common, but the provider should inform the patient of this use and the reasons behind the addition of compounded medications. Monotherapy with either morphine or baclofen is currently the only on-label treatment, and any addition of other medications or modifications of the single medications (including dilution) will reclassify the usage as off-label.

Compounding medications offer distinct advantages of being able to produce positive synergistic effects from the multiple medications. It also has the possibility of being able to produce more profound pain relief with fewer side effects. Most patients started on monotherapy have mixed pain states that can be difficult to successfully treat if monotherapy is utilized. Although compounding medications offer numerous advantages, it also has the potential for additional side effects or adverse outcomes. Specifically, the Medtronic Synchromed II pump, which is recommended for monotherapy only, can have a shorter pump life and can potentially be damaged when certain compounded medications are utilized (Deer et al. 2017; Rezai et al. 2013; Medtronic 2012; Kim 2011). Medtronic reported data that the stall rate for approved medications was 2.4% at 5 years and was 4.5% for unapproved medications. The Polyanalgesic Consensus Guidelines (PACC) state that compounding medications are the de facto standard of care, and peer-reviewed literature exists to support the use of both on-label and off-label medication use (Deer et al. 2017). The guidelines also state that intrathecal drug delivery essentially mandates the use of compounded medications.

The Flowonix Prometra II pump is also recommended for on-label monotherapy, but compounded medications do not seem to shorten the life expectancy of the Flowonix pump (Deer et al. 2017). When utilizing compounded medications, providers should use a compounding pharmacy that is credentialed, skilled, and experienced in producing these medications. The coordination

should also ensure that the medication preparation and delivery is done in a timely manner to coordinate with the patient's pump refill appointment.

3   Starting Dosages

After pump implantation, the patient should discontinue all systemic opioids. Clinicians who manage patients with IDDSs have various methodologies for stopping systemic opioid medications. Some clinicians will discontinue all systemic medications immediately following implantation of the IDDS. Other implanters will reduce the systemic dose and continue to titrate down to zero over a short period of time. Currently, these methods are both being used successfully and no real consensus opinion that exists for which protocol to utilize.

Regardless of whether monotherapy or a multi-medication mixture is used, the provider should always start at the lowest effective dose and titrate upward to treatment effect. The choice of first-line medications is almost always a single on-label agent with ziconotide and morphine considered as first-line treatments (Tables 1, 2, 3, and 4). The choice of which medication to use first and which medications follow is aided by the Polyanalgesic Consensus Guidelines (PACC) that offer guidance on medication choice and hierarchy (Tables 1, 2, 3, and 4) (Deer et al. 2017). The PACC guidelines provide given recommendations for medication selection for patients with both cancer and noncancer-related pain. The starting dosages recommended by the PACC guidelines assume that the patient is being dosed using the chronic continuous infusion method. It has been assumed that intrathecal medication is 300 times more potent than oral medications in a patient that is not tolerant to the medication being given. This assumption is based on previous experience and data that intravenous medication is three times stronger than oral medication, epidural medication is ten times stronger than intravenous medication, and intrathecal medication is ten times stronger than epidural medication (Foley 1985) (Table 5). The final ratio

Table 1 Noncancer-related pain with diffuse nociceptive or neuropathic pain

			Ziconotide[a]	
Line 1A	Morphine			
Line 1B	Hydromorphone		Morphine or hydromorphone + bupivacaine	
Line 3	Morphine or hydromorphone + clonidine		Fentanyl + bupivacaine	Ziconotide + morphine or hydromorphone
Line 4	Morphine or hydromorphone + bupivacaine + clonidine	Fentanyl + ziconotide	Sufentanil + bupivacaine or clonidine	Ziconotide + clonidine or bupivacaine or both
Line 5	Fentanyl or sufentanil + bupivacaine + clonidine		Sufentanil + ziconotide	
Line 6	Opioid + ziconotide + clonidine or bupivacaine			Baclofen

Adapted from: Deer T, Pope J, Hayek S, et al. The polyanalgesic consensus conference (PACC): recommendations on intrathecal drug infusion systems best practices and guidelines. Neuromodulation 2017;20(2):96–132

[a]Ziconotide should be the first choice in patients with >120 morphine equivalents or fast systemic dose escalation, in the absence of history of psychosis

Table 2 Noncancer-related pain with localized nociceptive or neuropathic pain

Line 1A	Ziconotide		Morphine	
Line 1B	Fentanyl		Fentanyl + bupivacaine	
Line 2	Fentanyl + clonidine	Morphine or hydromorphone + bupivacaine	Fentanyl + bupivacaine + clonidine	Bupivacaine
Line 3	Fentanyl + ziconotide + bupivacaine	Morphine or hydromorphone + clonidine	Ziconotide + clonidine or bupivacaine or both	Bupivacaine + clonidine
Line 4	Sufentanil + bupivacaine or clonidine	Baclofen	Bupivacaine + clonidine + ziconotide	
Line 5	Sufentanil + bupivacaine + clonidine		Sufentanil + ziconotide	

Adapted from: Deer T, Pope J, Hayek S, et al. The polyanalgesic consensus conference (PACC): recommendations on intrathecal drug infusion systems best practices and guidelines. Neuromodulation 2017;20(2):96–132

Table 3 Cancer or other terminal condition-related pain with diffuse nociceptive or neuropathic pain

Line 1A	Ziconotide			Morphine		
Line 1BA	Hydromorphone			Morphine or hydromorphone + bupivacaine		
Line 2	Morphine or hydromorphone + clonidine			Ziconotide + morphine or hydromorphone		
Line 3	Hydromorphone or morphine or fentanyl + bupivacaine + clonidine	Ziconotide + bupivacaine	Ziconotide + clonidine	Hydromorphone or morphine or fentanyl + bupivacaine + ziconotide	Sufentanil	
Line 4	Sufentanil + ziconotide	Baclofen	Sufentanil + bupivacaine	Sufentanil + clonidine	Ziconotide + bupivacaine + clonidine	Bupivacaine + clonidine
Line 5	Sufentanil + bupivacaine + clonidine		Sufentanil + bupivacaine + ziconotide		Sufentanil + clonidine + ziconotide	
Line 6	Opioid[a] + bupivacaine + clonidine + adjuvants[b]					

Adapted from: Deer T, Pope J, Hayek S, et al. The polyanalgesic consensus conference (PACC): recommendations on intrathecal drug infusion systems best practices and guidelines. Neuromodulation 2017;20(2):96–132

[a]Opioids (all known intrathecal opioids)

[b]Adjuvants include midazolam, ketamine, octreotide

Table 4 Cancer or other terminal condition-related pain with localized nociceptive neuropathic pain

Line 1A	Ziconotide				Morphine	
Line 1B	Fentanyl			Morphine or fentanyl + bupivacaine		
Line 2	Hydromorphone	Hydromorphone + bupivacaine		Hydromorphone or fentanyl or morphine + clonidine	Morphine or hydromorphone or fentanyl + ziconotide	
Line 3	Hydromorphone or morphine or fentanyl + bupivacaine + clonidine	Ziconotide + bupivacaine		Clonidine + ziconotide	Morphine or hydromorphone or fentanyl + ziconotide + bupivacaine	Sufentanil
Line 4	Sufentanil + ziconotide	Sufentanil + bupivacaine	Baclofen	Sufentanil + clonidine	Ziconotide + bupivacaine + clonidine	Bupivacaine + clonidine
Line 5	Sufentanil + bupivacaine + clonidine				Bupivacaine + clonidine	
Line 6	Opioid[a] + bupivacaine + clonidine + adjuvants[b]					

Adapted from: Deer T, Pope J, Hayek S, et al. The polyanalgesic consensus conference (PACC): recommendations on intrathecal drug infusion systems best practices and guidelines. Neuromodulation 2017;20(2):96–132

[a]Opioids (all known intrathecal opioids)

[b]Adjuvants include midazolam, ketamine, octreotide

of 300:1 is an assumption to provide guidance rather than rigid rule, but nevertheless, it is universally agreed that intrathecal medication is significantly more powerful than oral medication (Sylvester et al. 2004; Du Pen and Du Pen 2003).

Table 5 Equianalgesic dosing

Narcotic agent	Route	Equianalgesic dose (mg)
Morphine	IM	10
	PO	30
Hydromorphone	IM	1.5
	PO	7.5
Meperidine	IM	75
	PO	300
Methadone	IM	10
	PO	20

IM intramuscular, *PO* oral. The IM-PO morphine ratio of 1:3 is conventionally used during chronic dosing
Adapted from: Foley KM. Treatment of cancer pain. N Engl J Med 1985;313:84–95

Table 6 Recommended starting dosage ranges of intrathecal medications for long-term therapy delivery

Drug	Recommended starting dose
Morphine	0.1–0.5 mg/day
Hydromorphone	0.01–0.15 mg/day
Ziconotide	0.5–1.2 mcg/day (to 2.4 mcg/day per product labeling)
Fentanyl	25–75 mcg/day
Bupivacaine	0.01–4 mg/day
Clonidine	20–100 mcg/day
Sufentanil	10–20 mcg/day

Adapted from: Deer T, Pope J, Hayek S, et al. The polyanalgesic consensus conference (PACC): recommendations on intrathecal drug infusion systems best practices and guidelines. Neuromodulation 2017;20(2):96–132

Many practitioners that have significant experience with intrathecal therapy more often use a 100 to 1 as their conversion ratio. Following the recognition of the opioid crisis and with the current climate where the opioid medication doses are statutorily limited, there are fewer patients that present with excessive doses of systemic opioids. The conversion from systemic to intrathecal was more applicable when patients were on hundreds of milligrams equivalent of morphine daily (Centers for Disease control (CDC) 2011). This is rarely encountered in the current climate with the exception of some patients with cancer, especially those with metastatic osseous disease who survive longer than the typical patient. Most patients receiving an intrathecal pump are in the range of 90–150 mg of oral morphine equivalent. An example of oral to intrathecal conversion would be an opioid-tolerant patient on 100 mg of oral morphine equivalent where the starting intrathecal dose would be anywhere from 0.3–1 mg depending on which conversion ratio that you utilize. The PACC guidelines offer recommended starting doses of the various medications and maximum daily doses which are shown in Tables 6 and 7, respectively.

If the standard dosages are utilized and the systemic weaning of opioids is adhered to, there is a high degree of safety associated with TDD. Coffey et al. reported from the device registration and Social Security master file that intrathecal therapy mortality rate is 0.088% at 3 days after implantation, 0.39% at 1 month, and 3.89% at 1 year (Coffey et al. 2009). It was noted that each patient in that database had an initial

Table 7 Maximum concentrations and daily doses of intrathecal agents as recommended PACC 2012 and 2016

Drug	Maximum concentration	Maximum dose per day
Morphine	20 mg/mL	15 mg
Hydromorphone	15 g/mL	10 mg
Fentanyl	10 mg/mL	1000 mcg
Sufentanil	5 mg/mL	500 mcg
Bupivacaine	30 mg/mL	15–20 mg[a]
Clonidine	1000 mcg/mL	600 mcg
Ziconotide	100 mcg/mL	19.2 mcg

Adapted from: Deer T, Pope J, Hayek S, et al. The polyanalgesic consensus conference (PACC): recommendations on intrathecal drug infusion systems best practices and guidelines. Neuromodulation 2017;20(2):96–132
[a]May be exceeded in end-of-life care and complicated cases as determined by medical necessity

starting dose of more than 0.5 mg per day of morphine.

Most insurance carriers require a trial of intrathecal medication before permanent implantation of an IDDS, although many make an exception for patients with cancer-related pain (Malhotra et al. 2013). There are several studies to suggest trialing for intrathecal therapy is appropriate in the outpatient setting, but many clinicians perform intrathecal trials only when the patient can stay overnight (Deer et al. 2017). There is no general consensus on the optimal way to trial a patient or which medication and dose to use during the trial. Given this lack of consensus, trialing is more about determining the magnitude of pain relief and the ability of the patient to tolerate the medication used. During a trial, the clinician wants to ensure that the patient has an adequate analgesic response, usually determined by an 80% or more reduction of pain and that they do not have any significant adverse sequelae such as nausea or vomiting, urinary hesitancy, or unacceptable pruritus. It is important to discuss with the patient that they may not experience the same level of analgesia with the initial placement of the IDDS as they did during the trial. If a patient is pain-free with a trial, it is not expected that they will be completely pain-free after the initial placement of the pump. The expectation is that the dosage of the pump will have to be increased and titrated to a point where the patient will have better functionality, better sleep habits, and be able to engage in enjoyable activities. The starting dose with any medication should be a low dose that is increased slowly to the point where adequate analgesia is attained. As with trialing, initiation of the permanent device may safely be performed in the outpatient setting, but expert consensus and the PACC guidelines propose to start the initial pump dose at half of the trialing dose. The expert consensus also recommends an overnight admission if the medication is started at a dose higher than this recommendation.

In addition to the baseline continuous daily rate, most clinicians will also give the patient an option for intermittent bolus dosing separated by a predetermined amount of time. Both the Medtronic pump and the Flowonix pump allow for bolus dosing. The PACC guidelines suggest patient-controlled bolus doses to be in the range of 5–20% of the total daily dose. The Cleveland clinic review stated that up to 30% of the 24-h dose could be safely given up to four times per day (Bolash and Mikail 2015).

The greater the amount of weaning off of oral opioids prior to starting TTT, the greater the likelihood that the intrathecal therapy will be successful, and if patients are maintained on high doses of systemic opioids, the initial intrathecal monotherapy will almost certainly be suboptimally effective (Hayek et al. 2011b; Pope and Deer 2015; Kim et al. 2011; Kroin 1992). If a patient is on an adequate oral dose of opioid medication and doing poorly, an intrathecal equivalent of that dose cannot be expected to be more effective in regards to pain relief, but this similar amount of pain relief could be provided with significantly fewer medication side effects. This type of patient would benefit substantially from weaning down or off of the opioids and would also likely benefit from adding non-opioid pain relieving compounded medications such as bupivacaine or clonidine.

Medications used in TDD have various affinities for fat- and water-based environments. Hydrophilic, hydrophobic, and lipophilic drugs are utilized, and it is beneficial to know which category the medication fits into to optimize the efficacy of that medication. The steady-state delivery of intrathecal therapy provides a consistent dose of medication that allows for a diffusion gradient across the pia arachnoid and white matter of the spinal cord (Campos and Pope 2018). Diffusion across the pia matter is generally considered unimpeded because it is a single layer of cells without intracellular junctions (Kroin 1992). The receptor sites for most intrathecal medications are located in the dorsal horn of the spinal cord specifically the horizontal lamina II which is called the substantia gelatinosa. The spinal white cord matter is made up of myelinated axons making it hydrophobic due to the lipid-rich characteristics of the myelin. The gray matter consists of cell bodies in the various lamina and is hydro-

Table 8 Recommended doses for intrathecal bolus trialing

Drug	Recommended dose
Morphine	0.1–0.5 mg
Hydromorphone	0.025–0.1 mg
Ziconotide	1–5 mcg
Fentanyl	15–75 mcg
Bupivacaine	0.5–2.5 mg
Clonidine	5–20 mcg
Sufentanil	5–20 mcg

Adapted from: Deer T, Pope J, Hayek S, et al. The polyanalgesic consensus conference (PACC): recommendations on intrathecal drug infusion systems best practices and guidelines. Neuromodulation 2017;20(2):96–132

philic. Hydrophilic medications have longer half-lives than lipophilic medications, and although lipophilic medications have faster clearance, they also often penetrate more deeply into the cord. This medication can be useful for precise targeting of myelinated neural tissue.

The 2016 PACC guidelines recommend a starting dose range of intrathecal medication for long-term therapy delivery (Table 6), as well as recommended doses for intrathecal bolus trialing (Table 8). This can be helpful to clinicians when a standard and safe bolus trial dose is desired for patients especially when using a medication that is uncommonly used for trials. The initial starting dose for patients beginning their TDD therapy begins therapy at a low dose so it can be determined if the patient will respond early to relatively low medication doses.

4 Training and Education

Since the advent of IT therapy in the 1980s, there has been substantial advancement in the technology and management segments of IT drug delivery. There have been advancements in IT pump technology, the interfaces between the IDDS and the clinician, and pharmacologic knowledge of how different medications perform and metabolize in the intrathecal environment. The rapid pace of the clinical knowledge combined with the increased clinical need have driven the need for optimal and updated training of clinicians that

implant and manage IDDSs. The type of training and education that is needed to implant and manage intrathecal drug delivery systems depends on the scope of practice for the individual provider and the type of patients that are being treated. The training necessary to provide competence in these areas may come from academic medical programs, industry sponsored or related courses, or by didactic and cadaver labs. The credentialing for the treatment and management of all aspects of IDDS management is left to the discretion of the facility or hospital.

Physicians implanting and managing IDDSs should have an understanding of the pharmacology of the medications utilized and be well versed in potential complications (see chapters "Postoperative Care and Complication" and "Intrathecal Pump and Catheter Troubleshooting"). If the managing physician is also the primary implanter of the device, they should be skilled at placing implantable devices and be able to manage intraoperative and postoperative complications. The physician also needs to be able to recognize intraoperative issues during placement such as a malpositioned catheter, an epidural hematoma, or the signs of various neurological injuries. The treating physician needs to recognize a surgical site infection that requires treatment or explantation of the IDDS and should also be able to recognize catheter or pump malfunctions that require treatment or revision of the system. Not all managers of intrathecal pumps implant the IDDSs and vice versa. If this is the case, the two providers should be in close communication regarding the appropriate preoperative planning for placement of the pump and catheter and to determine the concentration and type of medication that will be initially used in the pump. The planning process should also include a predetermined decision regarding who will manage any immediate or long-term complications. After the pump placement and adequate healing has occurred, there are different types of complications that can potentially arise over the lifetime of the pump. These complications can include unexpected catheter migration, catheter kinking or fracturing, or failure of the pump itself. Each of these scenarios typically produces withdrawal-type symptoms in the patient. The patient will then need systemic pharmacotherapy to control their withdrawal symptoms and ultimately surgical revision to correct the problem. Catheter tip granulomas are another complication that is unique to intrathecal therapy, and if a granuloma is suspected, the patient should be imaged and the problem addressed as quickly as possible. The clinician managing the pump should be able to perform catheter contrast studies, rotor studies, and should be able to interpret fluoroscopic imaging as well as CT and MRI cross-sectional imaging. Another potential complication that is associated with the intrathecal pump refill process is that the patient can inadvertently receive excess of medication due to a pocket fill or, much more rarely, a pump failure. The managing clinician and the staff need to be trained to recognize these problems and treat and resuscitate the patient if necessary.

It has been estimated that for clinicians or fellows new to intrathecal drug delivery systems, it takes experience in the implantation and management of approximately ten implantable systems for the practitioner to be proficient (Deer et al. 2017). Ultimately, the local credentialing committees of each hospital decide the expertise needed to appropriately perform these duties.

It is important to have a support staff that is familiar with intrathecal drug delivery therapy. They will need initial and often continuing education and training on filling an intrathecal pump, using sterile technique, and in recognizing potential complications. An administrative staff that is able to schedule patients is also necessary as the initial visit or trial is only the beginning for a therapy that is associated with pump refills, dose adjustments, catheter and rotor studies, and pump replacements. The more familiar the administrative staff is with IT drug delivery and the various aspects of it, the more they will be able to help the patient with whatever they may need. It should always be kept in mind that there is a potential for severe withdrawal symptoms if a patient misses a pump refill or has an IDDS malfunction.

5 Opioid Tolerance and Its Effect on IT Opioid Therapy

There are several patterns of metabolism of opioids that are well defined. Most opioids are metabolized primarily through the hepatic system prior to entering the systemic circulation. The liver's blood supply comes primarily through the gastrointestinal tract and the portal venous system which accounts for about 75% of the blood flow entering the liver. Opioid pills are taken orally then absorbed in the small bowel and carried to the liver where they are metabolized. The metabolism is a process of converting a lipophilic opioid and making it more hydrophilic so as to enable its excretion in the urine.

There are two phases of opioid metabolism occurring within the liver. The first phase involves the cytochrome P450 (CYP) enzymes that alter the opioid and the second phase is hydrophilic and that is more easily excreted in the urine. The CYP enzymes can be dramatically upregulated which can contribute to an increasing tolerance to the medication along with the biotransformation processes which can lead to induced enzymatic expression and increased medication tolerance (Berkowitz 1976; Säwe 1986).

The result of the above described process is that the blood flow through the portal venous system can contain a high concentration of opioid that is distributed directly to the liver and then metabolized by the CYP enzymes that can contribute to upregulation and tolerance.

Before the statutory regulation of opioid doses, practices commonly saw patients on doses exceeding 100 mg equivalents of morphine or more daily. There were also patients on extremely high doses of 1000 mg equivalents or more of morphine daily. It has been our routine to use the 1:100 ratio when calculating the intrathecal to oral equivalent but doses that high prompted a reevaluation of the appropriate dose to use for a trial. Following a few underdosed trials, doses up to 8.0 mg of intrathecal morphine were occasionally given for those patients on extremely high doses of systemic narcotics.

There is obviously an increased risk of overdose when IT doses that high are given, but, in our experience, what we saw with these patients was a prominent decrease in their pain of 80% or more followed by a rapid recurrence of their pain within 3–6 h. This scenario was consistent in patients on very high doses of systemic opioids and highlighted to us the ability of the CYP system to upregulate to the degree that there is almost no large amount of intrathecal opioid that can be given which will adequately treat pain in a patient that has an extremely high tolerance to systemic opioids. Due to an extreme amount of upregulation that is possible with the CYP enzymes in patients on chronic opioids, we do not allow systemic opioids for more than 2 weeks following pump implantation because it can be a self-defeating therapy if allowed.

In addition to the enzymatic development of tolerance, there is evidence that neuroadaptation interferes with opioids ability to provide long-term analgesia (Rivat and Ballantyne 2016). One of the reasons for the extensive and unregulated use of opioids over the last couple of decades was the belief of some providers that if a patient was not experiencing adequate analgesia, it was due to an insufficient opioid dose (Smith 2020; Blendon and Benson 2018; King et al. 2005). This erroneous concept that dose escalation could overcome tolerance resulted in much higher daily opioid dosages. Providers did not understand the concept of opioid-induced hyperalgesia (OIH) that was inevitably propagated by high doses of opioids taken over an extended period of time (Fletcher and Martinez 2014). There were also new long-acting opioid medications that were developed that provided a sustained higher dose over the course of the day. This represented a shift from short-acting opioids that could exit the system and provide times during the day where the patient would have a low or absent systemic levels of opioid. The concept of treating breakthrough pain also contributed to daily dose escalation. Breakthrough pain was an adapted theory from palliative care that described severe pain that increases when the patient is already medicated with a long-acting pain medication (Portenoy et al. 2006). Because of the changes in treatment strategies, patients were maintained on much higher dosages of opi-oid analgesics for longer periods of time. Providers now understand that this can have chronic adverse long-term effects such as OIH and increased side effects from the opioids and can put the patient at a much higher risk of overdose.

Patients that take chronic opioids can develop their tolerance to the medication as well as OIH in a relatively short period of time (Angst et al. 2003). Opioid tolerance is a clinical lack of response to an opioid that can initially be overcome by increasing the dose. Hyperalgesia is a chronic sensitization process by which the long-term exposure to opioids can cause a paradoxical response where patients become more sensitive to painful stimuli (Angst et al. 2003; Lee et al. 2011). When patients reach the point of experiencing OIH, escalating the opioid dose will not resolve hyperalgesia and will make it worse. Hyperalgesia occurs after potent short-acting mu agonists such as fentanyl, remifentanil, and buprenorphine and also after potent long-acting mu agonists such as morphine (Roeckel et al. 2016). The main inhibitory effect of opioids on pain transmission is due to the stimulation of mu opioid receptors resulting in an inhibition of adenylyl cyclase and ion channels. The decreased analgesic effect over time is not only due to an alteration of the opioid receptor but is also associated with an activation of the pronociceptive systems that counteract opioid analgesic effects. Opiate-induced pronociceptive activity may also be present long after the opioid is discontinued (de Conno et al. 2001). There is also limited data to suggest that intrathecal opioids can cause opioid-induced hyperalgesia, albeit to a lesser degree (Loram et al. 2012). Augmenting therapy by introducing other intrathecal medications can help reduce opioid requirements in chronic pain patients. It seems that most preventive strategies have focused on NMDA receptor activation and glutaminergic systems which result in hyperalgesia. Medications such as ketamine and methadone, as well as gabapentinoids, alpha-2 receptor agonists (i.e., clonidine), have been shown to be effective at attenuating the hyperalgesia (Cooper et al. 1997). The best method to address tolerance and opiate-induced hyperalgesia, however, is to prevent the occurrence of this problem from the outset of the patient's treatment.

6 Conclusion

Intrathecal pumps have the ability to make patients more comfortable, to increase their functionality, and to diminish the untoward side effects from oral medications. Patient selection is important for success of the therapy, and practitioners need to carefully select and screen their patients before offering this therapy. Treating clinicians need to be well versed in intraoperative management, postoperative care, understanding of complications, and the appropriate use of the various medications utilized in intrathecal drug delivery systems. Clinicians also need an adequately trained and competent staff, including nurses, medical assistants, and administrative and scheduling personnel. In order to optimize the therapy, the expert clinician will also consider the other less well-known contributing factors to the success of the patient including their nutritional status, comorbidities, ongoing insurance status, and family support which all play an important role in the successful of the intrathecal therapy.

References

Angst M, Koppert W, Pahl I et al (2003) Short-term infusion of the mu-opioid agonist remifentanil in humans causes hyperalgesia during withdrawal. Pain 106:49–57

Befverud S, Mogilner A, Schulder M (2008) Review article intrathecal pumps. Neurotherapeutics 5(1):114–122

Berkowitz BA (1976) The relationship of pharmacokinetics to pharmacological activity: morphine, methadone and naloxone. Clin Pharmacokinet 1(3):219–230

Blendon R, Benson J (2018) The public and the opioid abuse epidemic. N Engl J Med 378:407–411

Bolash R, Mikail M (2015) Multi-center prospective analysis of on-demand intrathecal morphine bolus dosing among patients with targeted drug delivery systems. Poster presented at the North American Neuromodulation Society meeting; Las Vegas, NV

Brown K, Phillips T (2010) Nutrition and wound healing. Clin Dermatol 28(4):432–439

Bruel B, Burton A (2016) Intrathecal therapy for cancer related pain. Pain Med 17:2404–2421

Campos L, Pope J (2018) Chapter 66. Pharmacology of intrathecal therapy. In: Neuromodulation, 2nd edn. Comprehensive textbook of principles, technologies, and therapies, pp 819–828

Centers for Disease control (CDC) (2011) Vital signs: overdoses of prescription opioid pain relievers—United States, 1999–2008. Morb Mortal Wkly Rep 60:1–6

Chau D, Walker V, Pai L et al (2008) Opioids and elderly: use and side effects. Clin Interv Aging 3(2):273–278

Coffey R, Owens M, Broste S et al (2009) Mortality associated with implantation and management of intrathecal opioid drug infusion systems to treat non cancer pain. Anesthesiology 111:888–891

Cooper D, Lindsay S, Ryall D et al (1997) Does intrathecal fentanyl produce acute cross-tolerance to i.v. morphine? Br J Anaesth 78:311–313

de Conno F, Caraceni A, Martini C et al (2001) Hyperalgesia and myoclonus with intrathecal infusion of high dose morphine. Pain 47:337–339

Deer T, Caraway D, Kim C et al (2002) Clinical experience with intrathecal bupivacaine in combination with opioid for the treatment of chronic pain related to failed back surgery syndrome and metastatic cancer pain of the spine. Spine J 2(4):274–278

Deer T, Pope J, Hayek S et al (2017) The polyanalgesic consensus conference (PACC): recommendations on intrathecal drug infusion systems best practices and guidelines. Neuromodulation 20(2):96–132

Demartini L, Stocco E, Bonezzi C (2010) Failed back surgery syndrome and intrathecal drugs infusion. Eur J Pain Suppl 4(4):299–301

Doleys D (2003) Psychological evaluation for patients undergoing neuroaugmentative procedures. Neurosurg Clin N Am 14:409–417

Doleys D, Brown J (2001) MMPI profile as an outcome "predictor" in the treatment of noncancer pain patients utilizing intraspinal opioid therapy. Neuromodulation 4:93–97

Du Pen S, Du Pen A (2003) The dilemma of opioid conversion and intrathecal therapy. Semin Pain Med 1(4):260–264

FDA (2018) Understanding unapproved use of approved drugs "off label"

Fletcher D, Martinez V (2014) Opioid-induced hyperalgesia in patients after surgery: a systemic review and a metaanalysis. Br J Anaesth 112:991–1004

Foley KM (1985) Treatment of cancer pain. N Engl J Med 313:84–95

Gulati A, Puttanniah V, Hung J et al (2014) Considerations for evaluating the use of intrathecal drug delivery in the oncologic patient. Curr Pain Headache Rep 18(2):391

Hagedorn J, Atallah G (2017) Intrathecal management of complex regional pain syndrome: a case report and literature. Scand J Pain 14:110–102

Hassenbusch S, Paice J, Bedder M et al (1997) Clinical realities and economic considerations: economics of intrathecal therapy. J Pain Symptom Manag 14(3 Suppl):S36–S48

Hassenbusch S, Gunes S, Wachsman S et al (2002) Intrathecal clonidine in the treatment of intractable pain: a phase 1/2 study. Pain Med 3(2):85–91

Hayek S, Deer T, Pope J (2011a) Intrathecal therapy for cancer and non-cancer pain. Pain Physician 14(3):219–248

Hayek S, Veizi I, Narouze S et al (2011b) Age dependent intrathecal opioid escalation in chronic noncancer pain patients. Pain Med 12:1179–1189

Horlocker T (2011) Regional anesthesia in the patient receiving antithrombotic and antiplatelet therapy. Br J Anaesth 107(Suppl 1):i96–i106

Kienle R (2020) Sterile compounding safety: the pharmacist's responsibility. Am J Health Syst Pharm 77(11):811–813

Kim P (2011) Case series of distal catheter obstruction. Presented at: NANS annual meeting; Las Vegas, NV

Kim D, Sidov A, Mandhare V et al (2011) Role of pretrial systemic opioid requirements intrathecal trial dose and non-psychological factors as predictors of outcome of intrathecal pump therapy: one clinician's experience with lumbar postlaminectomy pain. Neuromodulation 14:165–175

King T, Ossipov M, Vanderah T et al (2005) Is paradoxical pain induced by sustained opioid exposure an underlying mechanism of opioid antinociceptive tolerance? Neursignals 14:194–205

Kroin J (1992) Intrathecal drug administration. Present use and future trends. Clin Pharmacokinet 22:319–326

Lee M, Silverman SM, Hansen H, Patel VB, Manchikanti L (2011) A comprehensive review of opioid-induced hyperalgesia. Pain Physician 14(2):145–161. PMID: 21412369

Loram L, Grace P, Strand K et al (2012) Prior exposure to repeated morphine potentiates mechanical allodynia induced by peripheral inflammation and neuropathy. Brain Behav Immun 26:1256–1264

Malhotra T, Root J, Kesselbrenner J et al (2013) Intrathecally pain pump infusions for intractable cancer pain and algorithm for dosing without a neuraxial trial. Anesth Analg 116(6):1364–1370

Mathur S, Chu S, McCormick Z et al (2014) Long-term intrathecal baclofen: outcomes after more than 10 years of treatment. PMR 6:506–513

Medtronic product bulletin: summary of approved drugs Medtronic's synchromed II infusion system. Medtronic plc, Minneapolis, 2012

Mekhail BR (2014) Intrathecal pain pumps: indications, patient selection, techniques, and outcomes. Neurosurg Clin N Am 25(4):735–742

Moryl N, Coyle N, Essandoh S et al (2010) Chronic pain management in cancer survivors. J Natl Compr Cancer Netw 8(9):1104–1110

Pope J, Deer T (2015) Intrathecal drug delivery for pain: a clinical guide and future directions. Pain Manag 5:175–183

Portenoy R, Bennett D, Rauck R et al (2006) Prevalence and characteristics of breakthrough pain and opioid-treated patients with chronic non cancer pain. J Pain 7:583–591

Przybyl J, Follet A, Caraway D (2003) Intrathecal drug therapy: general considerations. Semin Pain Med 1(4):228–233

Rezai A, Kloth D, Hansen H et al (2013) Physician response to Medtronic's position on the use of off label medications in the SynchroMed pump. Pain Physician 16:415–417

Rivat C, Ballantyne J (2016) The dark side of opioids in pain management: basic science explains clinical observation. Pain Rep 1(e570):1–9

Roeckel L, Le Coz G, Gaveriaus-Ruff C et al (2016) Opioid induced hyperalgesia: cellular and molecular mechanisms. Neuroscience 338:160–182

Saulino M, Ivanhoe C, McGuire J et al (2016) Best practices for intrathecal baclofen therapy: patient selection. Neuromodulation 19:607–615

Saunders K, Dunn K, Merrill J et al (2010) Relationship of opioid use and dosage levels to fractures in older chronic pain patients. J Genet Int Med 25:310–315

Säwe J (1986) High-dose morphine and methadone in cancer patients. Clinical pharmacokinetic considerations of oral treatment. Clin Pharmacokinet 11(2):87–106

Schiess M, Eldabe S, Konrad P et al (2020) Intrathecal baclofen for severe spasticity: longitudinal data from the product surveillance registry. Neuromodulation 23:996–1002

Serrano B, Cuenca E, Higuera E et al (2014) Anticoagulation and interventional pain management. Tech Reg Anesth Pain Manag 18(1–2):58–64

Smith H (2020) Ethics, public health, and addressing the opioid crisis. AMA J Ethics 22(8):E647–E650

Smith T, Staats P, Deer T et al (2002) Randomized clinical trial of an implantable drug delivery system compared with comprehensive medical management for refractory cancer pain: impact on pain, drug related toxicity, and survival. J Clin Oncol 20(19):4040–4049

Stearns L, Boortz-Marx R, Du P et al (2005) Intrathecal drug delivery for the management of cancer pain: a multidisciplinary consensus of best clinical practices. J Support Oncol 3(6):399–408

Sylvester R, Lindsay S, Schauer C (2004) The conversion challenge: from intrathecal to oral morphine. Am J Hosp Palliat Care 21(2):143–147

van der Plas A, Marinus J, Eldabe S et al (2011) The lack of efficacy of different infusion rates of intrathecal baclofen in complex regional pain syndrome: a randomized double blind crossover study. Pain Med 12:459–465

Wallace M, Lotz N, Pope J (2015) Perspectives in intrathecal therapy: patient selection, referral, and communication strategies. In: Medscape education neurology and neurosurgery

Wang P, Huang B, Horng H et al (2018) Review article wound healing. J Chin Med Assoc 81(2):94–101

Pump Management: Intrathecal Baclofen Pumps

Lissa Hewan-Lowe and Corey W. Hunter

Contents

L. Hewan-Lowe (✉)
Department of Rehabilitation and Human
Performance, Icahn School of Medicine at Mount
Sinai Hospital, New York, NY, USA
e-mail: lissa.hewan-lowe@mssm.edu

C. W. Hunter
Ainsworth Institute of Pain Management,
New York, NY, USA
e-mail: chunter@ainpain.com

© The Author(s), under exclusive license to Springer Nature Switzerland AG 2022
D. P. Beall et al. (eds.), *Intrathecal Pump Drug Delivery*, Medical Radiology Diagnostic Imaging,
https://doi.org/10.1007/978-3-030-86244-2_8

Abstract

For more than three decades, intrathecal baclofen (ITB) has been used to manage severe spasticity related to cerebral palsy, multiple sclerosis, spinal cord injury, and stroke. Spasticity, defined as a velocity-dependent increase of resistance to passive muscle stretch, can be severe enough to cause debilitating pain and contractures significantly reducing quality of life. ITB should be considered for patients who fail oral medications or cannot tolerate the often sedating side effects. ITB therapy utilizes a catheter placed within the intrathecal space and delivers medication directly into the cerebral spinal fluid (CSF). This method requires a significantly lower dose of baclofen to be administered and bypasses the blood-brain barrier (BBB), avoiding many unwanted side effects of high-dose oral medications. Catheter tip placement is a crucial step in ITB therapy and determines the concentration center given CSF's limited ability to distribute baclofen due to flow and baricity. Before the initiation of ITB therapy, patient goals and spasticity severity should be assessed. Prior to pump placement, a trial is generally performed to evaluate patient response and estimate initial dosing. After pump placement, initial dosing and titration to a steady therapeutic state should be achieved with the fewest number of adjustments and may be done outpatient or expedited in an inpatient setting. This chapter will address and define the appropriate clinical use and placement of intrathecal pumps in the management of severe spasticity as well as explore short- and long-term management of baclofen pumps including dosing adjustments, adverse events, and discontinuation of care.

Abbreviations

ADL	Activities of daily living
BBB	Blood-brain barrier
CNS	Central nervous system
CP	Cerebral palsy
CSF	Cerebrospinal fluid
DRG	Dorsal root ganglion
FES	Functional electrical stimulation
GABA	Gamma aminobutyric acid
IT	Intrathecal
ITB	Intrathecal baclofen
LE's	Lower extremities
MAS	Modified Ashworth scale
MS	Multiple sclerosis
NMJ	Neuromuscular junction
PO	Per os
ROM	Range of motion
SCI	Spinal cord injury
TENS	Transcutaneous electrical nerve stimulation
TID	Three times daily

1   Introduction

Intrathecal baclofen (ITB) has been used over the last three decades to manage severe spasticity. It has superior efficacy over oral medication and allows for significantly lower doses of baclofen to be used due to the delivery into the intrathecal space where the medication can bypass the blood-brain barrier and directly inhibit neurotransmitter activity thereby resulting in muscle relaxation. Intrathecal baclofen should be considered for patients who fail oral medications or cannot tolerate the often sedating side effects. Before initiation of this therapy, considerations including patient goals and spasticity severity should be assessed. After pump placement, initial dosing and titration to a steady therapeutic state should be achieved with the fewest number of adjustments that accomplish the goals. These dose adjustments may be done as an outpatient, but, if necessary, the process can be expedited by titrating the dose of ITB in an inpatient setting. The following chapter will address and define

these topics and explore what is needed for outpatient follow-up and long-term management of baclofen pumps including dosing adjustments, warning signs and symptoms of underdosing or overdosing, and intrathecal drug delivery (IDD) system troubleshooting.

2   Defining Spasticity: *Velocity Dependent*

Spasticity is defined as velocity-dependent increased resistance to passive muscle stretch (Kim and Shin 2018; Lance 1980a). It can be focal or diffuse and is often characterized by hyperreflexia, clonus, flexor and extensor spasms, primitive reflexes, and dystonia. Spasticity manifests most commonly in spinal cord injury (SCI), stroke, multiple sclerosis (MS), traumatic brain injury (TBI), and cerebral palsy (CP) (Lapeyre et al. 2010). In spinal cord origin spasticity, the spasticity is due to the removal of supraspinal control that results in increased excitability of motor neurons and primitive spinal reflexes that cause exaggerated responses to all afferent input, effecting flexor more than extensor muscle groups. Brain stem control is not altered, and hyperexcitability is not as severe as seen with some other types of pathology. In cerebral origin spasticity, abnormal supraspinal reflexes from lost descending inhibition or from an uncontrolled facilitatory descending pathway cause the increased neural activity leading to contraction.

3   Assessing Spasticity: *Modified Ashworth Scale (MAS)*

Clinicians' tools for measuring spasticity have existed for many years with few updates (Hugos and Cameron 2019). The Tardieu, Ashworth, and Modified Ashworth Scale (MAS) practically assess resistance to passive movement (Lapeyre et al. 2010). These scales are limited by interrater reliability and inability to assess spasticity with intentional movement. Biomechanical assessment tools are better at movement assessment, but these tools lack practicality (Li and Francisco 2019). There are more specific measurement tools for assessing both *spinal cord origin spasticity* and *MS* spasticity, but the most commonly used scale for all forms of spasticity is the modified Ashworth Scale (Table 1) (Lapeyre et al. 2010; Hugos and Cameron 2019; Li and Francisco 2019; Benz et al. 2005).

4 Setting Goals: *Baseline Function, Management of Expectations, Patient-Centered Focus*

Guiding principles in spasticity management include prevention of soft tissue contractures and maintenance or improvement of function and independence and hygiene maintenance. If effective treatment is not rendered, excessive muscle tone can cause pain, stiffness, joint subluxations, and decreased range of motion (ROM) and can contribute to peripheral neuropathy, pressure sores, and deformity that may significantly impair quality of life. Patients may lose functional ability to perform self-care and activities of daily life (ADLs) (Lapeyre et al. 2010). Spasticity may even

Table 1 Modified Ashworth Scale

Modified Ashworth Scale	Degree of muscle tone
0	No increase in tone
1	Slight increase in muscle tone, manifested by a catch and release or by minimal resistance at the end of the range of motion when the affected part(s) is moved in flexion or extension
2	Slight increase in muscle tone, manifested by a catch, followed by minimal resistance throughout the remainder (less than half) of the range of movement (ROM)
3	More marked increase in muscle tone through most of the ROM, but affect part(s) easily moved
4	Considerable increase in muscle tone passive, movement difficult
5	Affected part(s) rigid in flexion or extension

lead to weakness and involuntary movement disorders. Reducing spasticity without proper strengthening or alignment, however, often provides little functional benefit (Chang et al. 2013a). Muscle tone from spasticity may assist some patients with ADLs such as in transfers and with ambulation (Tilton et al. 2010). This benefit of spasticity could be taken away if the degree of spasticity is decreased which underlines the importance of proper assessment and goal setting in order to make the right treatment goals for the patient.

When setting spasticity management goals, the underlying cause of spasticity often guides treatment. Goals should aim to treat the spastic muscle(s) that are causing problems for the patient. The goals also typically include short-term goals such as improving ambulation, optimizing the ease of rehabilitation therapy, and creating a situation for better patient hygiene as well as long-term goals such as preventing or limiting joint contractures. Decreasing spasticity can allow for more normal muscle movement that can save caregivers time and effort.

Important consideration should be given to the patient's medical history, functional history, care provider(s), therapist recommendations, and their support system. A particular importance should be placed on the patient's functional history. The patient and caregivers' priorities should be assessed in relation to the patient's initial baseline functional status. Practitioners should aim for patient-centered goal setting with agreement by caregivers and other providers. Patient expectations may be unrealistic in terms of goal setting as they may hope to return to normal function. Thus it is important to have a thorough goal setting conversation prior to initiating treatment.

The goals will vary in regards to patients' specific clinical situation. For example, goals for stroke patients focus primarily on motor recovery. In addition to motor recovery, aims also include decreasing painful spasms, facilitating hygiene, preventing contractures and pressure sores, improving the patient's positioning in bed, decreasing the burden on the caregiver, improving the patient's ADLs, and whatever possible to improve their independence (Francisco et al. 2006; Sangari et al. 2019).

5   Treatment Options for Spasticity

Typically spasticity management requires a comprehensive approach including rehabilitative techniques and pharmacological treatments (Thibaut et al. 2013; Bakheit 2012) tailored to individual needs based on factors that aggravate spasticity and with functional goals in mind. Treatment aims to decrease spasticity and associated pain, to prevent contracture, and to improve function and independence. Treatment options include rehabilitative therapies, medications, surgical, and oral neuromodulatory interventions.

Overall, a stepwise approach to spasticity control should initiate with the least invasive therapies starting with the removal of noxious stimuli, followed by physical therapy, oral medications, and then ending up with chemodenervation and ITB therapy. Typically, the therapies are used in a synergistic manner and may be used concurrently.

Rehabilitative therapy aims to increase mobility, prevent deformity, and maximize function and endurance. Both inpatient and outpatient therapies often include strengthening of weak muscles, maintaining joint alignment, and contracture prevention through stretching, casting, tendon pressure heat/cold, vibration, taping, massage, and, in stroke, the promotion of motor learning.

Medications for generalized spasticity are administered via oral or intrathecal routes. Oral medications are more expensive in the short term; however, they provide ease of use and may prove better for patients with generalized spasticity (Thibaut et al. 2013; Chang et al. 2013b). Central acting medications include baclofen, tizanidine, clonidine, benzodiazepines, and gabapentin (Fig. 1). Baclofen, a GABA analog, is first-line medication, and spasticity and secondary

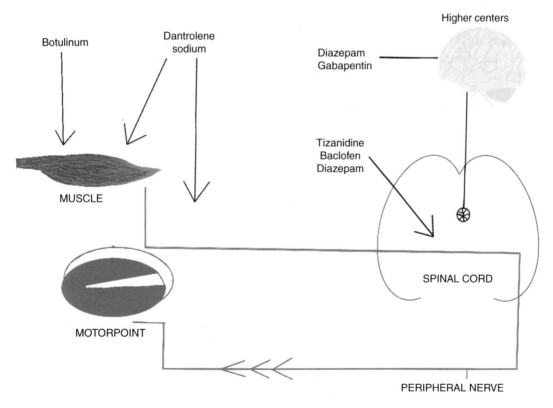

Fig. 1 Medications for spasticity and their locations of action (Adapted from: Lapeyre, Eric, Kuks, Jan B.M., and Meijler, Willem J. 'Spasticity: Revisiting the Role and the Individual Value of Several Pharmacological Treatments'. 2010: 193–200. (Lapeyre et al. 2010))

dystonia are its most common indications (Lance 1980b; Lake and Shah 2019). Clonidine and tizanidine are alpha-2 agonists and are typically used as adjunctive therapies. Both medications have hypotension as a side effect. Tizanidine can prolong the corrected QT interval (QTc). Benzodiazepines and gabapentin are both anticonvulsants with sedating effects. Benzodiazepines work at the GABA-A receptor, and diazepam in particular inhibits flexor more than extensors muscles coinciding with SCI pathology (Fig. 1). Gabapentin works on calcium channels inhibiting calcium current, mostly used for neuropathic-related pain (Chang et al. 2013b). The only peripheral acting medication is dantrolene, which works directly on muscles to uncouple excitation and contraction by inhibiting the release of calcium at the sarcoplasmic reticulum (Fig. 1) (Chang et al. 2013b).

Focal treatments avoid generalized weakness and have better tolerance and efficacy than oral medications. Focal spasticity is typically treated with chemodenervation with botulinum neurotoxin type A or Botox (Fig. 1) (Simpson et al. 2008; Esquenazi et al. 2013). Botox causes denervation via decrease in acetylcholine release at the neuromuscular junction. Botox is generally very effective, however temporary, and may not be adequate for controlling spasms over a long period of time or in patients with multifocal or severe spasticity.

Other therapies include Alcohol and Phenol, injected perineural, causing denervation, axonal degeneration, neurogenic atrophy, and local necrosis lasting months to years. Their side effects include chronic pain and paresthesias. This denervation is also painful as these are noxious substances and, as such, children and some pain-sensitive adults this have to be done under general anesthesia (Tilton et al. 2010; Chang et al. 2013b). Treatment of SCI-related spasticity with transcutaneous electrical nerve stimulation (TENS) and functional electrical stimulation (FES) has been shown to reduce spasticity (Sivaramakrishnan et al. 2018), and there is some evidence for the use of repetitive transcranial magnetic stimulation (Leszczyńska et al. 2020)

in patients with cervical and upper thoracic incomplete SCI, but no evidence exists that supports poststroke treatment of spasticity (Lake and Shah 2019; Fisicaro et al. 2019).

Spinal cord stimulation has been shown effective in managing spasticity from multiple origins (Simpson et al. 2008; Nagel et al. 2017). Neuroablation, neurectomy, and selective rhizotomy have also been shown to be effective for functional improvement (Lapeyre et al. 2010). However, rhizotomies are used more for pain syndromes rather than spasticity, and the removal of nerves can cause chronic pain syndromes (Chang et al. 2013b; Lin and Chay 2018). Surgical interventions for spasticity should only be considered in refractory cases where ITB therapy may be incompletely effective and if there is reasonable expectations for improvement of function, self-care, hygiene, or pain relief from contracture (Gart and Adkinson 2018).

6   Intrathecal Baclofen (ITB) Therapy: *Severe, Intractable, Problematic Spasticity*

Baclofen is a GABA analog that works at the GABA-B receptor to block the release of excitatory neurotransmitters and causes muscle relaxation. In order for oral baclofen to have this effect, large doses must be consumed creating a diffuse target and often unwanted and sedating side effects (Ethans 2007). Intrathecal baclofen bypasses the blood-brain barrier (BBB) by targeted delivery of liquid baclofen delivered directly into the cerebrospinal fluid (CSF) targeting spinal neurons (Fisicaro et al. 2019; Saulino 2018).

7   Indication to Initiate ITB: *Failed Oral Medication Management*

Oral medications, most commonly baclofen, are effective in treating mild or even moderate spasticity. However when treating severe spasticity, oral medications may produce suboptimal results or unacceptable side effects at therapeutic doses (Lance 1980b; Alexon 2005). Intrathecal baclofen (ITB) therapy is useful when oral baclofen is inadequate and is indicated for use in patients with severe, chronic spasticity of spinal or cerebral origin.

8 Contraindications to Baclofen and ITB

The absolute contraindications for ITB therapy include hypersensitivity to baclofen (rare), a patient body habitus that precludes pump implantation and the presence of an active and untreated infection (Saulino et al. 2016). The relative contraindications include poor health precluding general anesthesia and an inability to attend the necessary follow-up appointments (Lake and Shah 2019). Additionally, there are some psychosocial factors or mental health issues that preclude compliance including unrealistic patient goals or undue financial burdens (Saulino et al. 2016). Other items to consider prior to pump implantation or pump replacement surgery are whether the patient will be undergoing shunt surgery for hydrocephalus, whether they have abdominopelvic or spine surgery planned and whether or not they have a seizure disorder. All of these factors can affect the timing or technique of placing an intrathecal pump and catheter.

9 Efficacy

The effectiveness of ITB in controlling spasticity has been shown in controlled studies with cerebral palsy, multiple sclerosis, spinal cord injury, and stroke (Ertzgaard et al. 2017). In pharmacologic treatment, systemic medications should be initiated first, and the patient should "fail" systemic treatment before advancing to intrathecal baclofen. Intrathecal baclofen therapy can be used alone or in conjunction with other methods of managing spasticity described above.

10 Pharmacology and Drug Delivery

In ITB, a catheter is placed in the intrathecal space between the dura and arachnoid layers of the spinal cord where baclofen is then delivered directly into the CSF. This method of delivery provides alternative to oral medication as the intrathecal delivery bypasses the BBB. Intrathecal and plasma half-life are the same at 1–5 h. Baclofen is optimal for intrathecal delivery as it is slightly lipid soluble and remains in the CSF a moderate amount of time after administration (Hsieh and Penn 2006a). Baclofen is also slightly hydrophilic and generally will stay in the CSF after having been delivered there via the catheter (Heetla et al. 2014). This accounts for a lower baclofen dose necessary to produce the same effect compared to the medication given systemically (Meythaler et al. 2001a). The CSF administration is also associated with greater efficacy and, because of the lower dose, limited CNS side effects such as drowsiness, headaches, or sedation (Meythaler et al. 2001a). Intrathecal delivery directly to the neural axis allows for doses as low as 100–1000 times smaller than the comparable oral dose (Barnes and Johnson 2008).

10.1 Baricity

Baricity refers to the density of a substance in relation to CSF and helps to predict its behavior in the intrathecal space. Hyperbaric solutions will follow gravity, and hypobaric solutions rise against it. Baclofen on its own is hypobaric and tends to hold its position after infusion into CSF (Hejtmanek et al. 2011). Hyperbaric medication such as morphine or bupivacaine at higher concentrations will sink potentially away from the spinal cord. In the case of a posteriorly placed catheter, anytime a patient is supine, some hyperbaric medications have the potential to sink through arachnoid matter and into epidural space (Hejtmanek et al. 2011).

Baclofen has hypobaricity in relation to CSF allowing the medication to distribute against gravity in the CSF. As baclofen infuses into CSF, it binds directly to GABA-B receptors in the dorsal root ganglion (DRG) and spinal gray matter causing neuronal presynaptic inhibition and postsynaptic hyperpolarization, which inhibits neurotransmitter release thereby causing relaxation (Yang et al. 2001).

In the intrathecal space, there is a gradient in drug distribution between the cephalad and caudal portions of the spinal cord with a 4:1 concentration differential that is greater in the spinal and cauda equina region than it is in the brain (Kroin and Penn 1991). The concentration differential serves to decrease side effects and keeps the medicine near target (Kroin and Penn 1991). Pulsatile flow of CSF causes a concentration gradient after 48 h of continuous infusion of baclofen. This results in a mean lumbar to cisternal ratio of about 4:1 with a concentration decrease of about 0.9–1.5% per centimeter.

The CSF also has a "to-and-fro" oscillatory pattern along a rostrocaudal axis rather than the previously thought of circulatory pattern in a caudad-cephalad motion. These oscillatory cycles are primarily cardiac driven (Bernards 2006a; Flack and Bernards 2010). The CSF motion is limited as it is moved in opposite directions during cycles. The more caudad from the foramen magnum, the less movement is seen meaning drug delivery in a cervical region will have more movement than in the thoracic location (Heetla et al. 2014; Bernards 2006a; Flack and Bernards 2010).

11   Catheter Tip Placement

The location of the tip is critical given the limited capacity of CSF to distribute baclofen. As the dorsal horn is the target, posterior placement is key (Bernards 2006a). An intraventricular catheter tip placement may have a role in managing dystonia and spasticity although there are increased risks of CNS side effects. Care has to be taken in the case of CSF flow obstruction as regional toxic effects may be seen (Heetla et al. 2014). Animal studies show a gradient of baclofen during slow infusion so that most of the ITB

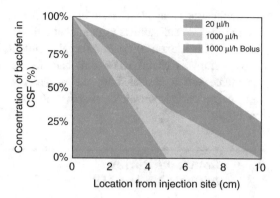

Fig. 2 The effects of baclofen flow rate and the distance from the injection site on the concentration of baclofen in the CSF (Adapted from: Heetla HW, Staal MJ, Proost JH, van Laar T. Clinical relevance of pharmacological and physiological data in intrathecal baclofen therapy. *Arch Phys Med Rehabil.* 2014;95(11):2199–2206. https://doi.org/10.1016/j.apmr.2014.04.030)

remains around the catheter tip (Fig. 2) (Heetla et al. 2014; Bernards 2006b). This implies that the position of the catheter tip is important in determining the clinical efficacy for the patient's specific condition. An example of this was shown by Grabb et al. when they determined that the placement of the tip of the intrathecal catheter at the T6–7 level was associated with greater relief of upper extremity spasticity than the same dosages administered at the T11–12 level without the loss of effect on the lower extremities (Grabb et al. 1999).

Considerations should be made for anatomical variants (i.e., postinfectious or postsurgical changes) or other causes that could effect flow and concentration gradient of baclofen within the CSF.

12   Cervical Vs Thoracic Placement

Location of catheter tip determines the concentration center. Theoretically, it should be placed near the lumbar enlargement (Th11-L1) for spasticity in the lower extremities and around the cervical enlargement (C3-Th2) for spasticity in the upper extremities (Heetla et al. 2014). In patients with both upper and lower spasticity, placement of the catheter tip closer to the lower extremities target with increased dose to cover upper extremities can cause hypotonia of the lower extremities. One solution is a double lumen catheter that would target both a cervical and thoracic site, but this catheter type currently does not yet exist.

Traditionally, catheters have been placed in lower thoracic level, but it has been shown that placement of the tip in the cervical region can effectively manage both upper and lower extremity spasticity. This disadvantage of a cervical placement is that it can potentially cause more central side effects. In one study, the technical aspects of tip placement were no different than thoracic placement, and adverse effects and overdose in rostral vs caudal placement were found to be similar (McCall and MacDonald 2006). Increasing the dose in a more caudally placed catheter to provide added coverage to upper extremities can decrease truncal rigidity needed for posture and increase frequency of pump refills. It has been also shown that placement of the catheter tip in cervical region around C5–7 provided a more equal distribution of spasticity reduction compared to a T6 placement which provides more coverage to lower extremities than the upper extremities (McCall and MacDonald 2006).

13   Optimal Timing

One study surmised that the timing of the pump placement may affect its efficacy (McCall and MacDonald 2006). In stroke, it is thought that early placement could improve the patients' discomfort and promote their rehabilitation goals if there is a concern that nonaggressive therapy will result in significant contracture. The additional of ITB must be balanced against possible or theoretical effects of slowed neurologic recovery poststroke (motor and cognitive). Overall, the timing of pump placement should be based on functional goals. The recommendation of placing the pump 3–6 months after a stroke is reasonable in the setting significant spasticity resulting in disability and pain/discomfort, especially if the patient has failed oral meds and/or chemodener-

vation/neurolytic therapies (Francisco et al. 2006). Additionally, ITB has been shown to have a favorable cost-effective analysis, especially when compared to other therapies (Tilton et al. 2010).

14   Adjunctive Therapies to ITB

Once ITB therapy is initiated, the patient may continue to be managed with adjunctive therapies as above. If the ITB is more effective for the lower extremities, focal spasticity management can still be attained with Botox for upper extremities. Once tone control is improved via ITB, the patient should be reassessed for new functional goals. These goals should again focus on improving the ROM, functional improvement, strengthening, and constraint induced movement therapy with treatments such as functional electrical stimulation, the treadmill, and applicable robotic therapies. Practitioners should coordinate their therapy goals with the beginning of a therapeutic ITB dose. Initial treatments such as limb elongation, serial casting and joint mobilization, core muscle strengthening, and muscle tone improvement will help the patient move toward functionally retraining their bodies after having benefitted from less muscular spasm. Experienced neurorehab therapists are important in attaining the patient's goals and for optimizing the therapy.

15   Oral Antispasmodics: Baclofen, Tizanidine, Diazepam

Baclofen has a half-life of 2–6 h. The usual oral dose of baclofen is 40–80 mg daily, not to exceed 80 mg daily (Ghanavatian and Derian 2020a). Patients are candidate for ITB when side effects of the oral medication become too difficult to manage or the baclofen is not sufficiently effective at the maximum recommended dosing.

Tizanidine has a half-life of 2.5 h. In treating spasticity, the medication should be taken three times daily with a maximum dose of 36 mg per day. Prolonged use at high doses will necessitate tapering of medication to reduce the risk of tachycardia and rebound hypertension (Ghanavatian and Derian 2020b). The tizanidine can be reduced by 2–4 mg daily prior to performing a baclofen trial to reduce the likelihood of cardiac effects due to the decrease in daily medication dose.

Diazepam is sometimes used as an adjective therapy, dosed between 2 and 10 mg, three to four times daily. It has a half-life of 46 hours and numerous potential side effects (Montané et al. 2004). Diazepam also creates physical dependence and should also be tapered prior to an ITB trial if the patient is taking higher doses (Joseph and Hack 2020).

15.1 Conversion from Oral to IT Baclofen

There is no direct conversion between oral and ITB as ITB is delivered to the spinal cord with greater efficacy at a dose approximately 100 times smaller than that of the oral route (Lim and Cunningham 2012; Ross et al. 2011; Boster et al. 2016a). Oral baclofen has a slower onset of action and peak time to effect than does ITB with oral baclofen not reaching peak efficacy for days as compared to hours for ITB (Boster et al. 2016a).

15.2 Prior to Trial

Currently, there are no specific guidelines to the management of a patient's oral antispasmodics prior to an intrathecal baclofen trial. The ITB Therapy Best Practices Expert Consensus Panel recommends giving thought to weaning patients prior to a trial but states that this should be tailored to each patient individually. Patients may be on more than one oral antispasmodic, in addition to oral baclofen. They do not comment on the order of which medications should be weaned first. They do however remark that careful consideration should be given to side effects and the dangers of withdrawal. The potential withdrawal symptoms should be factored into how far in advance baclofen should be weaned. Some

patients may be able to hold oral antispasmodics on the morning of the trial, but others may require a gradual weaning. After the trial is complete, the patients may gradually restart oral medications as their spasticity returns. Some patients, if necessary, may return to baseline medication doses the same day as the trial. Additionally, an ITB trial should be timed not to coincide with any injections for spasticity that may make the results of the trial difficult to interpret (Boster et al. 2016b).

The patient is ready for a trial when they can no longer tolerate oral medication side effects or the dose of oral medications necessary to provide adequate relief of spasm. In general, we recommend holding the morning dose of oral antispasmodics prior to an ITB trial. If the procedure is scheduled for the end of the day, however, the patient should be permitted to take the morning dose, and the mid-day dose may be held instead. Given that diazepam has a longer half-life, it can be tapered days before the ITB trial as the patient's condition allows. In general, the goal prior to the trial should be to taper the oral antispasm medications as much as possible while still allowing enough medication to mitigate unacceptable side effects such as moderate to severe painful spasms or withdrawal (Boster et al. 2016a; Connors and Hamilton 2020).

15.3 Approach to Baclofen Trials

An ITB trial prior to pump placement should appropriately identify candidates in regards to patients who respond favorably to the trial. The trial is also a useful basis upon which to discuss the patient's goals and to initiate an optimal starting dose. Prior to all trials, a baseline modified Ashworth score (MAS) measuring spasticity should be established. Trialing may be performed by giving a single bolus dose or by infusing continuous medication. Typically, a lumbar puncture is performed with a 25-gauge needle, a small amount of nonionic contrast is given to confirm the intrathecal location of the needle tip, and a bolus of 50 mcg of medication is given intrathecally (Boster et al. 2016b). In very small children and patients that utilize their spasticity for mobility, trial dosing may be reduced to 25 mcg (Boster et al. 2016b). Alternatively, some patients that have more severe spasticity or who do not have the ability to walk may require a larger dose of 75–100 mcg. Bolus dosing has an effect that begins within about 1 h and the maximum effect at approximately 3–4 h with trials last between 4 and 8 h (Pucks-Faes et al. 2019; Slonimski et al. 2004). Additional doses can be given, but the typical treatment approach is to allow 24 h to pass between bolus doses. During the beginning of an ITB trial, cardiopulmonary function should be closely monitored while observing the patient for loss of muscle tone, and the observation and intermittent physical examinations end when the patient's spasticity returns (Boster et al. 2016b). Bolus trials tend to have less of an effect on upper extremity spasticity, and if this is the primary clinical concern, a trial with placement of a catheter with the catheter tip in the cervical spine may be more optimal to test for upper extremity response to the ITB (Pucks-Faes et al. 2019). During the ITB trial, the practitioner should watch for adverse events such as headaches, nausea, vomiting, urinary retention, hypotension, seizures, sedation, respiratory depression, and even coma (Boster et al. 2016b).

If a patient fails single bolus trialing, or a more thorough assessment is required, a continuous approach can be used via an intrathecal catheter, or repeated bolus doses may be performed at a minimal interval of 24 h. Continuous trials are an off-label approach to trialing and are done at the treating physician's discretion almost always in an inpatient setting. A temporary subarachnoid catheter is placed in the desired area (Pucks-Faes et al. 2019) and connected to a programmable external pump. Continuous trials allow for patient observation for longer periods of time to better assess functional impact. One center has reported a protocol that adjusts dosing by 25 mcg increments based on twice daily assessments by a physical therapist until the desired effects are reached, making the first adjustment 24 h after placement (Vats et al. 2019). Additionally, continuous trials have the advantage of better mimicking the therapeutic effects of a permanent pump implant and may produce more reliable functional results.

15.4 Prior to Implantation

If the implantation is planned for a later date after the trial, we recommended continuing oral antispasmodics through the implantation date including the patient's morning dose. This helps to address and decrease uncontrolled spasticity that could interfere with the implantation procedure.

15.5 Oral Medications After Implantation

Once the pump is in place, intrathecal baclofen infusion may begin immediately at the effective continuous does that was found effective at the trial or at twice the effective trial bolus dose. At this point, oral medications may be weaned in stepwise fashion, one at a time, starting with baclofen (Boster et al. 2016c).

15.6 Compounding Baclofen with Other Agents

Intrathecal baclofen has been shown to have efficacy in treating pain syndromes both acute and chronic. It has additionally been shown to be effective in treating chronic pain in patients who have built tolerance to IT morphine (Hsieh and Penn 2006b; Meythaler et al. 2001b). This includes patients without motor dysfunction and is effective in both spastic and non-spastic pain (Hsieh and Penn 2006b; Meythaler et al. 2001b). In animal studies, it has been found to be antinociceptive and effective in treating sympathetic and supraspinal mediated pain and pain from muscle spasms. It may also have effects against neuropathic pain and centrally mediated pain in patients with stroke or MS (Slonimski et al. 2004; Meythaler et al. 2001b).

Adding clonidine to baclofen has been shown to decrease spasticity. Combining baclofen and clonidine is also effective in treating pain

(Slonimski et al. 2004). In the setting of severe pain related to spasticity, IT baclofen can be compounded with morphine or combined with morphine and clonidine to provide pain sustainable pain relief (Gatscher et al. 2002). Morphine combined with baclofen is stable for at least 30 days in the pump (Meythaler et al. 2001b). Baclofen, however, is not recommended as a first-line agent in treating pain due to higher cost (Meythaler et al. 2001b). In animal studies, coadministration of ineffective doses of both morphine and baclofen demonstrates increased analgesia (Slonimski et al. 2004), and authors recommend starting IT baclofen on patients who already have IT devices and either cannot tolerate the opioid side effects or who have had waning pain relief over time presumed to be related to the tolerance of the IT opioid (Hsieh and Penn 2006b). If pain is present at time of baclofen trial, one can consider adding single bolus dose of morphine to the trial.

16   ITB Pump Management

Previously pumps came in two types, mechanical and programmable. Mechanical pumps were gas driven and had a preset flow rate but now are no longer produced. Programmable pumps are battery operated with batteries that can last from 7 to 10 years (https://www.medtronic.com/us-en/patients/treatments-therapies/drug-pump-severe-spasticity/living-with-itb-therapy/pump-management.html n.d.). For practical application purposes, only programmable pumps will be discussed in this chapter. The pump is surgically attached to the anterior abdominal wall after having constructed a pocket in either the right or left lower quadrant. This position is optimal for patient comfort and makes it accessible for periodic refills of the pump's reservoir.

17   Dosing Options

In general, there are three recognized modes for infusion: *continuous*, *flex mode*, and *bolus*. Continuous dosing is liquid medication infused at a constant speed. It is typically the initial mode that is started after placement of the patients pump, and the steady state of that dose is reached at the conventional time as determined by the medication (baclofen reaches a steady state in 24 hours which is approximately five half-lives of the medication). The patient's evaluation for appropriate dosing and for considering a dose change is done after a steady state is reached.

Flex mode is continuous with differing dosage rates during the course of the day with periods of higher and lower dosing depending on the severity of the patient's spasticity. It is best used in patients with a predictable pattern of spasticity who have increased need for spasticity that aids in certain activities such as transfers or standing but who need relief of their spasticity to be able to rest or sleep at night. In patients with an increased need for evening or nighttime dose, practitioners may increase the dose before bed, not to exceed 10–15% of the baseline dose (Boster et al. 2016d). Flex dosing cannot be used effectively to lower daily dose in baclofen-tolerant patients, and that any increased dose takes several hours to arrive at a new steady state. Patients should be warned that time changes (i.e., travel to new time zones or daylight savings) may affect dosing.

Bolus dosing involves taking the daily dose and dividing it into a certain number of doses that will be given over a shorter period of time repeated over a 24-h period. Of note, in one type of pump (SynchroMed II pump, Medtronic Inc., Dublin, Ireland), there is always a low basal rate flowing between the bolus doses as the pump cannot be stopped completely, but in the other commonly used pump (Prometra Pump, Flowonix, Mt. Olive, NJ, USA), there is no baseline dose between administration of the bolus doses. Patients may receive better distribution with bolus dosing as compared to that of continuous mode dosing (Heetla et al. 2014) as there is some element of forward propulsion and mixing of the medication liquid with the CSF when bolusing (Bernards 2006a; Flack and Bernards 2010). In one study examining bolus dosing, the bolus group had evidence of fewer differences in average peak concentration, and a more uniform distribution in the bolus group as compared to the infusion group (Bernards 2006a; Flack and Bernards 2010).

Maximal clinical effect is seen with bolus dosing at 4–6 h which lasts 6–8 h as compared to a slow infusion which maximizes the effect at 6–8 h and lasts 12–24 h (Heetla et al. 2014). In another study of ITB therapy for stroke patients, no difference was found between continuous and bolus dosing (Francisco et al. 2006).

Overall, there is a time delay between increased or decreased dosing and the pharmacologic effect and that time delay is typically 2 h in most patients, although a certain degree of patient variability exists.

18   Initial Dosing: *Commonly Available Dosing Concentrations*: 500, 1000, and 2000 mcg/mL. Starting Concentration Is Typically 500 mcg/mL

Initial dosing adjustments require multiple adjustments done over the course of a few days to weeks so it is recommended that the pump be filled and the dosing start during time of surgery, with patient monitored for at least 8 h following pump implantation. A "back table prime" or pre-implant priming bolus can be done prior to implantation or a post procedure priming bolus can be done all the way to the tip of the measured catheter. Typically, the starting dose is initiated at the initial dose of choice using a 500 mcg/mL concentration of baclofen. That dose is recommended to be twice the effective bolus dose during the trial unless there was a prolonged response or negative reaction to the medication, then the starting dose is same or even less than the trial dose at the discretion of the managing physician taking into account the type of negative reaction the degree of prolonged response (https://www.medtronic.com/us-en/patients/treatments-therapies/drug-pump-severe-spasticity/living-with-itb-therapy/pump-management.html n.d.).

If the patient is on oral antispasmodics, a tapering of these medications should be started beginning with oral baclofen, and the oral doses should be decreased or eliminated as the ITB dosing is increased. Oral baclofen, however, should remain available to patients in case of ITB delivery system failure and the subsequent appearance of withdrawal symptoms (Boster et al. 2016d).

19   Dose Adjustments

Dosing may be effected by etiology of the initial injury and the chronicity of the patients' condition (McCall and MacDonald 2006). Overdose is usually caused by programing/refill errors but can also be seen apart from egregious dosing miscalculations. Overdose is slightly more common in patients with catheters placed in a more rostral vs caudal placement and may also be seen more commonly in patients undergoing concomitant oral and IT baclofen dosing (McCall and MacDonald 2006). Signs of overdose include areflexia, flaccidity, respiratory depression, severe sedation, coma, or even death.

20   Dose Increases

According to at least one manufacturer of ITB, for spasticity of spinal origin, it is recommended to increase the daily dose by 10–30% every 24 h and continue this to titrate to effect. In cerebral origin spasticity and in pediatric spasticity, the daily dose should be increased by 5–15% every 24 h (https://www.medtronic.com/us-en/patients/treatments-therapies/drug-pump-severe-spasticity/living-with-itb-therapy/pump-management.html n.d.). Patients on a lower dose should receive adjustments toward the higher range of the dosing increase, and patients on higher doses should receive adjustments toward the lower limit of the percentage dose adjustment range.

Inpatient vs *outpatient*: The initial dose adjustments may take place in an inpatient environment when necessary to allow for rapid daily titration under close monitoring. This is indicated when expeditious treatment is necessary and can be beneficial for patients who cannot communicate accurately. Outpatient dosing adjustment is appropriate if patients can reliably return to clinic without undue difficulty, and they may return as frequently as every 24 h to quickly up-titrate dose (Boster et al. 2016d).

21   Arriving at Therapeutic State

The optimal therapeutic state is dependent on goals and may be related to the patient's diagnosis. Typically, the dose is adequately therapeutic when additional increases do not give more benefit or start to produce undesirable side effects. The initial portion of the titration is complete when the patient is weaned off of oral antispasmodics and the optimal dose is reached. In some cases, there may be a need to continue oral medications for unpredictable or intermittent spasticity or in patients who experience episodic painful nocturnal spasms and pain (Boster et al. 2016d).

22   Tolerance

Baclofen causes both physical dependence and tolerance. Tolerance to ITB can range from 3 to 20%. If tolerance to ITB develops to the point where it impedes optimal treatment, an inpatient drug holiday may be considered. This drug holiday involves an in-patient stay during which morphine is used to replace the baclofen. This technique can be used to reset the tolerance to baclofen and has been reported as effective in some cases.

23   Complications of the ITB
         Delivery System

Before placing an intrathecal pump and even before the ITB trial, there should be a discussion of the risks of pump placement and ITB therapy. The safety profile of the SynchroMed II pump has been documented in a yearlong study where the adverse events (AEs) were reported and identified as either device related or not device related

(Wesemann et al. 2014). Device-related AEs were all those related to the pump, pump refills, the catheter, or the surgery itself. Adverse events not related to the device included those related to the patients underlying health condition, medications, or the intrathecal medication. Serious AEs in this study primarily included events that resulted in hospitalization, life-threatening situations, permanent damage to the body, persistent disability, the need for surgical intervention, and patient death.

The investigators found the pumps were measured to have delivered within 1–2.5% of the programmed delivery volume. Additionally, there were no permanent injuries, unanticipated adverse device effects, or patient deaths. Adverse events were similar in character and severity to those described previously (Hayek et al. 2011; Atli et al. 2010; Flückiger et al. 2008). In this study, complications requiring surgical intervention were experienced by 14% of subjects, but the remainder of the system-related AEs resolved following medical intervention. Most of the AEs were due to implant site swelling or a spinal headache due to CSF leak, and most of the AEs relative to the device were catheter complications such as catheter kinking or rupture. Since the time of that manuscript, the pump manufacturer has introduced a new catheter designed to prevent the previously noted catheter complications.

In general, risks of ITB and intrathecal drug delivery include failure of the pump, loss of catheter integrity, and infection of the pump or the catheter. The rate of pump failure and catheter-related issues is not insubstantial, but the most common complications are related to surgical site infection. The medication treatment-related safety issues are primarily due to inadequate patient monitoring for conditions like respiratory depression and issues associated with the IT drug delivery such as an inflammatory granulomatous mass surrounding the catheter tip. Clinicians must also realize that sudden cessation of ITB can be life threatening. During the preimplant conversation with the patient, these known risks must be taken into consideration before proceeding to intrathecal pump implantation.

24   Outpatient Follow-Up for Pump Refill

Pump Refills: Once optimal dose is reached, the concentration should be increased to prolong time between refill appointments as much as possible with the target being 6 months between pump refills. It is recommended to that the optimal time to increase the concentration of the medication is at the time of the patient's next refill so the medication with the increased concentration is ordered prior to the patient's next pump refill. When increasing the concentration of the medication, a bridge bolus must be used. A bridge bolus pumps the old medication with the old rate and starts the new medication, with a different concentration, at the new rate. It should be noted that with an increased concentration, there is a decreased flow rate. As mentioned previously, a lower flow rate translates to lesser movement of baclofen in the intrathecal space which can mean less medication effect. Practitioners and patients are advised to watch for worsening spasticity when the concentration of the medication is increased. If this occurs, then the dosage of the ITB may be increased.

Technical difficulties in accessing the pump can be addressed by using the template that is designed to be placed over the pump as a guide to the central port where the pump reservoir may be accessed. In larger patients with an increased body mass index, they may be repositioned into a pump side up position or ultrasound may be used to identify the central port that is easily seen using this imaging modality. The operative report should include the direction of the pump's apex which can make accessing the catheter port easier given its location within the center of the pump apex.

25   Optimal Time to Schedule Refill Appointments

Pump refills typically occur every 3–6 months depending on the concentration of medication and its delivery rate (https://www.medtronic. com/us-en/patients/treatments-therapies/drug- pump-severe-spasticity/living-with-itb-therapy/ pump-management.html n.d.). It is recommended to reinforce importance of refill appointments in writing and communicate to the patients that noncompliance with their pump refill appoints can be dangerous as it can lead to symptoms of baclofen withdrawal and that if the patient is noncompliant, this will result in discontinuation of therapy. In patients who chronically miss appointments, the low-reservoir alarm can be reset from 2 to 3 mL which will audibly alert the patient that their pump needs to be refiled at a residual volume one-third more than the typical alarm volume. The scheduled refill appointments for these patients are optimally placed at 1 week before the low-reservoir alarm date (Boster et al. 2016d). Low-reservoir alarm dates should be charted and written down for both patients and caregivers.

26   Ongoing Management

Intrathecal baclofen has been shown to be effective for the long-term management of spasticity of various origins.

27   Maintenance: Use the Lowest Dose Possible

The goal of ITB is to maintain muscle tone and minimize the frequency and severity of muscle spasms while minimizing the side effects of the medication. Dosing should be titrated to optimize muscle function, while patients adjust to their new functional capabilities and reduced spasticity. Dosing decreases of 10–20% are typically employed to reduce side effects. Sudden changes in patient's symptomatology typically indicate a catheter malfunction (i.e., catheter kink, rupture, disconnection, or granuloma). Depending on the type of pump, it will need to be replaced about every 7–10 years, and the patient should be scheduled for replacement 3–4 months prior to their elective replacement indicator (ERI) alarm to avoid having an unexpected delay that cause a sudden cessation in pump function and drug delivery.

28   General Dosing Rules of Thumb

Spasticity of Spinal Cord Origin: Do not increase the daily dose more than 40% during the periodic pump refills. An average daily dose typically ranges from 300 to 800 mcg/day.

Spasticity of Cerebral Origin: Do not increase daily dose more than 20% during the periodic pump refills. An average daily dose typically ranges from 90 to 703 mcg/day.

Pediatric patients under 12 may require a lower trial dose than the typical 50 mcg ITB dose. The average daily dose in pediatric patients varies widely and can range from 24 to 1199 mcg/day. In patients on chronic ITB, tolerance can develop, and about 5% of patients may become refractory to increasing doses (https://www.medtronic.com/us-en/patients/treatments-therapies/drug-pump-severe-spasticity/living-with-itb-therapy/pump-management.html n.d.).

29   How to Provide Ongoing Monitoring: *Assess for New Adverse Effects*

Considerations for making dose adjustments depend on the patient's ambulatory status, the physician's clinical assessment, and the patient's progress related to the previously determined therapy goals. At each visit, a subjective assessment for changes in spasticity, function, and ease of ADLs should be performed along with an assessment for the presence of adverse side effects including nausea, hypotonia, weakness, sedation, headaches, dizziness, and bowel or bladder dysfunction). Objective assessments should also be performed including assessing the patient's spasticity according to the MAS and performing manual muscle testing, ROM, and functional assessments.

In all new patients, a discussion for the impending treatment should include a review of the goals for ITB therapy and making the patient aware of the practice's standards for scheduling appointments, whom to contact, signs of over- or underdose, importance of adhering to the refill schedule, and when therapy would need to be discontinued due to noncompliance of the patient. At each appointment, the practice should provide each patient with documentation of their daily dose, their dosing schedule (if applicable), the low-reservoir alarm date, and, if they are on a flex schedule, the times of their daily dose changes (Boster et al. 2016d).

30   Discontinuing Care

As mentioned previously, abrupt cessation of baclofen can cause serious side effects and even death, and so in the case of discontinuing baclofen given by either the oral or IT route, it should be slowly titrated down. Mild acute withdrawal side effects can be managed with oral medications including benzodiazepines, but in the case of a severe withdrawal symptoms, other medications may need to be employed such as cyproheptadine, propofol, dantrolene, or intravenous benzodiazepines (Ertzgaard et al. 2017).

In the situations of a baclofen pump infection, it has been shown that continuation of ITB therapy using an external pump has been shown to be an effective bridge that will allow a downward titration to a dose that can be effectively replaced with oral baclofen (Hwang et al. 2019).

31   Conclusion

Intrathecal baclofen has been increasingly used over 30 years to manage severe spasticity and is a superior option over oral medications as it allows for significantly lower doses of baclofen to be used. This chapter has presented information and discussion related to appropriate use of ITB therapy in patients with severe spasticity. In it, we define spasticity, treatment options, and how to assess for an appropriate candidate for intrathecal baclofen delivery, and we further discuss the contraindications to baclofen and ITB therapy. An important concept in intrathecal delivery, baricity, is introduced along with its relationship to baclofen and catheter tip placement. Prior to placement, a trial is recommended, which we discuss along with medication management prior to implantation. After pump placement, initial dosing and steady-state titration should be achieved with fewest number of dose adjustments and largely take place outpatient. The chapter goes on to discuss ITB pump management including dose adjustments and how to account for tolerance. Patients will require long-term monitoring and scheduled refill appointments which we discuss including complications with ITB therapy and outpatient management and ongoing monitoring and when to discontinue care. The hope is this chapter will benefit patients who are candidates for ITB by contributing to the appropriate identification, treatment, and management of these patients.

Acknowledgments Figure 1 was made by with the help of Anna Di Franco, and Figure 2 was made with the help of Viola Di Franco.

References

Alexon WH (2005) Signs of muscle thixotropy during human ballistic wrist joint movements. J Appl Physiol 99:1922–1929

Atli A, Theodore BR, Turk DC, Loeser JD (2010) Intrathecal opioid therapy for chronic nonmalignant pain: a retrospective cohort study with 3-year follow-up. Pain Med 11:1010–1016

Bakheit AM (2012) The pharmacological management of post-stroke muscle spasticity. Drugs Aging 29:941–947

Barnes MP, Johnson GR (2008) Upper motor neurone syndrome and spasticity: clinical management and neurophysiology. Cambridge University Press, Cambridge

Benz EN, Hornby TG, Bode RK, Scheidt RA, Schmit BD (2005) A physiologically based clinical measure for spastic reflexes in spinal cord injury. Arch Phys Med Rehabil 86(1):52–59. https://doi.org/10.1016/j.apmr.2004.01.033

Bernards CM (2006a) Cerebrospinal fluid and spinal cord distribution of baclofen and bupivacaine during slow intrathecal infusion in pigs. Anesthesiology 105(1):169–178. https://doi.org/10.1097/00000542-200607000-00027

Bernards CM (2006b) Cerebrospinal fluid and spinal cord distribution of baclofen and bupivacaine during slow intrathecal infusion in pigs. Anesthesiology 105:169–178

Boster AL, Bennett SE, Bilsky GS et al (2016a) Best practices for intrathecal baclofen therapy: screening

test. Neuromodulation 19(6):616–622. https://doi.org/10.1111/ner.12437

Boster AL, Bennett SE, Bilsky GS et al (2016b) Best practices for intrathecal baclofen therapy: screening test. Neuromodulation 19(6):616–622. https://doi.org/10.1111/ner.12437

Boster AL, Adair RL, Gooch JL et al (2016c) Best practices for intrathecal baclofen therapy: dosing and long-term management. Neuromodulation 19(6):623–631. https://doi.org/10.1111/ner.12388

Boster AL, Adair RL, Gooch JL et al (2016d) Best practices for intrathecal baclofen therapy: dosing and long-term management. Neuromodulation 19(6):623–631. https://doi.org/10.1111/ner.12388

Chang E, Ghosh N, Yanni D, Lee S, Alexandru D, Mozaffar T (2013a) A review of spasticity treatments: pharmacological and interventional approaches. Crit Rev Phys Rehabil Med 25(1–2):11–22. https://doi.org/10.1615/CritRevPhysRehabilMed.2013007945

Chang E, Ghosh N, Yanni D, Lee S, Alexandru D, Mozaffar T (2013b) A review of spasticity treatments: pharmacological and interventional approaches. Crit Rev Phys Rehabil Med 25(1–2):11–22. https://doi.org/10.1615/CritRevPhysRehabilMed.2013007945. PMID: 25750484; PMCID: PMC4349402

Connors NJ, Hamilton RJ (2020) Withdrawal principles. In: Nelson LS, Howland M, Lewin NA, Smith SW, Goldfrank LR, Hoffman RS, eds. Goldfrank's toxicologic emergencies, 11th edn. McGraw-Hill. https://accessemergencymedicine-mhmedical-com.eresources.mssm.edu/content.aspx?bookid=2569&sectionid=210259091. Accessed 16 Aug 2020

Ertzgaard P, Campo C, Calabrese A (2017) Efficacy and safety of oral baclofen in the management of spasticity: a rationale for intrathecal baclofen. J Rehabil Med 49(3):193–203. https://doi.org/10.2340/16501977-2211

Esquenazi A, Albanese A, Chancellor MB et al (2013) Evidence-based review and assessment of botulinum neurotoxin for the treatment of adult spasticity in the upper motor neuron syndrome. Toxicon 67:115–128

Ethans K. (2007) Intrathecal baclofen therapy: indications, pharmacology, surgical implant, and efficacy. In: Sakas D.E., Simpson B.A., Krames E.S. (eds) Operative neuromodulation. Acta Neurochirurgica Supplements, vol 97/1. Springer, Vienna

Fisicaro F, Lanza G, Grasso AA et al (2019) Repetitive transcranial magnetic stimulation in stroke rehabilitation: review of the current evidence and pitfalls. Ther Adv Neurol Disord 12:1756286419878317. Published 2019 Sep 25. https://doi.org/10.1177/1756286419878317

Flack SH, Bernards CM (2010) Cerebrospinal fluid and spinal cord distribution of hyperbaric bupivacaine and baclofen during slow intrathecal infusion in pigs. Anesthesiology 112(1):165–173. https://doi.org/10.1097/ALN.0b013e3181c38da5

Flückiger B, Knecht H, Grossmann S, Felleiter P (2008) Device-related complications of long-term intrathecal drug therapy via implanted pumps. Spinal Cord 46:639–643

Francisco GE, Yablon SA, Schiess MC, Wiggs L, Cavalier S, Grissom S (2006) Consensus panel guidelines for the use of intrathecal baclofen therapy in poststroke spastic hypertonia. Top Stroke Rehabil 13(4):74–85. https://doi.org/10.1310/tsr1304-74

Gart MS, Adkinson JM (2018) Considerations in the management of upper extremity spasticity. Hand Clin 34(4):465–471. https://doi.org/10.1016/j.hcl.2018.06.004

Gatscher S, Becker R, Uhle E, Bertalanffy H (2002) Combined intrathecal baclofen and morphine infusion for the treatment of spasticity related pain and central. Acta Neurochir Suppl 79:75–76

Ghanavatian S, Derian A (2020a) Baclofen. [Updated 2020 Apr 20]. In: StatPearls [Internet]. StatPearls Publishing, Treasure Island. https://www.ncbi.nlm.nih.gov/books/NBK526037/

Ghanavatian S, Derian A (2020b) Tizanidine. [Updated 2020 Apr 21]. In: StatPearls [Internet]. StatPearls Publishing, Treasure Island. https://www.ncbi.nlm.nih.gov/books/NBK519505/DhaliwalJS, Rosani A, Saadabadi A. Diazepam. [Updated 2020 May 18]. In: StatPearls [Internet]. Treasure Island (FL): StatPearls Publishing; 2020. https://www.ncbi.nlm.nih.gov/books/NBK537022/

Grabb PA, Guin-Renfroe S, Meythaler JM (1999) Midthoracic catheter tip placement for intrathecal baclofen administration in children with quadriparetic spasticity. Neurosurgery 45:833–837

Hayek SM, Deer TR, Pope JE, Panchal SJ, Patel V (2011) Intrathecal therapy for cancer and non-cancer pain. Pain Physician 14:219–248

Heetla HW, Staal MJ, Proost JH, van Laar T (2014) Clinical relevance of pharmacological and physiological data in intrathecal baclofen therapy. Arch Phys Med Rehabil 95(11):2199–2206. https://doi.org/10.1016/j.apmr.2014.04.030

Hejtmanek MR, Harvey TD, Bernards CM (2011) Measured density and calculated baricity of custom-compounded drugs for chronic intrathecal infusion. Reg Anesth Pain Med 36(1):7–11. https://doi.org/10.1097/AAP.0b013e3181fe7f29

Hsieh JC, Penn RD (2006a) Intrathecal baclofen in the treatment of adult spasticity. Neurosurg Focus 21:e5

Hsieh JC, Penn RD (2006b) Intrathecal baclofen in the treatment of adult spasticity. Neurosurg Focus 21:e5

https://www.medtronic.com/us-en/patients/treatments-therapies/drug-pump-severe-spasticity/living-with-itb-therapy/pump-management.html

Hugos CL, Cameron MH (2019) Assessment and measurement of spasticity in MS: state of the evidence. Curr Neurol Neurosci Rep 19(10):79. Published 2019 Aug 30. https://doi.org/10.1007/s11910-019-0991-2

Hwang RS, Sukul V, Collison C, Prusik J, Pilitsis JG (2019) A novel approach to avoid baclofen withdrawal when faced with infected baclofen pumps. Neuromodulation 22(7):834–838. https://doi.org/10.1111/ner.12873

Joseph S, Hack J (2020) Baclofen. Excerpts from the toxic matter newsletter. Division of Medical Toxicology, Brown University. https://www.acep.org/how-we-serve/sections/toxicology/news/september-2015/baclofen/. Accessed 16 Aug 2020

Kim H, Shin MR (2018) Special considerations in pediatric assessment. Phys Med Rehabil Clin N Am 29(3):455–471. https://doi.org/10.1016/j.pmr.2018.03.002

Kroin JS, Penn RD (1991) Cerebrospinal fluid pharmacokinetics of lumbar intrathecal baclofen. In: Lakke JPWF, Delhaas EM, Rutgers AWF (eds) Parenteral drug therapy in spasticity and Parkinson's disease. Parthenon Publishing, Camforth, pp 67–77

Lake W, Shah H (2019) Intrathecal baclofen infusion for the treatment of movement disorders. Neurosurg Clin N Am 30(2):203–209. https://doi.org/10.1016/j.nec.2018.12.002

Lance JW (1980a) The control of muscle tone, reflexes, and movement. Robert Wartenbeg Lecture Neurol 30(12):1303. https://doi.org/10.1212/WNL.30.12.1303

Lance JW (1980b) Symposium synopsis. In: Feldman RG, Young RR, Koella WP (eds) Spasticity: disordered motor control. Year Book Medical Publishers, Chicago, pp 485–494

Lapeyre E, Kuks JBM, Meijler WJ (2010) Spasticity: revisiting the role and the individual value of several pharmacological treatments. NeuroRehabilitation 27(2):193–200

Leszczyńska K, Wincek A, Fortuna W et al (2020) Treatment of patients with cervical and upper thoracic incomplete spinal cord injury using repetitive transcranial magnetic stimulation. Int J Artif Organs 43(5):323–331. https://doi.org/10.1177/0391398819887754

Li S, Francisco GE (2019) Spasticity. Handb Exp Pharmacol. https://doi.org/10.1007/164_2019_315

Lim CA, Cunningham SJ (2012) Baclofen withdrawal presenting as irritability in a developmentally delayed child. West J Emerg Med 13(4):373–375. https://doi.org/10.5811/westjem.2011.2.11460

Lin J, Chay W (2018) Special considerations in assessing and treating spasticity in spinal cord injury. Phys Med Rehabil Clin N Am 29(3):445–453. https://doi.org/10.1016/j.pmr.2018.03.001

McCall TD, MacDonald JD (2006) Cervical catheter tip placement for intrathecal baclofen administration. Neurosurgery 59(3):634–640. https://doi.org/10.1227/01.NEU.0000227570.40402.77

Meythaler JM, Guin-Renfroe S, Law C, Grabb P, Hadley MN (2001a) Continuously infused intrathecal baclofen over 12 months for spastic hypertonia in adolescents adults with cerebral palsy. Arch Phys Med Rehabil 82:155–161

Meythaler JM, Guin-Renfroe S, Law C, Grabb P, Hadley MN (2001b) Continuously infused intrathecal baclofen over 12 months for spastic hypertonia in adolescents adults with cerebral palsy. Arch Phys Med Rehabil 82:155–161

Montané E, Vallano A, Laporte JR (2004) Oral antispastic drugs in nonprogressive neurologic diseases: a systematic review. Neurology 63(8):1357–1363. https://doi.org/10.1212/01.wnl.0000141863.52691.44

Nagel SJ, Wilson S, Johnson MD et al (2017) Spinal cord stimulation for spasticity: historical approaches, current status, and future directions. Neuromodulation 20(4):307–321. https://doi.org/10.1111/ner.12591

Pucks-Faes E, Matzak H, Hitzenberger G et al (2019) Intrathecal baclofen trial before device implantation: 12-year experience with continuous administration. Arch Phys Med Rehabil 100(5):837–843. https://doi.org/10.1016/j.apmr.2018.09.124

Ross JC, Cook AM, Stewart GL et al (2011) Acute intrathecal baclofen withdrawal: a brief review of treatment options. Neurocrit Care 14:103–108. https://doi.org/10.1007/s12028-010-9422-6

Sangari S, Lundell H, Kirshblum S, Perez MA (2019) Residual descending motor pathways influence spasticity after spinal cord injury. Ann Neurol 86(1): 28–41. https://doi.org/10.1002/ana.25505

Saulino M (2018) Intrathecal therapies. Phys Med Rehabil Clin N Am 29(3):537–551. https://doi.org/10.1016/j.pmr.2018.04.001

Saulino M, Ivanhoe CB, McGuire JR, Ridley B, Shilt JS, Boster AI (2016) Best practices for intrathecal baclofen therapy: patient selection. Neuromodulation 19(6):607–615

Simpson DM, Gracies JM, Graham HK et al (2008) Assessment: botulinum neurotoxin for the treatment of spasticity (an evidence-based review): report of the therapeutics and technology assessment subcommittee of the American Academy of Neurology. Neurology 70:1691–1698

Sivaramakrishnan A, Solomon JM, Manikandan N (2018) Comparison of transcutaneous electrical nerve stimulation (TENS) and functional electrical stimulation (FES) for spasticity in spinal cord injury—a pilot randomized cross-over trial. J Spinal Cord Med 41(4):397–406. https://doi.org/10.1080/10790268.2017.1390930

Slonimski M, Abram SE, Zuniga RE (2004) Intrathecal baclofen in pain management. Reg Anesth Pain Med 29(3):269–276. http://p2048-eresources.library.mssm.edu.eresources.mssm.edu/login?url=https://search-proquest-com.eresources.mssm.edu/docview/205167944?accountid=41157

Thibaut A, Chatelle C, Ziegler E et al (2013) Spasticity after stroke: physiology, assessment and treatment. Brain Inj 27:1093–1105

Tilton A, Vargus-Adams J, Delgado R (2010) Pharmacologic treatment of spasticity in children. Semin Pediatr Neurol 17(4):261–267. https://doi.org/10.1016/j.spen.2010.10.009

Vats A, Amit A, Cossar M, Bhatt P, Cozens A (2019) Intrathecal baclofen trial using a temporary indwelling intrathecal catheter—a single institution experience. J Clin Neurosci 68:33–38. https://doi.org/10.1016/j.jocn.2019.07.073

Wesemann K, Coffey RJ, Wallace MS, Tan Y, Broste S, Buvanendran A (2014) Clinical accuracy and safety using the SynchroMed II intrathecal drug infusion pump. Reg Anesth Pain Med 39:341–346

Yang K, Wang D, Li YQ (2001) Distribution and depression of the GABA(B) receptor in the spinal dorsal horn of adult rat. Brain Res Bull 55(4):479–485. https://doi.org/10.1016/s0361-9230(01)00546-9

Postoperative Care and Complication

Daniel R. Kloster

Contents

Abstract

Intrathecal drug delivery has expanded since the inception of this technology in the 1980s and is utilized for a number of different conditions including pain control and management of spasticity. The use of intrathecal pumps is less common than most other techniques for interventional pain management but is essential in such conditions as refractory pain, cancer pain, multifocal pain, severe spasticity, and in patient who are not candidates for surgical correction of their underlying condition. Intrathecal drug delivery is usually considered when analgesics or antispasmodics administered via the oral, transdermal, or intravenous routes are ineffective or are associated with unacceptable side effects. The intrathecal delivery of medications bypasses the blood-brain barrier, which produces much higher concentrations of medication within the cerebrospinal fluid. This higher concentration can serve to dramatically reduce the effective dose of the medication and can be associated with higher rates of pain and spasm reduction compared to other routes of medication delivery. Although intrathecal drug delivery has been

D. R. Kloster (✉)
Crimson Pain Management, Overland Park, KS, USA

shown to be effective and cost-effective, this less utilized pain management tool is less well understood regarding its implantation and management than other technologies. This chapter will serve to highlight postoperative care and complications.

Abbreviations

BBB	Blood-brain barrier
CMM	Conventional medical management
CP	Cerebral palsy
CSF	Cerebrospinal fluid
CT	Computed tomography
CVA	Cerebrovascular accident
FDA	Food and Drug Administration
ITB	Intrathecal baclofen
MRI	Magnetic resonance imaging
MS	Multiple sclerosis
PSS	Poststroke spasticity
ROM	Range of movement
SCI	Spinal cord injury
SCS	Spinal cord stimulator
TBI	Traumatic brain injury
TDD	Targeted drug delivery

Intrathecal pumps can provide profound relief from pain and spasticity. Although intrathecal (IT) therapy is highly effective, the invasive nature of the pump and catheter implantation along with the potency of the intrathecal medications can occasionally result in various types of complications that may be seen in the patients that are treated with targeted drug delivery (TDD) (Staats 2008; Follett and Naumann 2000; Noreika and Fabbro n.d.; Deer et al. 2017a; Flückiger et al. 2008). The published rates of complications vary according to the various types and severity of the complications being evaluated but generally range from 10 to 20% annually in the patients undergoing TDD. A thorough knowledge of intrathecal medication pharmacology and intrathecal drug delivery troubleshooting are needed to manage and treat patients with implantable intrathecal pumps.

1 Infection

Device infections are well documented in the literature (Deer et al. 2017a; Follett et al. 2004; Engle et al. 2013; Carlson 2020). Any implantable device has the risk of becoming infected. Patients that require an intrathecal pump are generally in a higher-risk group than other patients requiring implantable devices. Most patients have been on chronic opioids which result in endocrine dysfunction including suppressing the immune system (Katz and Mazer 2009). This suppression of the immune system will not abate with the change in delivery of the opioids to an intrathecal route, and this should be explained to the patient (Duarte et al. 2013). Patients may also be on immunosuppressive therapies for an underlying disease process such as rheumatoid arthritis, systemic lupus erythematous, Crohn's disease, etc., or they may have an active cancer diagnosis such as a blood cell dyscrasias that can adversely affect the immune system. Additionally, common underlying comorbidities such as obesity (Pull ter Gunne and Cohen 2009), tobacco use (Sorensen 2012), diabetes, or poor nutrition can weaken what would otherwise be a normal immune system (Pull ter Gunne and Cohen 2009).

The rate of infection varies widely in the published literature but is generally quoted in the 2–9% range (Follett et al. 2004). Infection is higher in patients requiring replacement of the device compared to their first implant. The hypothesis for this increased rate of infection is reduced vascular flow due to the fibrous scar tissue that forms in the pump pocket (Abd-Elsayed et al. 2020).

Careful planning and strategy are needed to mitigate the risk of infection, and there should also be a well thought-out plan for treating infections once they present (Deer et al. 2017b). Preoperative planning should include controlling blood glucose, smoking cessation, improving nutrition, and testing for methicillin-resistant *Staphylococcus aureus* (MRSA) (Burgher et al. 2007). The preoperative planning specifics are discussed in greater detail in chapter "Targeted Drug Delivery Perioperative Planning Considerations".

There is general agreement in the literature regarding the need for perioperative antibiotics (Bowater et al. 2009; Alexander et al. 2011; Forse et al. 1989). Antibiotic coverage for the most likely infectious pathogens should be given prior to the incision. Intraoperative strategies such as limiting foot traffic in the operating room, double gloving, using local anesthetic without epinephrine, using ioban, and limit handling of the implant are also common and well supported in the literature (Deer et al. 2017b).

When closing the incisions, it is important to obtain a tight closure to minimize new tissue formation within the wound and to optimize skin healing (Essebag et al. 2016; Sridhar et al. 2016). It is also important to have fastidious attention to achieving hemostasis which will minimize or prevent hematoma and seroma formation (Essebag et al. 2016; Sridhar et al. 2016). After wound closure, an occlusive dressing should be applied.

Ideal wound management combined with perioperative antibiotics and good surgical technique will serve to decrease the risk of an infection. There is no consensus opinion regarding postoperative antibiotics, but most physicians implanting IT drug delivery systems will give a 3- to-7-day course of antibiotics following the procedure. Many clinicians implanting pumps are also using 500 mg–1 g of vancomycin powder in the pocket site during implantation (Molinari et al. 2012). This has been adapted from the neurosurgical and orthopedic literature and is not commonly applied during pump implantation (Kanj et al. 2013; Mallela et al. 2018).

It is also important to discuss home care with the patient including good hygiene as well as limiting exposure to other home contaminants such as pet dander. Discharge instructions should be provided to the patient that includes the limits to their postoperative physical activity.

An abdominal binder or other compression garment is necessary to secure the pump to the anterior abdominal wall. This will limit the motion of the pump in the pocket and will facilitate healing in the appropriate position and can limit seroma formation. There is no consensus as to the use of an abdominal binder, but they are used by experienced practitioners especially in obese patients as repetitive traction on the anterior abdominal wall by a large pannus may contribute to detachment of the pump and may cause the sutures that anchor the pump to pull through Scarpa's fascia. The binder also contributes to the security of the catheter and can promote healing of intrathecal drug delivery system in the intended location. Patients can shower immediately after pump implantation provided an occlusive dressing is utilized, but any submersion of the surgical wounds should be avoided until the incisions are completely healed.

Patients should have a routine follow-up visit in 1–3 weeks for an evaluation of the incisions and for consideration of a medication dose adjustment. Most pump site infections are caused by gram-positive bacteria with *Staphylococcus aureus* and *S. epidermidis* being the most common pathogens. If vancomycin powder is used in the pocket, a gram-negative pathogen such as *Escherichia coli* or *Pseudomonas aeruginosa* is more common. Wound cultures are necessary to appropriately treat the patient as less common pathogens may also cause infection including *Streptococci*, *Enterococci*, fungi, and anaerobic bacteria (Döring et al. 2018).

Infections are considered postsurgical if they occur within 1 year of system implantation and appear to be related to the surgery. Superficial infections can generally be treated with a course of antibiotics and superficial wound care with a good outcome expected. Deeper infections that involve any portion of the intrathecal drug delivery system will almost inevitably require explantation except in rare instances. Infections of implanted systems most often involve the pump site (Fig. 1). Swelling and redness are certainly signs of infection, but if present early, within 1–2 weeks after the implant, it is likely to be a noninfectious reaction to something that was applied to the skin's surface such as the antiseptic skin preparation, the subcuticular sutures, or the occlusive wound dressing. Pump site infections tend to manifest clinically 3–5 weeks after surgery and can be associated with a wound dehiscence. This scenario is diagnostic of a surgical site infection and requires removal of the pump.

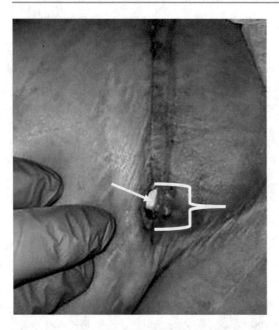

Fig. 1 Photograph of the pump implantation site showing wound dehiscence (white bracket) with an exposed pump (white arrow). This dehiscence was caused by an infection that presented seven weeks after pump implantation

If there is a suspicion of infection without dehiscence, a needle aspiration can be obtained and sent for culture. Noninfectious swelling can occur around the catheter insertion site or around the pump, and needle aspiration of this fluid will be helpful as a seroma (Deer et al. 2017a) will appear serosanguinous in appearance and a hematoma will be dark red (Deer et al. 2017a). Swelling from a bacterial infection will appear cloudy and purulent. Generally, patients with surgical site infections are stable, and explantation of the pump and catheter can be planned on a non-emergent basis unless there are meningeal signs that would indicate the possibility of meningitis and spread of the infection to the intrathecal space. If any meningeal signs such as a severe headache, neck stiffness, photophobia, and seizures are present, the explantation must be done emergently.

When an infection is encountered, a culture should be sent for laboratory analysis and sensitivity testing in preparation for antibiotic treatment. The sample should also be sent for a KOH prep assessing for the presence of a fungal infection which would necessitate the use of an antifungal rather than an antibiotic. In non-emergent cases, explantation can be performed on an outpatient basis, but if the patient is toxic or shows meningeal signs than an emergent intrathecal system, explant is needed. An infectious disease consultation may occasionally be needed, and the patient should be admitted to the hospital until they are clinically stable. In either case, all components of the intrathecal drug delivery system are removed, and an epidural blood patch should be performed unless a catheter insertion site infection is suspected. Systemic medications that are intended to replace the intrathecal medications will be needed to mitigate withdrawal symptoms since intrathecal therapy will be stopped (Lee et al. 2016; Ross et al. 2011; Hu et al. 2002). One or both of the incisions will need to be copiously irrigated and closed with an absorbable suture and/or skin staples. Either a loose wound closure that allows for wound drainage is performed or a tight closure is done along with a stab incision made at the inferior portion of the pocket site and a surgical site drain placed for postoperative drainage. The drain can be removed after the wound drainage has stopped. At the follow-up visit, 1–2 weeks after the system explantation, the incision and infection should be greatly improved. There is no consensus in the literature as far as when to replace the pump if the patient desires, but, if a replacement system is considered, a new pocket site should be chosen. Depending on the clinical circumstances, the replacement can be placed with days to weeks after explantation of the previous system.

In patients with a paucity of subcutaneous soft tissue, pumps can erode through the skin over time (Fig. 2), and the pump site should be inspected at the time of each pump refill. Cachectic patients as well as patients with spasticity and neuromuscular disorders are at highest risk. Skin erosion over the pump is most common in areas of higher friction such as when the pump is placed at the belt line or at a place that is subject to pressure erosion. In some patients, it can be difficult to find an anatomic location that decreases this risk. Placement in alternative subcutaneous locations such as the pectoral region or overlying the anterior thigh can be done if necessary, and surgical

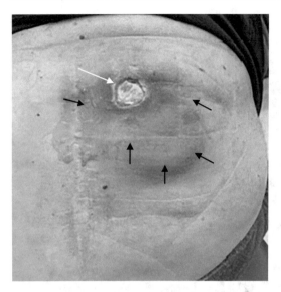

Fig. 2 Photograph of the pump site showing erythema (black arrows) of the skin and a pressure erosion (white arrow) of the skin where the overlying clothing progressively eroded through the skin to expose the underlying pump. (Photo courtesy of Dawood Sayed, M.D.)

site creation with soft tissue expanders in preparation for pump implantation is an option if no other site is available that reasonably avoids erosion through the integument.

2 Catheter Issues

When a Tuohy introducer needle is placed into the cerebrospinal fluid, there is generally a robust return of cerebrospinal fluid. While this is the typical scenario, it is not always the case. In patients that have low CSF pressure, have extensive spinal stenosis, obstruction to CSF flow or significant previous surgery, the CSF flow can be sparse. The catheter may still be able to be advanced without significant resistance, but the confidence of proper placement will need to be confirmed by aspirating CSF through the catheter once it is placed in a location with less obstruction to the flow of CSF.

Intrathecal catheters are blunt tipped and contain an internal wire to increase the stiffness and to augment the radiopacity of the catheter to make it easier to guide and to see, respectively. The catheter cannot be advanced with impunity,

however as it can penetrate structures within the spinal canal including the parenchyma of the spinal cord when advancing the catheter without the appropriate care (Fig. 3) (Fitzgibbon et al. 2016; Deer et al. 2017c). If the catheter is located in a location without fluid including the dura, outside of the spinal canal or even within the parenchyma of the spinal cord, cerebrospinal fluid will not be returned. If the catheter penetrates the spinal cord, the patient will most likely experience unilateral or bilateral lower extremity pain and weakness. Since the catheter is blunt tipped, more extensive traumatic injury to the spinal cord is generally not seen, but is possible.

The most common presenting symptom of a neural injury associated with catheter placement is new onset unilateral severe pain beginning immediately in the postoperative period combined with motor weakness on physical exam. The possibility of neural injury is increased with insertion above the L2 level, but the L3, L4, L5, and S1 dermatomes are the most commonly involved because of the conventional entry point of the stylet at or below the L3 level along with the common scenario of coexisting spinal stenosis. If neural injury is suspected, advanced imaging, such as MRI or CT myelography, should be immediately ordered.

An epidural hematoma (Fig. 4), when it occurs, will often be more devastating to neurologic function as it can involve higher levels including the thoracic spine which can result in spinal cord compression if the hematoma is large enough (Horlocker et al. 2018; Narouze et al. 2018). If an epidural hematoma occurs, the catheter can be left in place or removed, but if the catheter is removed when the spinal cord is being tightly compressed by a hematoma, there is a possibility of additional injury to the spinal cord. A symptomatic thoracic epidural hematoma will require surgical evacuation, and, if this is performed within minutes to hours after the appearance of the neurologic symptoms, patients will typically have a very good recovery but generally require skilled nursing or rehabilitation for their lower extremity weakness until it resolves.

Catheters intended for an intrathecal location may be improperly placed in the epidural space.

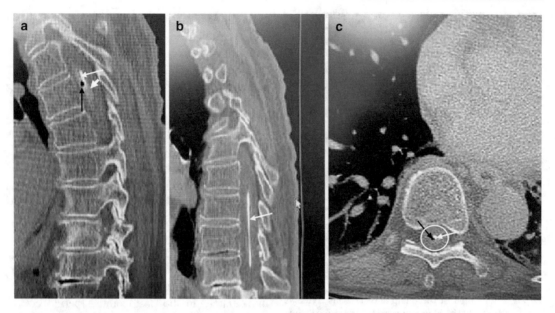

Fig. 3 Sagittal Computed Tomographic reconstructions (**a** and **b**) and an axial CT slice (**c**) showing the intrathecal catheter (white arrows in **a**–**c**) within the spinal cord (white circle in **c**). A small amount of contrast (white arrowhead in **a**) and air (black arrows in **a** and **c**) can be seen adjacent to the catheter resulting from a previous catheter injection test

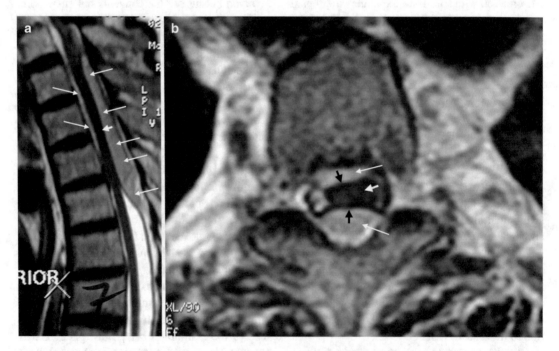

Fig. 4 Sagittal (**a**) and axial (**b**) T2-weighted Magnetic Resonance images showing an upper thoracic epidural hematoma (white arrows in **a** and **b**) extending from the T1–2 level to the T5–6 level surrounding the anterior and posterior portions of the spinal cord (white arrows in **a**). The spinal cord (white arrowheads in **a** and **b**) shows evidence of compression both anteriorly and posteriorly (black arrowheads in **b**) by the epidural hematoma

The position within the spinal canal and the lack of cerebrospinal fluid return when the catheter is aspirated are two of the indicators that the catheter is not in an intrathecal location. If contrast is injected into the catheter access port, an epidurogram will be seen versus a myelogram. Generally, the epidural space is easily distinguished from an intrathecal catheter location, but the visualization can be difficult in patients who have challenging anatomy such as those with severe degenerative scoliosis or patients with extensive hardware in the area of interest. Postoperative CT imaging can confirm catheter placement in the correct location. If the catheter is discovered to be epidural, the pump can still be utilized but a tenfold increased medication dose is typically needed to provide the same degree of analgesia compared to medication delivery intrathecally. Given the size of the reservoir, clinicians employing an epidural dosing technique usually use a higher concentration of the medication, and, even then, the pump needs to be refilled much more often as the medication is used much more quickly as compared to if it were used intrathecally (Zenz et al. 1985).

Epidural hematomas can occur with any neuraxial interventional procedure and have been described extensively in the literature (Staats 2008; Deer et al. 2017a; Abd-Elsayed et al. 2020). Delayed hematomas are much less common and, although possible, are rare. Epidural hematomas will most often present in the immediate or very recent postoperative period. Patients typically complain of profound limb heaviness, weakness, and they will often report varying degrees of pain. Compression of the neural elements by the hematoma may also cause bowel or bladder issues. If an epidural hematoma is suspected, immediate imaging is needed and should be obtained along with a surgical consultation. If a neuraxial anesthetic such as a spinal or epidural block is utilized in the interventional procedure, lingering effects of the anesthetic may be difficult to distinguish from a compressive hematoma. This similarity in presentation can lead to delayed diagnosis and treatment and worse outcomes. The usual anesthesia for placement of an intrathecal pump is deep sedation or general anesthesia, and neither of these types of anesthesia should adversely affect the strength or sensation of the extremities and therefore should not cloud the diagnosis. Restarting anticoagulant therapy following placement of a pump depends on several factors (Horlocker et al. 2018; Narouze et al. 2018). There are numerous anticoagulant medications in use, with the number and variety of these anticoagulants continuously changing. Some medications such as nonsteroidal anti-inflammatories and antidepressants have blood-thinning qualities without being cardiac, peripherally or cerebrally protective. Different patients will have different degrees of risk depending on their underlying pathology and their anticoagulation medication and will therefore have different lengths of time necessary for them to be off of their anticoagulant medication prior to a procedure (additional information on anticoagulation guidelines can be found in chapter "Targeted Drug Delivery Perioperative Planning Considerations"). It is important to have an updated resource such as the anticoagulation recommendations based on the current American Society of Regional Anesthesia and Pain Medicine guidelines for review prior to suspending and restarting anticoagulant therapy. It is also recommended to coordinate care with the prescribing physician of the anticoagulant medication. Unrecognized hematomas can have permanent and severe sequela, but with urgent care and optimal treatment, a good recovery is expected.

Intraoperative neuromonitoring has not been routinely utilized when placing intrathecal drug delivery systems, but it is becoming more commonplace especially when the invasive procedures require general anesthesia for patient comfort. The monitoring can help avoid or diminish neural injuries by early detection of nerve-related perturbations which can alert the physician of a potential impending injury (Fehlings et al. 2010; Gonzalez et al. 2009).

Out of all of the components of an implanted intrathecal drug delivery system, the most prone to failure is the intrathecal catheter. Even properly placed catheters can ultimately fail for various reasons. Catheter aspiration procedures

(CAPs) will confirm the integrity and patency of the intrathecal catheter but only test the catheter and do not provide information about the functionality of the pump itself. Both the Medtronic SynchroMed II pump and the Flowonix Prometra pump have a dedicated catheter aspiration port (CAP) procedure kit. A CAP procedure should be done if the patient presents with signs and symptoms of withdrawal in the absence of decreasing the intrathecal medication dose or if adequacy of the therapy is questioned (Deer et al. 2017a; Skalsky et al. 2020; Delhaas et al. 2020). The catheter aspiration procedure can be performed with or without fluoroscopy, but fluoroscopy is preferred as the port can be seen and the needle guided into the correct position under fluoroscopic guidance. Without fluoroscopy and contrast to test the catheter integrity and to look for locations of catheter disruption, the integrity of the catheter cannot be adequately assessed. Studying the catheter during a catheter aspiration procedure will give a quick answer as to the patency of the catheter. If the catheter is patent, CSF will be easily aspirated into the syringe connected to the CAP. If the catheter is severed, kinked, blocked, or has migrated out of the intrathecal space (Figs. 5, 6, and 7), no CSF will be returned. The exception to this is a properly working catheter that has been in place a long time. Over time, debris can be in the lumen, and inflammatory changes can surround the catheter tip (Fig. 8) such that forward flow is allowed but

with negative aspiration during a CAP, no aspirate is obtained. It is also possible that the catheter holes can be blocked with aspiration if the

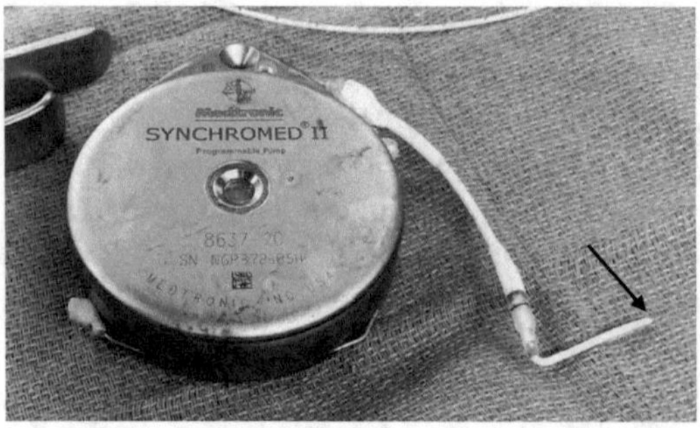

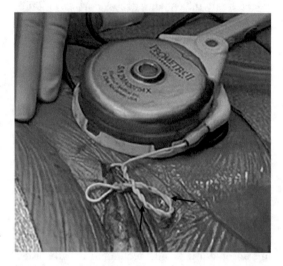

Fig. 6 Photograph of an explanted pump shows the catheter is twisted (black arrows) and was found to be kinked and the flow through the pump was obstructed. The pump had pulled loose from it's attachment to the anterior abdominal wall and was free to flip within the pump pocket

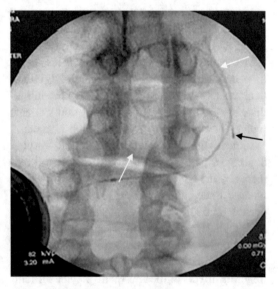

Fig. 7 Anteroposterior fluoroscopic image showing coiling of the intrathecal catheter (white arrows) with the catheter tip located outside of the spinal canal (black arrow). The catheter had migrated proximally into the catheter insertion location and was found coiled subcutaneously in this location

Fig. 5 Explanted pump and proximal catheter due to catheter disruption found when performing a catheter aspiration study shows the fractured catheter that was disrupted (black arrow) just a few centimeters distal to the proximal catheter connection

distal portion of the catheter is in close contact with the dura. Unintentional subdural placement of the catheter is also possible once the tip of the Tuohy needle or the catheter tip pierces the dura mater (Fig. 9). A granuloma can also form at the catheter tip, especially in patients undergoing intrathecal medication therapy with a highly con-

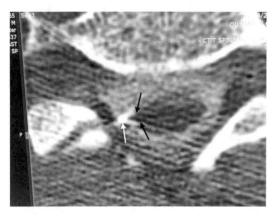

Fig. 8 Axial CT slice taken through the upper thoracic spine at the level of the tip of the intrathecal catheter shows the radiopaque catheter tip (white arrow) and asymmetric deformity of the spinal cord (black arrows) indicating an intradural adhesion connecting the right side of the spinal cord to the dura in the location of the intrathecal catheter tip

centration medication (Figs. 10 and 11). In cases of granuloma formation at the catheter tip, aspiration of CSF can also be limited or nonexistent and the granuloma can also block the infusion of the medication into the intrathecal space. If this is suspected, the pump daily dose can be diminished by 20–30% to test for a patient response to the decreased dose. If the catheter has been nonfunctional, the patient will not notice a dose change and should not experience worsening symptoms. If the patient was indeed receiving therapy through a functioning catheter, a 20–30% reduction of medication should be enough of a dose decrease to result in worsening pain scores. The catheter injection test is performed with fluoroscopy and after aspiration of fluid contrast may be injected through the catheter access port. This will confirm a normal appearing myelogram as well as help to identify the catheter position. If no aspirate is obtained, contrast should not be injected. The catheter lumen contains highly concentrated drug, and if contrast is injected before aspirating the catheter, the medication within the catheter can be injected rapidly into the intrathecal space and put the patient at risk for an overdose. This overdose risk depends on the type and concentration of the medication, the length of the

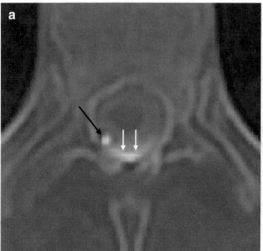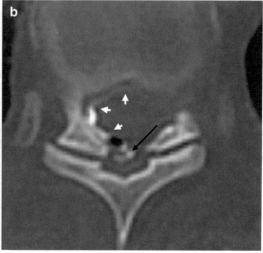

Fig. 9 (**a** and **b**) Axial CT images demonstrating the catheter (black arrows in **a** and **b**) and contrast layering in the intrathecal space (white arrows in **a**) with a normal appearance after contrast injection through the catheter access port as compared to the contrast located outside of its expected position within the dura and epidural space (white arrowheads in **b**)

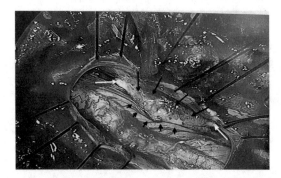

Fig. 10 Intraoperative photograph taken during surgical removal of a catheter tip granuloma shows the dura reflected by the sutures revealing the intrathecal catheter (white arrows), the catheter tip granuloma (black arrows) positioned next to and displacing the spinal cord (black arrowheads). Photo courtesy: Richard Morgan, MD

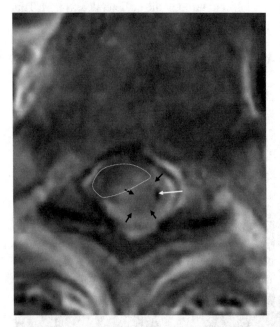

Fig. 11 Axial T1-weighted image near the catheter tip (white arrow) of a patient with an intrathecal drug delivery system showing a catheter tip granuloma (black arrows) that is compressing the spinal cord (outlined in white dashed line)

catheter, and the patient tolerance to the medication or medications. An exception of the general rule not to inject through an obstructed catheter can be made according to the clinical judgment of the clinician managing the pump if they deem it safe to proceed with injection of contrast into the catheter injected port in an attempt to unblock

the catheter. Sediment or precipitation present within the catheter may be forced through the lumen to unblock the obstruction by injecting contrast but planning and caution need to be exercised and a potential overdose anticipated. An informed consent is necessary prior to a catheter injection test and resuscitative equipment, and naloxone should be immediately available. A longer more planned out approach can be undertaken by filling the reservoir with saline and then forcing fluid through at a later date, with all the same precautions taken, but there is no guarantee that the lumen will become patent with either approach. Going to the operating room and revising the catheter have surgical risks, but the risk of overdose is eliminated. If the catheter is completely blocked, kinked, or twisted, an operative solution may be needed no matter the approach (Fig. 6). If there is a tear in the catheter, contrast material will be observed along the path of the catheter, and outside the intrathecal space with a focal collection of contrast at the location of the tear. If the catheter is found to be abraded or torn, revision of the catheter is needed (Fig. 12). The CAP procedure is performed under relatively high pressure, and the contrast is forced through the side port. The Medtronic SynchroMed II pump is a low pressure peristaltic pump that produces less pressure than is present within the CSF so if a disruption of the catheter is present, the CSF will flow retrograde through the catheter to the location of the disruption. The Flowonix Prometra pump has a piston that pumps the fluid

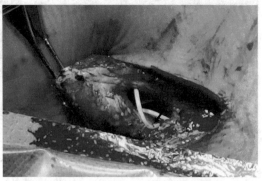

Fig. 12 Photograph of catheter insertion site showing a small nick in the catheter (black arrow) that was found to be leaking cerebrospinal fluid

under a higher pressure than the CSF so the medication can be pumped intrathecally during the forward cycle, but medication can also be lost between cycles.

Over time with the pulsations of the CSF, the catheter can migrate out of the intrathecal space (Fig. 7) (Deer et al. 2017a; Abd-Elsayed et al. 2020). When this occurs, the catheter will slowly migrate caudally into the catheter insertion site and is most often located subcutaneously just beneath the incision. The anchor is usually still properly secured, but the cephalad portion of the catheter most often retracts out of the intrathecal space. When this occurs, the patient will experience withdrawal symptoms. On plain film imaging, or fluoroscopy, the catheter will appear coiled in the anterior posterior view (Fig. 7). On the lateral view, it will be located posterior to the lamina and often at the level of the catheter insertion site. When this occurs, the catheter will require replacement, and care must be taken to place as much catheter length intrathecally as possible with an insertion angle as parallel to the spinal column as possible. These techniques along with a secure anchor should serve to hold the catheter as securely as possible within the intrathecal space. Both Flowonix and Medtronic have catheter splice kits, and a new catheter may be placed into the intrathecal space and spliced to the retained but trimmed catheter. With this approach, the pump site does not need to be opened. Unfortunately, there is not a current good solution to splice a catheter from one company to another, and if the decision has been made to change from one vendor to another, it is best to replace the entire catheter system.

3   Granuloma

A catheter tip granuloma is an aseptic inflammatory mass that can arise from the arachnoid tissue at the distal portion of the catheter (Fig. 10). Granulomas are well described in the literature and have been reported in 0.04% of patients within the first year after catheter insertion, and the overall incidence is thought to be less than 3% (Deer et al. 2017a; Abd-Elsayed et al. 2020;

Kratzsch et al. 2015; Shields et al. 2005; Yaksh et al. 2013; Ramsey et al. 2008; Deer et al. 2007). The histologic examination of these catheter tip masses often shows central necrosis with a periphery if fibrotic and inflammatory cells originating from the arachnoid and possessing substantial vascularity (Kratzsch et al. 2015; Shields et al. 2005; Yaksh et al. 2013; Ramsey et al. 2008; Deer et al. 2007). They are classically described as granulomas but usually do not meet the histologic criteria for a granuloma (Deer et al. 2007). The most common medications associated with catheter granulomas are opioids with morphine being the most commonly associated. Rarely, non-opioid medications have been linked to granulomas, including ziconotide, baclofen, clonidine, and bupivacaine. The first presenting signs of a granuloma are typically worsening pain control or medication withdrawal symptoms. An increase in pump doses is commonly tried when the pain control worsens and the usual response in the presence of a catheter granuloma is the lack of improvement in the patient's painful symptoms. If left unrecognized or unchecked, granulomas can increase in size and encroach on the spinal cord or cauda equina and cause neural symptoms corresponding to the level of the catheter tip. Eventually, spinal cord involvement or compression can result in neurological deficits including leg weakness or paraparesis. Risk factors for development of catheter granulomas include the location of the catheter tip where the CSF volume is the lowest and the flow is the slowest which is located in the thoracic spine. Other risk factors include highly concentrated intrathecal medications, opioid medications, high daily doses of intrathecal medication, low infusion rates, and low velocity of infusion at the catheter tip all increase the chance of forming a catheter tip granuloma. The difference in pump infusion may also play a role with the Flowonix intrathecal pump having a higher exit velocity from the catheter than the Medtronic pump given its piston injection mechanism as compared to the rotary peristaltic injection method that is utilized by Medtronic. In a Flowonix post approval registry of 414 patients, only 1 patient had a granuloma.

As mentioned previously, the incidence of catheter granuloma formation is thought to be less than 3% overall, and most implanters have had at least a granuloma patient with one. Although catheter granulomas can form in just a few weeks, the vast majority that are reported in the literature form over several years. If a granuloma is suspected, MR imaging of the thoracic and lumbar spine with contrast should be ordered for diagnostic purposes. If the presence of the granuloma is confirmed, the intrathecal opiate needs to be decreased or stopped, and the catheter should be pulled caudally. Once the opiate infusion is removed from the site of the granuloma, the granuloma typically resolves. Therapy can be resumed at the new catheter location, and surgical intervention is rarely required.

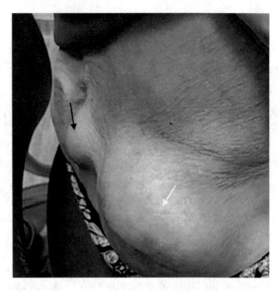

Fig. 13 Photograph of the patient's low back showing rounded prominences under the skin at the catheter insertion site and the pump site (white arrow and black arrow respectively) representing accumulation of cerebrospinal fluid (CSF) in these locations. This has progressively collected at these sites to form a CSFoma. Photo Courtesy of Dawood Sayed, MD

4   Cerebrospinal Fluid Leak

A persistent cerebrospinal fluid leak can occur following placement of an intrathecal catheter (Follett and Naumann 2000; Abd-Elsayed et al. 2020; Singh et al. 2008). This can cause a collection of CSF typically in the location of the catheter insertion site and around the pump and can occur either with or without a post-dural puncture headache (Grant et al. 1991). When they occur, the headaches generally are usually short lived and resolve over several days without intervention. If the symptoms persist, an epidural blood patch can be performed. Care needs to be taken to inject blood in the epidural space around the catheter entry point and to avoid needle trauma to the intrathecal catheter. The longer the CSF leak persists, the more likely it is to become chronic with the CSF fluid typically accumulating in the pocket site (Fig. 13). This can be difficult to distinguish from a postoperative hemorrhage or, later in the postoperative course, a seroma or lymphocele. The risk of the patient developing a headache after pump placement increases with multiple passes of the Tuohy needle. The risk of leaking around the catheter increases in patients with increased intracranial pressure. It is also increased if the catheter is placed through a site of prior surgery as there can

be substantial scarring present that may compromise the integrity of the soft tissue around the dura. It is recommended the needle be placed through tissue that has not been previously disrupted so normal healing can take place around the catheter. If the entry site is through existing scar tissue or if patients have a condition that compromises the quality of their soft tissue (i.e., Ehlers-Danlos syndrome), the risk of chronic CSF leak is increased. Patients undergoing a pump and catheter replacement are also at increased risk for a persistent CSF leak. A detailed informed consent should include this possibility for all patients but should be verbally emphasized in patients at higher risk. The patient may require multiple epidural blood patches or treatment with fibrin glue or a dural sealant. Persistent leaks can necessitate hospitalization and placement of a lumbar drain for resolution or even surgical closure of the dura and surrounding soft tissue. A collection of CSF at the catheter insertion site or within the pocket may be the presenting physical finding in a patient whose catheter is damaged or has migrated out of the intrathecal space. This will typically be accompanied by symptoms of medication withdrawal and poor pain control. When revising a intrathecal drug delivery system and placing a new catheter, a nonabsorbable suture should be used at the catheter entry site to ensure that this closure is as secure as possible around the catheter and that there is no leaking fluid at the time of wound closure. Despite all precautions and even with a dry field intra operatively, a persistent CSF leak is still possible. The efficacy of the therapy can be decreased or lost with a spinal leak but if the patient still has adequate benefit from their intrathecal drug delivery system, however, a revision of their system may not be necessary.

5   Seroma

A seroma is a collection of serous fluid that builds up under the skin at previous surgical sites (Deer et al. 2017a; Gunn et al. 2016). This can develop within days to weeks of the surgery and can cause swelling and surgical site discomfort. Seromas occur in areas of tissue disruption and can cause a discharge of clear fluid from the incisional site. The seroma is fluctuant and, unlike an abscess, generally non-tender and can be chronic. The goal of closure during pump placement is to perform a tight closure thereby minimizing the amount of free space and securing the pump in a tight pocket. Anchor loops are present on the outside of the intrathecal pump that should be used for suturing the pump to the underlying tissue. This is effective at securing the pump to the soft tissue in the pocket and can facilitate postoperative healing and allows the pump to adhere to the tissue. A binder should also be utilized postoperatively to diminish free space around the pump and to help hold the pump securely in place so it can heal in good position against the underlying soft tissue. A seroma can lead to a compromise of the tissue surrounding the pump and can contribute to loosening of the pump attachments and can predispose to an infection and other postoperative complications. A seroma can also be present directly over the pump and can make the refill process difficult often necessitating drainage of the seroma prior to

accessing the pump for a refill. Similar to CSF surrounding the pump at the implantation site, a seroma can be located at the site of pump implantation and can compromise the soft tissue thereby predisposing to pump detachment and free movement of the pump within the pocket. If the pump flips with the posterior portion facing the skin, a refill is not possible. When this situation occurs, the pump can usually be easily flipped back to its original position for the refill. If this occurs repeatedly, however, the catheter can become excessively twisted and kinked or fractured (Figs. 5 and 6). If a seroma is encountered, it should be drained, and a binder applied to help mitigate against the reformation of the seroma. If the seroma continues to persist, the pump site may need revision. Revision may not be necessary if the refill process can be successfully continued, the targeted drug delivery system continues to function normally, and the patient remains satisfied with the therapy.

6   Pump Complications

The intrathecal pump is a programmable device that communicates by standard wireless communication between a communicator placed over the pump and a clinician programmer. This way the patient data and therapy details can be viewed, and information may be manually entered via the programmer. When entering the data, it is necessary to have a dedicated checks and balance system in place to confirm accurate data was entered into the clinician programmer (Deer et al. 2017a; Abd-Elsayed et al. 2020). Incorrect data entry can lead to over or underdosing which can have devastating outcomes. When targeted drug delivery system is initially placed, the length of the catheter is entered. With both Medtronic and Flowonix intrathecal pumps, the proximal portion of the catheter is trimmed to the desired length. This final catheter length is then entered into the programmer. The catheter length and the lumen size are used to determine the volume of medication that is held by the catheter, and this information is needed for calculating various portions of the therapy including priming boluses, bridge boluses, and future catheter revisions. The concentrations of the drugs also need to be entered as this has a direct and substantial effect on determining the daily intrathecal medication dose. If more than one medication is present within the pump reservoir, the software will only allow a calculation of the daily infusion rate based on a single drug only. Both vendors allow for very flexible dosing regimens which can add additional complexities to programming. Correct data entry is essential, and errors can cause clinically important issues. For example, if an incorrect volume is entered, the refill date will be incorrect which can likely result in a missed refill date and subsequent withdrawal symptoms. Any volume discrepancy between the expected pump volume and the encountered volume needs to be evaluated. If more than the expected amount of medicine is found within the pump at the time of refill, the differential diagnosis would include pump failure, catheter occlusion, motor stall, programming error, or impending pump failure. If too little medicine is found, the differential diagnosis is over infusion of the pump, a programming error, or a prior unrecognized partial pocket fill.

During the pump refill process, if the pump refill port is not properly accessed and the needle is errantly placed outside of the pump, the entire contents of the refill medication can be delivered into the pocket outside and surrounding the pump. This is a serious treatment error and is termed a pocket fill (Maino et al. 2017). The intrathecal pump medication is highly concentrated and expected to be infused over several weeks. If the medication is injected into the pocket and outside of the pump, an acute overdose results. If this happens, the patients should be monitored with serial vital signs for at least 30 min following the pump refill, and if an overdose is expected, resuscitative and supportive measures should be immediately implemented with transfer to an acute care setting if needed. The pump should be emptied to determine the amount of medication delivered into the pocket. If a limited amount was delivered to the pocket, patients can have subtle or moderate symptoms but may be stable. If the patient is observed over

the course of a few hours, they may be either discharged to home if they have been deemed to be stable or may be have to be admitted for supportive therapy with medications that vary depending on the contents of the pump. When the effects of the medication abate, the patient may be discharged.

Intrathecal pumps can also have mechanical failures and may malfunction (FDA news release 2018a, b). The pump can over infuse medications as well as under infuse them and if the pump over infuses, overdosing may occur. If under infusing, withdrawal symptoms will typically occur. Pump failures can occur for various reasons including battery failure, mechanical failure of the pumping components, and a motor stall. The most common cause of pump failure is a motor stall, and this malfunction is readily detected when the pump is interrogated. If the medication within the pump contains medications that produce physical dependency such as opioids, clonidine, or baclofen, a pump failure with decreased intrathecal medication dosing can produce withdrawal symptoms, and these symptoms will be consistent with the medications being infused. Depending on the medication and the dose previously given intrathecally, an abrupt decrease in medication can lead to an emergent situation. The three medication types can be associated with significant withdrawal syndromes and require rescue strategies in the event the IT TDD system is interrupted. The rescue strategies for all three medications include oral medications, but for higher doses of IT baclofen, intravenous baclofen may need to be given in the case of an abrupt cessation of the IT dosing. Opiate withdrawal symptoms can be divided into early and late symptoms with early symptoms including agitation, myalgias, anxiety, runny nose, diaphoresis, insomnia, and yawning. Late symptoms include nausea and vomiting as well as abdominal cramping, tachycardia, hypertension, dilated pupils, and diarrhea. Clonidine withdrawal symptoms include headache, tremor, delirium, uncontrolled hypertension, and tachycardia that can lead to stress-induced cardiomyopathy (Bowcock et al. 2016). Baclofen withdrawal can be profound with such symptoms as spasticity, neuroleptic malignant syndrome, sepsis, serotonin syndrome, malignant hyperthermia, autonomic dysreflexia, seizure, and autonomic storming (Riordan and Murphy 2015). These withdrawal symptoms can be severe enough to produce a fatal outcome (Riordan and Murphy 2015).

The risk of pump failure increases with the use of off-label medications and compounded medications. Most of the motor stalls occur spontaneously and have been shown to happen at a rate of 2.4% when on-label medications are present within the pump and at a rate of 7% with off-label medications (FDA news release 2018a, b). The FDA released a safety communication in November 2018 addressing this issue of off-label medication use and pointed out that medications are prescribed off label across all specialties, but an informed consent needs to be obtained. The Polyanalgesic Consensus Guidelines show that most practitioners use multiple intrathecal medications (Deer et al. 2017b). Multiple medications or off-label medications are used to improve pain control or to mitigate intolerable side effects. If there has been any compromise of pump function or pump failure, there will be more medication in the pump at the time of refill because less of it will have been pumped into the intrathecal space. This volume discrepancy detected at the time of refill will be obvious if enough time has elapsed between failure and refill; the volume discrepancy will be a larger volume and will be more obvious. A discrepancy in pump reservoir volume at the time of pump refill is often the first indication of a pump failure. There are also times when the pump is still functional but slowing down due to an end-of-life battery. When serial volume discrepancies are noted, it is recommended to go ahead and replace the pump regardless of the chronologic age of the implant. A CAP procedure should always be performed to confirm that the catheter is not the culprit for the volume discrepancy. If the catheter is still viable, the existing catheter can be utilized with the new pump. When replacing any portion of an IT drug delivery system, the clinician must keep in mind that the patient has not been receiving the desired dose of medication and is therefore no longer as tolerant to the medication so a new starting dose

should be chosen that is lower than the previous amount to avoid an overdose situation.

7   Baclofen

Intrathecal pumps implanted in patients to control their dystonia and spasticity can potentially have severe consequences if the pump fails as described above (Deer et al. 2017b; Riordan and Murphy 2015). Baclofen is a derivative of gamma-aminobutyric acid (GABA) an inhibitory neurotransmitter, and sudden removal from the central nervous system (CNS) can result in neural excitation. In properly working intrathecal pumps, a therapeutic dose of baclofen decreases muscle tone and spasms (Duarte et al. 2016). When the inhibitory action of baclofen is removed, withdrawal symptoms will typically begin within 24–48 hours of drug cessation. Presenting signs and symptoms are those of CNS depressant withdrawal. In addition to the symptoms of baclofen withdrawal, patients will generally have mental status changes, including confusion, obtundation, and hallucinations. Their spasticity predictably worsens, sometimes severely, and patients may have malignant hyperthermia necessitating treatment with dantrolene. Because the signs and symptoms of baclofen withdrawal can be mimicked by other causes of CNS withdrawal, it is important to exclude other possible causes for the patient's symptoms. There is no specific diagnostic test for baclofen withdrawal, but patients on a therapeutic intrathecal dose of baclofen for almost any duration will consistently experience withdrawal symptoms if this intrathecal dose is stopped. Supportive care should be started immediately with transfer to an acute care facility and intensive care monitoring. Benzodiazepines and propofol may be needed to treat the CNS irritability and hypertension, and intravenous baclofen may need to be given if the symptoms are sufficiently severe. Patients can have substantial fluid loss from fever and diaphoresis, increased respiratory rate, and significant muscle spasms. With recurrence of the patient's dystonia and spasticity, the severe muscle contractions can produce rhabdomyolysis which can lead to renal dysfunction and multisystem failure. Intrathecal pump and catheter troubleshooting algorithms should be implemented to assess the functionality of the device and system (Delhaas et al. 2020). This includes interrogating the pump to make sure a refill date was not missed, plain film or fluoroscopic evaluation to rule out catheter dislodgement, accessing the pump to confirm medication is still present in the reservoir, and performing a catheter aspiration procedure to confirm patency of the catheter. Unfortunately, oral baclofen has little value in the setting of severe withdrawal as adequate CNS levels are not achieved. It is important to reestablish intrathecal administration if possible. If the catheter is intact, baclofen can be administered via the side port of the pump, but if the catheter has failed, intrathecal medication can only be administered via lumbar puncture or insertion of another intrathecal catheter.

8 Miscellaneous

Ziconotide is a recommended first-line treatment (see chapter "Intrathecal Drug Delivery Trialing" for intrathecal medication recommendations and like all pharmacological products, there are unique side effects associated with its use (Deer et al. 2017b; Pope and Deer 2013)). Mental status changes can develop either acutely or at any time point in the therapy including with chronic use. These changes can include hallucinations, confusion, aphasia, and memory impairment (Rauck et al. 2006). A lesser-known complication is creatinine kinase elevation, but this can be seen in up to 40% of the patients receiving the medication, and more than 10% will have levels more than three times the upper limit of normal (Deer et al. 2017a). When these levels are very high, rhabdomyolysis can occur. If a patient receiving ziconotide intrathecal therapy experiences motor weakness, serial testing for rhabdomyolysis is recommended.

All patients receiving chronic opioids either systemically or intrathecally will experience endocrine dysfunction (Katz and Mazer 2009). Signs and symptoms of this include amenorrhea, decreased testosterone, hypothyroidism, worsening depression, weight gain, immune suppression, osteoporosis, and adrenal suppression. The patient should be informed of the inevitability of some endocrine issues, and the primary care physician should receive correspondence to alert them of this possibility. Another very common side effect seen with intrathecal opioid therapy is urinary hesitancy and/or urinary retention (Hustad et al. 1985). Older men are the most susceptible to urinary retention, and although this side effect is most pronounced with morphine, it can occur with all intrathecal opioids. Intrathecal opioids are known to cause dose-dependent suppression of the detrusor contractility and to decrease the sensation of urge. The urinary retention symptoms generally resolve but can persist and sometimes will necessitate the removal of the opioid from the mixture of infused intrathecal medicine.

Peripheral edema is another common physical finding after initiating intrathecal opiate therapy (Deer et al. 2017a). The proposed mechanism is opioid stimulation of postpituitary secretion of vasopressin and water retention, but most cases of peripheral edema will be in patients who already had some degree of lower extremity edema prior to the initiation of the intrathecal opioid therapy (Deer et al. 2017a). This finding will often ease over time, but if persistent or severe, changing to a lipophilic opiate such as fentanyl may be beneficial. Edema can also be observed with clonidine and bupivacaine secondary to vasodilation caused by these medications.

9 Magnetic Resonance Imaging

Both Flowonix and Medtronic implantable intrathecal pumps are labeled as MRI conditional and may be safely scanned under the conditions of safe use. Each company provides current information regarding the recommendations and limitations of MRI scanning (Deer et al. 2017a, b). Their respective websites at www.flowonix.com and www.medtronic.com contain updated information for imaging patients with implanted targeted drug delivery systems. The pumps differ in the requirements prior to the patient undergoing an MR imaging examination. The Flowonix pump requires removing all the medication from the reservoir prior to the MRI. The scan is then performed, and the medication is placed back into the pump. The pump has a flow activation valve that limits forward flow if rapid emptying of the pump is detected. This flow activation valve is triggered by the MRI scan and needs to be reset. If the pump is not emptied, the reservoir has the potential to empty its entire contents into the intrathecal space resulting in overdose and death if the flow activation valve happens to fail. Resetting the flow activation valve is similar to a refill procedure and should occur after the patient completes the MR imaging examination. The Flowonix pump is FDA approved for MR scanning under the specific conditions of safe use in a 1.5 T magnet.

The Medtronic pump is conditionally approved for up to a 3 T magnet. The roller ball driving the pump will stop when placed in a strong magnetic field and will be temporarily stagnant. Once the patient is clear of the field, the pump will resume rotating. Motor stalls also occur frequently after MR imaging exams, and sometimes the motor stall can be prolonged. Because of this, pumps should always be interrogated after the exam to make sure it is functioning normally.

Both manufacturers recommend limiting scanning times to avoid withdrawal symptoms. For the vast majority of MR imaging scans, this will not be an issue but if a patient on moderate-to high-dose IT baclofen requires an MRI with a very long scan time, caution should be used, and the patient should be observed for signs and symptoms of baclofen withdrawal.

10 Conclusion

Intrathecal pumps provide profound pain and spasticity relief in patients that have failed more conservative treatment options. It allows the application of medications at a lower dose and with significantly less side effects and allows the delivery of medications that are limited systemically by the blood-brain barrier. This form of delivery allows more rapid titration in patients with quickly worsening disease such as with some forms of metastatic cancer. Overall, it has an incredibly low risk of opioid overdose compared to systemic opioid medications. Despite the reduced complication risk from overdose, there are possibilities for surgical complications and medication withdrawal difficulties that need to be treated in an informed manner to optimize the patient's postoperative care. The knowledge of what can happen and the best way to treat it will help the patient to benefit from this unique and highly effective therapy.

References

Abd-Elsayed A, Karri J, Michael A et al (2020) Intrathecal drug delivery for chronic pain syndromes: a review of considerations in practice management. Pain Physician 23:E591–E617

Alexander J, Solomkin J, Edwards M (2011) Updated recommendations for control of surgical site infections. Ann Surg 253:1082–1093

Bowater R, Stirling S, Lilford R (2009) Is antibiotic prophylaxis in surgery a generally effective intervention? Testing generic hypothesis over a set of meta-analyses. Ann Surg 249:551–556

Bowcock E, Morris I, Lane A (2016) Dexmedetomidine for acute clonidine withdrawal following intrathecal pump removal: a drug beginning to find its expanding niche. J Intensive Care Soc 17(3):271–272

Burgher A, Barnett C, Obray J et al (2007) Introduction of infection control measures to reduce infection associated with implantable pain therapy devices. Pain Pract 7(3):279–284

Carlson J (2020) Checklist for detecting and managing implant infection. ASRA and Pain Medicine

Deer T, Raso L, Garten T (2007) Inflammatory mass of an intrathecal catheter in patients receiving baclofen as a sole agent: a report of two cases and a review of the identification and treatment of the complication. Pain Med 8(3):259–262

Deer T, Pope J, Hayek S et al (2017a) The polyanalgesic consensus conference (PACC): guidance for improving safety and mitigating risks. Neuromodulation 20(2):155–176

Deer T, Pope J, Hayek S et al (2017b) The polyanalgesic consensus conference (PACC): recommendations on intrathecal drug infusion systems best practices and guidelines. Neuromodulation 20(2):96–132

Deer T, Lamar T, Pope J et al (2017c) The neurostimulation appropriateness consensus commit (NACC)

safety guidelines for the reduction of severe neurological injury. Neuromodulation 20(1):15–30

Delhaas E, Harhangi B, Frankema S et al (2020) Catheter access port (computed tomography) myelography in intrathecal drug delivery troubleshooting: a case series of 70 procedures. Neuromodulation 23:949–960

Döring M, Richter S, Hindrick G (2018) The diagnosis and treatment of pacemaker-associated infection. Dtsch Arztebl Int 115:445–452

Duarte R, Raphael J, Southall J et al (2013) Hypogonadism and low bone mineral density in patients on long-term intrathecal opioid delivery therapy. BMJ Open 3:e002856

Duarte R, Raphael J, Eldabe S (2016) Intrathecal drug delivery for the management of pain and spasticity in adults: an executive summary of the British Pain Society's recommendations for best clinical practice. Br J Pain 10:67–69

Engle M, Vinh B, Harun N et al (2013) Pain Physician 16:251–257

Essebag V, Verma A, Healey J et al (2016) Clinically significant pocket hematoma increases long-term risk of device infection: Bruise control infection study. J Am Coll Cardiol 67(11):1300–1308

FDA news release (2018a) FDA alerts doctors, patients about risk of complications when certain implanted pumps are used to deliver pain medications not approved for use with the devices

FDA news release (2018b) Use caution with implanted pumps for intrathecal administration of medicines for pain management: FDA safety communication

Fehlings M, Brodke D, Norvell D et al (2010) The evidence for intraoperative neurophysiological monitoring in spine surgery: does it make a difference? Spine 35(9S):S37–S46

Fitzgibbon D, Stephens L, Posner K et al (2016) Injury and liability associated with implantable devices for chronic pain. Anesthesiology 124:1384–1393

Flückiger B, Knecht H, Grossman S et al (2008) Device-related complications of long-term intrathecal drug therapy via implanted pumps. Spinal Cord 46:639–643

Follett K, Naumann C (2000) A prospective study of catheter-related complications of intrathecal drug delivery systems. J Pain Symptom Manag 19(3):209–215

Follett K, Boortz-Marx R, Drake J et al (2004) Prevention and management of intrathecal drug delivery and spinal cord stimulation system infections. Anesthesiology 100:1582–1594

Forse R, Karam B, MacLean L et al (1989) Antibiotic prophylaxis for surgery in morbidly obese patients. Surgery 106:750–756; discussion 756–757

Gonzalez A, Jeyanandarajan D, Hansen C et al (2009) Intraoperative neurophysiological monitoring during spine surgery: a review. Neurosurg Focus 27(4):E6

Grant R, Condon B, Hart I et al (1991) Changes in intracranial CSF volume after lumbar puncture and their relationship to post-LP headache. J Neurol Neurosurg Psychiatry 54:440–442

Gunn J, Gibson T, Li Z et al (2016) Symptomatic axillary seroma after sentinel lymph node biopsy: incidence and treatment. Ann Surg Oncol 23: 3347–3353

Horlocker T, Vanderdeuelen E, Kopp S et al (2018) Regional anesthesia in the patient receiving antithrombotic or thrombolytic therapy. Reg Anesth Pain Med 43:263–309

Hu K, Connelly N, Viera P (2002) Withdrawal symptoms in a patient receiving intrathecal morphine via an infusion pump. J Clin Anesth 14(8): 595–597

Hustad S, Djurhuus J, Husegard H (1985) Effect of postoperative extradural morphine on lower urinary tract function. Acta Anaesthesiol Stand 29:183

Kanj W, Flynn J, Spiegel D et al (2013) Vancomycin prophylaxis of surgical site infection in clean orthopedic surgery. Orthopedics 36(2):138–146

Katz N, Mazer N (2009) The impact of opioids on the endocrine system. Clin J Pain 25:170–117

Kratzsch T, Stienen M, Reck T et al (2015) Catheter-tip granulomas associated with intrathecal drug delivery-a two-center experience identifying 13 cases. Pain Physician 18:E831–E840

Lee H, Ruggoo V, Graudins A (2016) Intrathecal clonidine pump failure causing acute withdrawal syndrome with 'stress-induced' cardiomyopathy. J Med Toxicol 12(1):134–138

Maino P, Perez R, Koetsier E (2017) Intrathecal pump refills, pocket fills and symptoms of drug overdose: a prospective, observational study comparing the injected drug volume vs. the drug volume effectively measured inside the pump. Neuromodulation 20:733–739

Mallela A, Abdullah K, Brandon C et al (2018) Topical vancomycin reduces surgical-site infections after craniotomy: a prospective, controlled study. Neurosurgery 83(4):761–767

Molinari R, Khera O, Molinari M (2012) Prophylactic intraoperative powdered vancomycin and postoperative deep spinal wound infection: 1,512 consecutive surgical cases over a 6-year period. Eur Spine J 21(Suppl 4):S476–S482

Narouze S, Benzon H, Provenzano D et al (2018) Interventional spine and pain procedures in patients on antiplatelet and anticoagulant medications (second edition). Reg Anesth Pain Med 43:225–262

Noreika D, Fabbro E Complications of intrathecal pump therapy in malignancy-related pain. J Clin Oncol 3(26 suppl):102

Pope J, Deer T (2013) Ziconotide: a clinical update and pharmacologic review. Expert Opin Pharmacother 14:957–966

Pull ter Gunne A, Cohen D (2009) Incidence, prevalence, and analysis of risk factors for surgical site infection following adult spinal surgery. Spine 34(13):1422–1428

Ramsey C, Owen R, Witt W et al (2008) Intrathecal granuloma in a patient receiving high dose hydromorphone. Pain Physician 11(3):369–373

Rauck R, Wallace M, Leong M (2006) A randomized, double-blind, placebo-controlled study of intrathecal ziconotide in adults with severe chronic pain. J Pain Symptom Manag 31:393–406

Riordan J, Murphy P (2015) Intrathecal pump: an abrupt intermittent pump failure. Neuromodulation 18(5):433–435

Ross J, Cook A, Stewart G et al (2011) Acute intrathecal baclofen withdrawal: a brief review of treatment options. Neurocrit Care 12(1):103–108

Shields D, Palma C, Khoo L et al (2005) Extramedullary intrathecal catheter granuloma adherent to the conus medullaris presenting as cauda equina syndrome. Anesthesiology 102:1059–1061

Singh P, Jain R, Mishra S et al (2008) Management of pericatheter cerebrospinal fluid leak after intrathecal implantation of a drug delivery system. Am J Hosp Palliat Care 25(3):237–239

Skalsky A, Dalal P, Le J et al (2020) Screeing intrathecal baclofen pump systems for catheter patency via catheter access port aspiration. Neuromodulation 23(7):1003–1008

Sorensen L (2012) Wound healing and infection in surgery. The clinical impact of smoking and smoking cessation: a systematic review and meta-analysis. Arch Surg 147(4):373–383

Sridhar A, Yarlagadda V, Kanmanthareddy A et al (2016) Incidence, predictors and outcomes of hematoma after ICD implantation: an analysis of a nation-wide database of 85,276 patients. Indian Pacing Electrophysiol J 16:159–164

Staats S (2008) Complications of intrathecal therapy. Pain Med 9(S1):S102–S107

Yaksh T, Allen J, Veesart L et al (2013) Role of meningeal mast cells in intrathecal morphine-evoked granuloma formation. Anesthesiology 118:664–678

Zenz M, Piepenbrock S, Tryba M (1985) Epidural opiates: long-term experiences in cancer pain. Klin Wochenschr 63:225–229

Intrathecal Pump and Catheter Troubleshooting

Anjum Bux and Pooja Chopra

Contents

Abstract

Intrathecal drug delivery has been widely used for over four decades to treat symptoms of spasticity as well as those related to chronic malignant and nonmalignant pain. Intrathecal drug delivery systems safely and effectively deliver medication to the cerebrospinal fluid, allowing for better relief of pain or spasticity symptoms with less side effects than other routes of administration. Despite the safety of these pumps, there are complications that can occur, leading to serious morbidity and even mortality for the patient. The morbidity and mortality associated with pump therapy can result from several sources including complications from implant procedures, drug reactions or side effects, device malfunction, programming errors, or pump refill errors (Deer et al. 2012). Device registration and social security analyses from 2009 showed an intrathecal opioid mortality rate of 0.088% at 3 days after implantation, 0.39% at 1 month, and 3.89% at 1 year (Coffey et al. 2009). Physicians that are managing these pumps should be knowledgeable in the potential complications of this system and how to manage them. This chapter will focus on troubleshooting device-related complications and the appropriate management of catheter and pump-related issues.

A. Bux (✉)
Ephraim McDowell Regional Medical Center, Harrison Memorial Hospital, Danville, KY, USA

Bux Pain Management, Danville, KY, USA

P. Chopra
Henry Ford Hospital, Detroit, MI, USA

Abbreviations

CSF	Cerebrospinal fluid
IDDS	Intrathecal drug delivery system
IV	Intravenous
MRI	Magnetic resonance imaging
N-type	Neuronal type
PSI	Pound force per square inch

There are currently two commercially available intrathecal drug delivery systems on the market, the Flowonix Prometra II and the Medtronic Synchromed II (Figs. 1 and 2). Each of these pumps has a unique mechanism of delivering medication into the intrathecal space. The Prometra II is a positive pressure, valve-gated pump system that delivers medication through a precision dosing system with micro-boluses and the Synchromed II pump utilizes a low pressure,

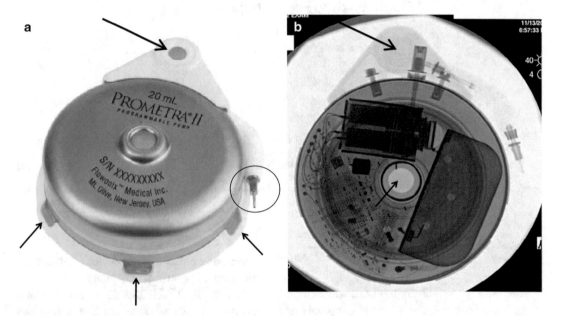

Fig. 1 The Prometra II pump by Flowonix. The external view of the pump shows the catheter access port (large black arrow in **a**) and the catheter attachment site (within black circle) as well as the loops to connect the pump to the underling fascia (smaller black arrows in **a**). An x-ray of the Prometra pump shows the catheter access port (large black arrow in **b**) as well as the refill port (smaller black arrow in **b**)

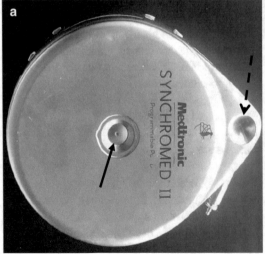
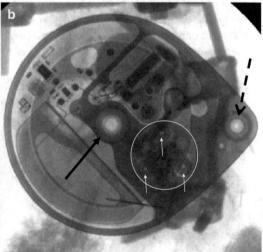

Fig. 2 (**a** and **b**) Photographic (**a**) and fluoroscopic (**b**) views of the Medtronic SynchroMed II Intrathecal Pump demonstrates the rollers (small white arrows in **b**) within the pump rotor (white circle in **b**) as well as the pump refill port (black arrows in **a** and **b**) and the catheter access port (dashed black arrows in **a** and **b**)

roller geared rotor system in which medication is delivered via a peristaltic pumping mechanism.

The Flowonix Prometra® II Pump uses a system of valves and positive pressure to regulate the flow of medication into the cerebrospinal fluid (CSF). A pressure of 22.5 PSI surrounds the reservoir (Prometra 2019). This displaces the drug from the reservoir through a filter into the precision dosing system. This system consists of an inlet valve, an accumulator, and an outlet valve (Fig. 1). The accumulator has a fixed capacity of 2–3 mcL surrounded by a pressure of 11 PSI (Prometra 2019). The pressure in the accumulator chamber ejects the medication, through the intrathecal catheter, once the outlet valve opens. After the chamber is cleared, the outlet valve closes. Immediately following this, the inlet valve opens allowing medication to refill the accumulator chamber from the reservoir. This is facilitated by the pressure of 22.5 PSI within the reservoir. Once the chamber is filled, the volume of medication remains there until the next programmed activation of valves. The flow activated valve is a safety mechanism designed to safeguard against over infusion at times such as during a magnetic resonance (MR) imaging exam. The flow activated valve has a free-floating pin that allows the drug to pass through under normal flow conditions, but if rapid flow (40 µL/s) is detected, however, the pin will close the fluid pathway, effectively stopping the flow of medication (Prometra 2019). This occurs when the inlet and outlet valve open simultaneously during exposure to magnetic fields such as those in an MRI unit. Because of the pressurized system, it has been shown that the medication effect is enhanced due to the dispersion of drug in the cerebrospinal fluid (Tangen et al. 2017). Clinical accuracy of the Prometra® II pump has been shown to be up to 97.7% and battery life is 10 years at a flow rate of 0.25 mL/day (Prometra 2019). The accuracy of the pump is independent of normal operating environmental conditions. This includes altitude, temperature, and reservoir volume, allowing people to enjoy activities such as skiing, flying, saunas, and scuba diving without any effect on the delivery of medication.

The Medtronic Synchromed II Pump (Fig. 2) consists of a roller geared rotor system in which medication is delivered through an internal catheter via a peristaltic system (Pope and Deer n.d.). It consists of a low-pressure reservoir (3−5 psi) with multiple points at which the plastic catheter tubing is occluded by rollers in order to control flow of reservoir fluid. The medication lies within the metal bellows reservoir and surrounding these bellows is pressurized gas, which exerts pressure (3–5 psi) on the bellows. Because this system relies on low pressure in the reservoir, there is a potential for variability in drug delivery especially with various environmental pressure changes including hyperbaric chambers, scuba diving, and high altitudes (Wilkes 2014). This intrathecal drug delivery system is MRI conditional for closed, open, standing, or sitting imaging systems, but the magnetic field from an MR imaging examination usually results in a motor stall. It can take several hours until the motor begins functioning again, and it is recommended that patients have their pump checked within 24 h of a MRI to confirm proper functioning and recovery from the MRI-induced motor stall. Battery life for this intrathecal drug delivery system (IDDS) will range between 5 and 7 years depending on how much medication the patient is programmed to receive each day (Pope and Deer n.d.).

Regardless of the pump system, the patient presentation is much the same in regards to device-related complications. Most of these patients initially present with loss of efficacy and increased pain or spasticity symptoms. Depending on the medication and their daily intrathecal dose, they may even present with withdrawal symptoms. Rarely, patients may present with symptoms of overmedication, which usually occurs with malfunction of the pump itself. In general, pump complications are less frequent as catheter complications are a majority of the device-related complications that occur with intrathecal drug delivery systems. In a report from Sterns and colleagues, the annual rate for device-related complications was reported to be 10.5%, with the majority being catheter-related (65%) versus pump-related (35%) (Sterns et al.

2005). These catheter-related complications can include dislodgement at the connection to the pump, kinking or fracture of the catheter, or dislodgement from the catheter anchor leading to displacement of the catheter out of the intrathecal space. If there is dislodgement of the catheter at the point of its connection to the pump, then the intrathecal medication will be deposited into the subcutaneous pocket as opposed to the intrathecal space. The patient will more than likely have a sudden increase in pain symptoms and/or withdrawal symptoms and may notice a fullness or swelling around the pump. The same symptoms of increased pain and/or withdrawal also occur if there is dislodgement of the catheter from the anchor leading to displacement of the catheter out the intrathecal space. Again, medication would be deposited in the subcutaneous tissues, thereby resulting in the patient experiencing increased pain and/or medication withdrawal. Medication is most potent when delivered into the intrathecal space, and when the catheter is malpositioned and medication is no longer being delivered to the CSF, patients are much more susceptible to experiencing withdrawal symptoms and increased pain instead of symptoms associated with overmedication.

The symptoms of overmedication commonly occur with errors in programming or in refilling the pump. Rarely these symptoms are caused by over infusion of medication because of pump malfunction.

The specific overdose and withdrawal symptoms from intrathecally delivered medications vary depending on which medication is utilized. Overdose of intrathecal baclofen can be a medical emergency and may present with drowsiness, dizziness, hypotension, hypotonia, cardiac abnormalities, and respiratory depression (Leung et al. 2006). There is no specific antidote for intrathecal baclofen overdose, but treatment consists of stopping the infusion of baclofen and supportive care until the symptoms resolve (Watve et al. 2012). Baclofen withdrawal, much like baclofen overdose, can be a medical emergency and may be life threatening. The symptoms of baclofen withdrawal usually present with increased spasticity, tachycardia, hypertension, autonomic dys-

reflexia, delirium/hallucinations, seizures, and rhabdomyolysis (Watve et al. 2012). Treatment for acute baclofen withdrawal consists of inpatient supportive care and supplementation of oral baclofen, benzodiazepines, or propofol infusion until symptoms resolve (Watve et al. 2012). In severe cases, it may be necessary to inject baclofen intrathecally or infuse it intravenously to adequately mitigate prominent withdrawal symptoms (Watve et al. 2012).

Opioid withdrawal or overmedication symptoms can also occur with complications of intrathecal drug delivery systems containing opioids. The most common symptoms of opioid overdose include somnolence, nausea, vomiting, itching, pinpoint pupils, confusion, delirium, and respiratory depression. These symptoms can be life threatening and may need to be treated in the hospital setting with IV naloxone and symptomatic management. Because of the short duration of action of IV naloxone relative to some opioids, these patients may need to be placed on a continuous infusion of naloxone and observed in the ICU until all symptoms of overmedication have resolved. Symptoms of withdrawal include agitation, restlessness, runny nose, anxiety, tachycardia, hypertension, increased pain, dilated pupils, abdominal cramping, and diarrhea. These symptoms again can be life threatening and need to be treated acutely with administration of short-acting opioids and management of symptoms with antiemetics and clonidine.

Ziconotide is the only nonnarcotic medication that is FDA approved for use in intrathecal drug delivery systems for the treatment of chronic pain. Ziconotide, as a non-opioid presynaptic N-type calcium channel blocker, has its own specific side effects related to overdose. These side effects include nausea, abdominal pain, anxiety, forgetfulness, change in speech, confusion, delusions, hallucinations, unsteadiness, nystagmus, and paranoia (Mayo Clinic drugs and supplements 2020). Interestingly, symptoms of ziconotide overdose are more related to the rate of dose increase rather than the final dose. If a patient experiences these side effects, it is recommended to reduce the dose and uptitrate more gradually, thereby contributing to the resolution of adverse effects (Mayo Clinic drugs and supplements 2020).

Bupivacaine and clonidine are also non-opioid medications that can be utilized intrathecally for the purposes of pain relief. Overdose symptoms of bupivacaine include hypotension, syncope, extreme motor and sensory neurological changes, urinary retention, and bradycardia. These symptoms are usually treated with supportive management. If the patient experiences symptoms of toxicity, then IV intralipid (a 20% intravenous fat emulsion liquid) may be administered which binds free bupivacaine and helps to reduce the symptoms of toxicity. Meanwhile, effects due to clonidine overdose include hypotension, bradycardia, drowsiness, fatigue, dizziness, and shivering (Manzon et al. 2020). Clonidine overdose symptoms are primarily treated with supportive management. Naloxone has shown some efficacy in treatment of overdose symptoms, but this treatment is controversial and continues to be debated (Manzon et al. 2020). It is equally important to recognize withdrawal symptoms for these non-opioid medications, and signs of withdrawal from bupivacaine may include increased pain, while clonidine withdrawal results in tachycardia, headache, hypertension, palpitations, nausea/vomiting, and tremors (Geyskes et al. 1979).

1 Catheter and Rotor Study

Whenever a patient presents with either a sudden increase in their pain symptoms, has a discrepancy in the amount of medication remaining in the pump at the time of refill, and/or has symptoms of overdose or withdrawal, it is prudent to check the pump and catheter for malfunction. Since most device-related complications are catheter related, checking of the catheter for patency and proper placement is the first step in troubleshooting complications of intrathecal drug delivery systems. When looking for catheter-related complications, the clinician needs to examine the catheter under fluoroscopy and perform a catheter contrast study. The Medtronic Ascenda catheter may be difficult to visualize under fluoro except for its titanium tip which can

be easily seen under fluoroscopy but is less radiopaque than barium or tungsten. The Flowonix catheter is more radiopaque and has a tungsten-coated tip making it easier to visualize under X-ray. The steps to performing a catheter contrast study in the Medtronic pump are slightly different from performing a contrast study in the Flowonix pump. When performing a catheter contrast study in the Medtronic pump, the pump is interrogated to determine the reservoir volume, medication dose, and concentration, and then the patient is placed under fluoroscopy to visualize the pump and tip of the catheter. It is important to visualize the tip of the catheter in the intrathecal space to confirm proper placement. After the pump and catheter are visualized under fluoro, the catheter access port of the pump is accessed with a 25-G needle provided in the Medtronic catheter access kit. After accessing the catheter access port, it is important to remove approximately 1–2 mL of medication and CSF from the catheter before attempting to inject contrast to visualize the catheter. While injecting nonionic contrast that is compatible for intrathecal use, it is important to visualize the entire catheter as it exits from the pump and travels to the intrathecal space. While visualizing the catheter, it is critical to note any extravasation of contrast indicating the possibility of a catheter fracture, disruption, or malposition. It is also important to observe contrast coming out of the tip of the catheter with spread throughout the intrathecal space while documenting placement of the tip in compared to the initial placement to check for migration of the catheter.

The Flowonix pump catheter contrast study is very similar to the procedure for the Medtronic pump, except that a larger 20-G specialized needle with a side port is used to access the catheter access port. This specialized needle is provided in the Flowonix catheter access kit. Again it is important to withdraw approximately 1–2 mL of medication and CSF from the catheter access port before injecting any contrast. Also, when injecting contrast, it is important to visualize the entire catheter from the pump to the intrathecal space to confirm catheter tip position and patency of the intrathecal catheter. Any extravasation of contrast could indicate possible fracture, disruption, or malposition of the catheter.

When performing a catheter contrast study in either pump, if the catheter is intact and patent, it is typical that the practitioner will be able to aspirate more than 1 ml of medication and CSF from the catheter access port. If this is accomplished, then it is safe to say that the catheter is within the intrathecal space. However, if medication and CSF cannot be extracted from the catheter access port, catheter dislodgement or disruption should be suspected, and the patient should be scheduled for a catheter revision. Moreover, if medication and CSF are unable to be withdrawn from the catheter access port, then it should be noted that injecting contrast will result in an inadvertent intrathecal bolus administration of medication to the patient when the catheter contents are flushed through the catheter by the contrast. This could be clinically detrimental depending on the concentration of medication that is present in the catheter. It is left up to the clinician to decide whether it is safe for the patient to receive a bolus of medication through the catheter or not. If catheter issues are suspected as the result of a failed intrathecal catheter contrast study, then consideration should be given to revision or replacement of the intrathecal catheter as soon as possible while providing replacement therapy to the patient with oral or IV medication.

Another potential catheter complication that may prevent withdrawal of medication or CSF from the catheter access port includes granuloma formation around the tip of the intrathecal catheter. A granuloma is the result of an inflammatory reaction with histologic findings of granuloma tissue formed by histiocytes and granulocytes usually with necrotic areas and hemorrhagic residues. These granulomas are typically seen forming a mass around the tip of the catheter. This inflammatory reaction is usually caused by pooling of highly concentrated medication around the tip of the catheter. If these masses become large enough, they may impinge on the spinal cord, conus medularis, or cauda equina depending on the catheter tip location and result in sudden increases in pain along with neurological changes that may be irreversible. Patients who have been diagnosed with intrathecal catheter tip granuloma formation typically present with sudden worsening pain, bowel and bladder dysfunction, and sensory and/or motor deficits (Deer et al. 2017). Granuloma formation can potentially occur with any intrathecal medication, but historically it has been associated with highly concentrated morphine and hydromorphone. The incidence of granuloma formation ranges from 0.04% at 1 year up to 1.15% at 6 years although reports of these rates are variable (Follett 2003). Despite the low incidence of this complication, it is prudent to do an appropriate workup if a catheter tip granuloma is suspected because of its detrimental consequences if left undiagnosed. Anytime a patient presents with a sudden increase in pain or a change in neurological status, a thorough history and physical including a neurological exam should be performed and followed by a contrast-enhanced MRI or a CT myelogram to rule out granuloma. If a granuloma is diagnosed, it may be prudent to consult neurosurgery to urgently explant the intrathecal catheter to minimize risk of permanent neurological damage.

If the catheter contrast study is successful and catheter complications have been ruled out, then we turn toward troubleshooting possible pump malfunction. In general, pump malfunctions or pump failures occur rarely, but, if suspected, it is prudent to access the reservoir to compare the actual (measured) volume to expected or predicted volume based on the previous pump volume, the medication concentration, and the daily dose. A volume discrepancy outside the labeled accuracy specification for each specific pump, either too large or too small of an infused volume, may suggest a pump malfunction (Wesemann et al. 2014). The volume discrepancies that may indicate malfunction are usually greater than 5–10%.

In the Medtronic Synchromed II pump, the etiology of a malfunction is typically due to a motor stall or issues of over- or under-infusion. Motor stalls that occur spontaneously have been documented to occur at the rate of 2.4% with use of on-label medications and up to 7% with the use of non-FDA-approved off-label medications (Riordan and Murphy 2015). Additionally, cases of over- and under-infusion have been documented and reported, but in a study of 82 subjects done by Coffey et al., it was found that the Medtronic Synchromed II pump accurately and safely delivered intrathecal medications with small variances (less than 1–2%) in infusion (Wesemann et al. 2014).

As part of troubleshooting the pump, it is necessary to interrogate it using the clinician programmer. The information that is obtained includes the pump function logs that show any pump errors, stalls, or malfunctions. If the pump interrogation is done first, after checking the pump logs, the catheter access port should be accessed to aspirate approximately 1–2 mL of medication and CSF from the catheter. The catheter aspiration should be done before performing a rotor movement study as—during a rotor study, the patient will receive a bolus of 0.01 mL over 1 min. If CSF is able to be aspirated into the catheter, the bolus will be the patient's own CSF, but if aspiration is not possible, the patient may receive a bolus of the contents of the catheter which includes the intrathecal medication. This bolus could be significant for the patient depend-

ing on concentration and volume of medicine in the catheter. As demonstrated in Fig. 3, the pump rotor needs to be visualized under fluoroscopy and the roller arm with the radiopaque tungsten marker needs to be identified as a reference point (Figs. 3 and 4). At that point, the pump is programmed to conduct a rotor study bolus. After waiting 2 min to allow the rotor study bolus to be completed, a new image is taken to analyze movement of the rotor arms and rollers. The entire three roller pump mechanisms should have moved counterclockwise approximately 60° from its previous position (Figs. 4 and 5). Failure of movement of the pump rotor during the rotor study bolus indicates pump failure. If the rotor has stalled, the pump needs to be replaced and the patient is provided with replacement oral or IV medication until the pump is replaced.

The Flowonix Prometra pump does not have a rotor and roller pumping mechanism but rather a series of valves and positive pressure to regulate the flow of medication into the CSF. When troubleshooting the Flowonix pump, again it is prudent to interrogate the pump and run the logs to identify any errors or pump malfunction. Since

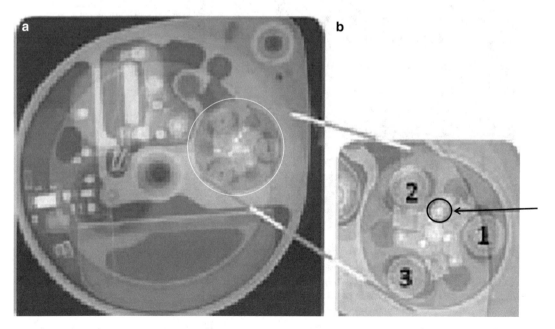

Fig. 3 An x-ray image of the Medtronic Synchromed II pump shows the circular rotor (white circle in **a**). The magnified view (**b**) shows the rollers (numbered 1, 2, and 3 in **b**) and the radiopaque markers (one marker is shown within the black circle indicated by the arrow in **b**) on the roller arms

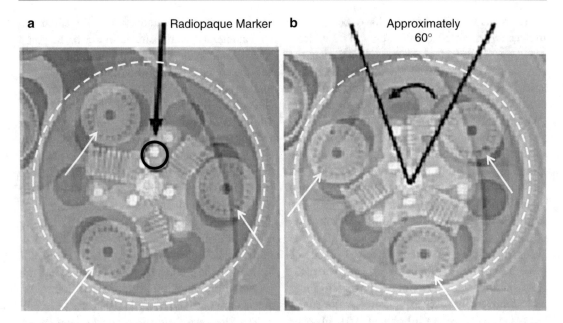

Fig. 4 An x-ray image of the Medtronic Synchromed II pump with a magnified view of the circular rotor (white dashed circle in **a** and **b**) shows the radiopaque markers on the roller arms (one marker is shown within the black circle indicated by the arrow in **a**). During the rapid bolus the rotor arms move counterclockwise and are see to move approximately 60° from the original position of the rotor arm seen in a to the final position as is indicated by the angle in (**b**)

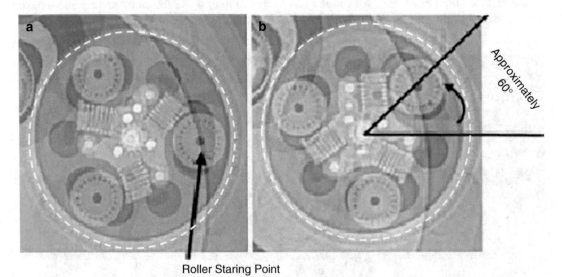

Fig. 5 An x-ray image of the Medtronic Synchromed II pump with a magnified view of the circular rotor (white dashed circle in **a** and **b**) shows the roller on the right side of the pump starting out at the 3 o'clock position (black arrow indicating starting position in **a**) and rotates approximately 60° (angle and degree of movement shown in **b**) during a rapid bolus with the rotors moving counterclockwise

the pump does not have a motor or any rollers to follow, one way to assess proper functioning of the Flowonix pump is to run a bolus while contrast is in the catheter and watch under live fluoro as the contrast is expelled from the tip of the catheter. Additionally, a stethoscope can be used to listen to the opening and closing of the inlet and outlet valves as identified by clicking sounds as the valves open and close during a bolus. If there are no clicking sounds identified or the bolus through the catheter does not show contrast expelled from the tip of the catheter, then pump failure should be considered. If there is failure of the intrathecal pump, it should be replaced, and the patient should be provided with replacement oral or IV medication until replacement takes place.

2   Conclusion

Intrathecal drug delivery systems are very safe, and with increased utilization, there will be more patients treated safely while improving their symptoms of pain and spasticity. Physicians managing these systems must be knowledgeable in identifying and troubleshooting potential complications as it can lead to serious morbidity and even mortality for patients. Complications may arise from various origins including those secondary to implant procedures, medication reactions or side effects, device malfunction, programming errors, or refill errors (Deer et al. 2012). When a patient presents with symptoms of increased pain and/or withdrawal or overmedication, being familiar with pump mechanics and a problem-solving algorithm (Fig. 6) will help to systematically rule out possible causes (Rez 2017). Once the pump and/or catheter have been identified as the source of the difficulty, early troubleshooting can minimize harm to the patient by allowing for early identification of the problem

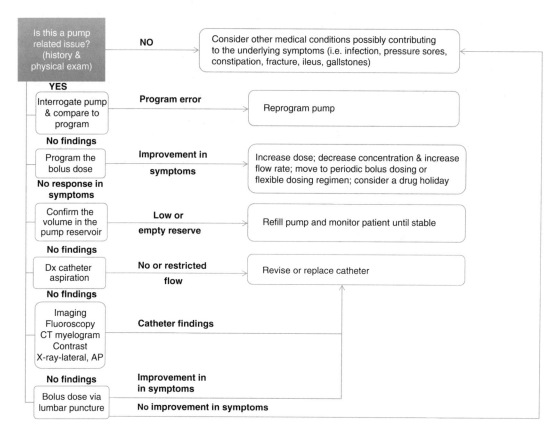

Fig. 6 Loss of intrathecal pump efficacy troubleshooting algorithm. *Dx* diagnostic, *AP* anterior-posterior, *CT* computed Tomography (Adapted from: Farid R. Problem- Solving in Patients with Targeted Drug Delivery Systems. *Mo Med.* 2017;114(1):52–56)

and execution of optimal management strategies. Although catheter and pump issues are not a common occurrence, vigilance in identifying and managing these complications will minimize untoward outcomes for these patients and will help to promote the safety and efficacy of this therapy.

References

Coffey RJ, Owens ML, Broste SK, Dubois MY, Ferrante FM, Schultz DM, Stearns LJ, Turner MS (2009) Mortality associated with implantation and management of intrathecal opioid drug infusion systems to treat noncancer pain. Anesthesiology 111:881–891

Deer TR, Levy R, Prager J, Buchser E, Burton A, Caraway D, Cousins M, De Andrés J, Diwan S, Erdek M, Grigsby E, Huntoon M, Jacobs MS, Kim P, Kumar K, Leong M, Liem L, McDowell GC II, Panchal S, Rauck R, Saulino M, Sitzman BT, Staats P, Stanton-Hicks M, Stearns L, Wallace M, Willis KD, Witt W, Yaksh T, Mekhail N (2012) Polyanalgesic consensus conference—2012: recommendations to reduce morbidity and mortality in intrathecal drug delivery in the treatment of chronic pain. Neuromodulation 15:467–482

Deer TR, Pope JE, Hayek SM, Lamer TJ, Veizi IE, Erdek M, Wallace MS, Grider JS, Levy RM, Prager J, Rosen SM, Saulino M, Yaksh TL, De Andrés JA, Abejon Gonzalez D, Vesper J, Schu S, Simpson B, Mekhail N (2017) The polyanalgesic consensus conference (PACC): recommendations for intrathecal drug delivery: guidance for improving safety and mitigating risks. Neuromodulation 20(2):155–176. https://doi.org/10.1111/ner.12579. Epub 2017 Jan 2. PMID: 28042914

Follett KS (2003) Intrathecal analgesia and catheter-tip inflammatory mass. Anesthesiology 99:5–6

Geyskes GG, Boer P, Dorhout Mees EJ (1979) Clonidine withdrawal. Mechanism and frequency of rebound hypertension. Br J Clin Pharmacol 7(1):55–62

Leung NY, Whyte IM, Isbister GK (2006) Baclofen overdose: defining the spectrum of toxicity. Emerg Med Australas 18:77–82

Manzon L, Nappe TM, Delmaestro C, et al. (2020) Clonidine toxicity. [Updated 2020 Jun 30]. In: StatPearls [Internet]. StatPearls Publishing, Treasure Island

Mayo Clinic drugs and supplements (2020) Ziconotide (intrathecal route)

Pope J, Deer T (n.d.) Intrathecal drug delivery: available technologies. In: Treatment of chronic pain conditions: a comprehensive handbook, pp 191–192

Prometra II (2019) Programmable pump instructions for use. https://flowonix.com/sites/default/files/pl-21611-00-prometra_ii_programmable_pump_ifu_us_commercial.pdf. Accessed 22 Mar 2019

Rez F (2017) Problem solving in patients with targeted drug delivery systems. Mo Med 114(1):52–56

Riordan J, Murphy P (2015) Intrathecal pump: an abrupt intermittent pump failure. Neuromodulation 18:433–435

Sterns L, Boortz-Marx R, Du Pen S, Friehs G, Gordon M, Halyard Herbst L, Kiser J (2005) Intrathecal drug delivery for the management of cancer pain: a multidisciplinary consensus of best practices. J Support Oncol 3(6):399–408

Tangen KM, Leval R, Mehta AI, Linninger AA (2017) Computational and in vitro experimental investigation of intrathecal drug distribution: parametric study of the effect of injection volume, cerebrospinal fluid pulsatility, and drug uptake. Anesth Analg 124:1686–1696

Watve SV, Sivan M, Raza WA, Jamil FF (2012) Management of acute overdose or withdrawal state in intrathecal baclofen therapy. Spinal Cord 50:107–111

Wesemann K, Coffey RJ, Wallace MS, Tan Y, Broste S, Buvanendran A (2014) Clinical accuracy and safety using the synchromed II intrathecal drug infusion pump. Reg Anesth Pain Med 39(4):341–346

Wilkes D (2014) Programmable intrathecal pumps for the management of chronic pain: recommendations for improved efficiency. J Pain Res 7:571–577

Current Intrathecal Pump Costs, Coding, and Reimbursement

Clarisse F. San Juan and Amitabh Gulati

Contents

Abstract

Intrathecal drug delivery systems (IDDS) have evolved to become an important component in the management of chronic pain. Substantial costs are incurred with IDDS at the time of surgical implantation, pump or catheter revision, or at the event of any complications, but studies have shown that it decreases overall health utilization and is cost-effective compared to conventional medical management. This chapter compares the costs of IDDS to other interventional procedures based on the 2019 CPT codes and Medicare Physician Payment Schedule payment information and reviews the data on cost-effectiveness of IDDS.

C. F. San Juan (✉)
Physical Medicine and Rehabilitation, SUNY
Downstate Medical Center, Brooklyn, NY, USA

A. Gulati
Memorial Sloan Kettering Cancer Center,
New York, NY, USA
e-mail: Gulatia@mskcc.org

D. P. Beall et al. (eds.), *Intrathecal Pump Drug Delivery*, Medical Radiology Diagnostic Imaging,
https://doi.org/10.1007/978-3-030-86244-2_11

Abbreviations

CMM   Conventional medical management
IDD   Intrathecal drug delivery
IDDS   Intrathecal drug delivery system

1   Introduction

Management of chronic pain with an intrathecal pump incurs an upfront cost for pump and catheter placement as it requires surgical implantation. Additional costs are incurred at the time of revision when the batteries are at the end of life (Bolash et al. 2015). Expected battery life varies per device and ranges anywhere from 3–10 years (Bolash et al. 2015). One study conducted in 2015 looking at the longevity and cost of IDDS had a median longevity of 5.9 years for pumps explanted at the end of battery life and a median cost per day of $9.26 (Bolash et al. 2015). The cost per day goes up to $44.59 per day for premature explantations due to other complications (Bolash et al. 2015). These costs were calculated based on the 2013 fee schedule of the Centers for Medicare & Medicaid Services and do not include the pump refills, intrathecal medication costs, or the savings due to decreased utilization of other medical services (Bolash et al. 2015).

2   Intrathecal Drug Delivery Versus Conventional Pain Therapy: Evidence-Based Approach to the Cost-Effectiveness of Intrathecal Drug Therapy

Although IDDS have a larger upfront cost, patients with IDD for cancer and noncancer pain have decreased medical utilization post-implant. A 2013 study looking at the cost projections over 30 years of IDD used for noncancer pain showed lower costs compared to conventional pain therapy, with financial breakeven occurring 2 years post-implant, and a lifetime analysis savings of $3111 per patient per year compared to conventional pain therapy (Guillemette et al. 2013).

A critical point of emphasis to consider when comparing the cost of IDDS to conventional medical management (CMM) is the assumption that the more effective delivery of the drug allowed for the elimination or near elimination of systemic medications like transdermal or oral opioids. A 2016 study on IDD for cancer patients resulted in a $3195 total cost savings when considering the costs of IDDS medications, implants, and pharmacy charges when compared to CMM over a 1-year duration post-implant (Stearns et al. 2016). This study also showed that the point where IDD began to show cost-effectiveness when compared to high cost CMM was between 7 and 8 months (Fig. 1).

A later study by Stearns et al. evaluated the healthcare costs for pain relief in patients with cancer-related pain that were treated with CMM alone as compared to those patients that were treated with IDD and CMM (Stearns et al. 2019). This consisted of an evaluation of insurance claims data for 536 patients that were evaluated retrospectively using a propensity score-matched analysis. The authors found that the use of IDD and CMM was associated with a significant cost savings of $15,142 ($p = 0.01$) at 2 months and $63,498 ($p = 0.03$) at 12 months and concluded that IDD is cost saving and should be considered in patients with cancer pain for whom CMM is inadequate or produces untenable side effects (Fig. 2). The authors also concluded that IDD should be expanded as healthcare systems transition to value-based models (Stearns et al. 2019). When expanding the usage or the indications for IDD, cost-effectiveness must be kept in mind along with the other options for patient treatment as well as the patient's indication for treatment. These indications will vary far beyond just whether the patient has cancer or noncancer-related pain, and the use of IDD must be compared to the advantages and disadvantages and

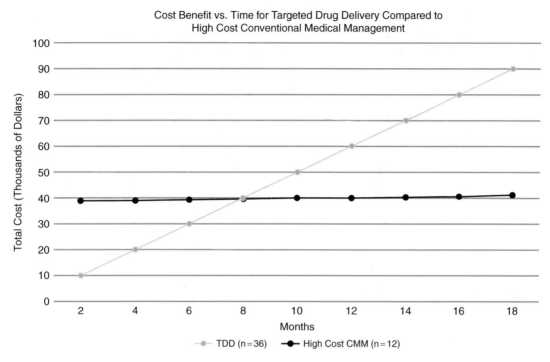

Fig. 1 Line graph showing the cost benefit over time for Targeted Drug Delivery (TDD) (black line) as compared to high cost Conventional Medical Management (CMM) (gray line). The crossover time point where the TDD began to show better cost effectiveness than CMM was between 7 and 8 months

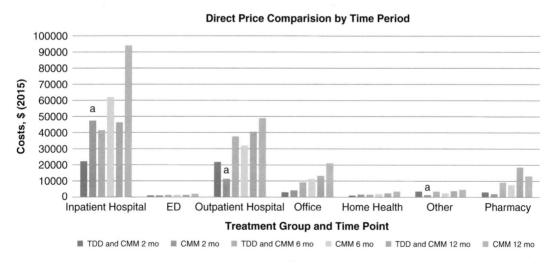

Fig. 2 Costs for Targeted Drug Delivery (TDD) and Conventional Medical Management (CMM) Group as compared to the CMM Only Group. *ED* Emergency Department, *IP* Inpatient, *OP* Outpatient. [a]Statistically significant differences for TDD and CMM compared with CMM. (Adapted from: Stearns LJ, Narang S, Albright RE, Jr, et al. Assessment of health care utilization and cost of targeted drug delivery and conventional medical management vs conventional medical management alone for patients with cancer-related pain. JAMA Netw Open. 2019;2:e191549)

costs of other treatment types. In the next section, the process of patient selection will be discussed, and the costs of various treatment types will also be presented.

2.1 Patient Selection for IT Therapy

Earlier utilization of IDD earlier in the treatment algorithm has been discussed earlier in chapter "Intrathecal Pump Management". This has been both cost-effective and efficacious

when used in this manner rather than using it only as a salvage therapy (Pope et al. 2015). Intrathecal therapy is most often used after other modalities have failed, but, as we have seen in chapters "Targeted Drug Delivery Perioperative Planning Considerations" and "Intrathecal Pump Management", there are algorithmic recommendations from the Polyanalgesic Consensus Conference (PACC) for the use of IDD in patients with refractory pain either due to cancer or nonneoplastic causes (Figs. 3 and 4) (Deer et al. 2017) (Tables 1, 2, 3, 4, 5, 6, and 7).

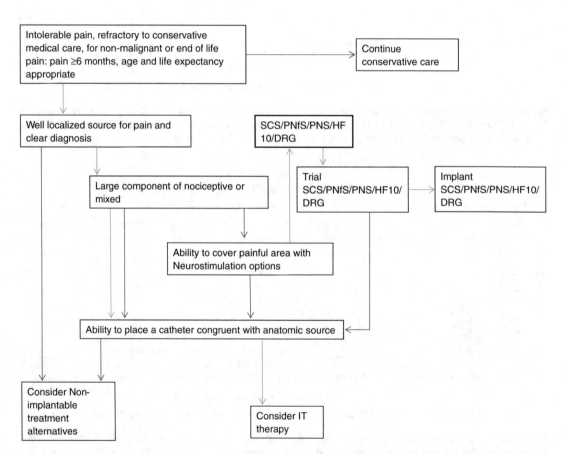

Fig. 3 Algorithm for device placement within the pain care algorithm for non-cancer patients or patients with pain not at the end of life. *DRG* dorsal root ganglion, *HF10* high frequency stimulation, *PNfS* peripheral nerve field stimulation, *PNS* peripheral nerve stimulation, *SCS* spinal cord stimulation. Blue arrows indicate an affirmation or positive response; red arrows signify a negative response. (Adapted from: Deer TR, Pope JE, Hayek SM, Bux A, Buchser E, Eldabe S et al. The Polyanalgesic Consensus Conference (PACC): Recommendations on Intrathecal Drug Infusion Systems Best Practices and Guidelines. Neuromodulation. 2017;20(2):96–132. https://doi.org/10.1111/ner.12538)

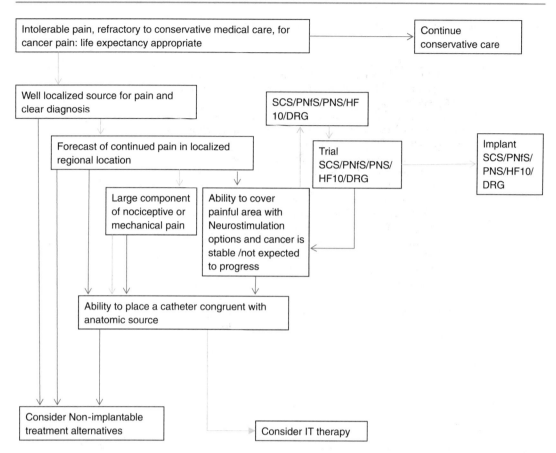

Fig. 4 Algorithm for cancer-related pain. *DRG* dorsal root ganglion, *HF10* high frequency stimulation, *PNfS* peripheral nerve field stimulation, *PNS* peripheral nerve stimulation, *SCS* spinal cord stimulation. Blue arrows indicate an affirmation or positive response; red arrows signify a negative response. (Adapted from: Deer TR, Pope JE, Hayek SM, Bux A, Buchser E, Eldabe S et al. The Polyanalgesic Consensus Conference (PACC): Recommendations on Intrathecal Drug Infusion Systems Best Practices and Guidelines. Neuromodulation. 2017;20(2):96–132. https://doi.org/10.1111/ner.12538)

As shown in Figs. 3 and 4, IDD is considered after neuromodulation. Although neuromodulation has been shown in multiple trials to be safe and effective (North et al. 2005; Kumar et al. 2007; Kumar et al. 2006), this effectiveness may wane over time with the patient becoming tolerant to neurostimulation (Kumar et al. 2006), and IDD may need to be applied. Intrathecal therapy has been shown to be durable but is more costly over time given the additional patient visits for pump refills, dose adjustments, and catheter and rotor studies and is more time intensive for the clinician managing this therapy given these additional visits. As discussed in this chapter, there are reimbursements associated with nearly everything that is done related in IDD pump management, and although the therapy is more time intensive than many other treatments, the overall reimbursements can be greater than for typical interventional pain management procedures (Table 8) and for neuromodulation (Table 9).

Table 1 CPT codes applicable to intrathecal drug delivery systems

CPT code	Description	Medicare payment	
		Non facility	Facility
62362	Implantation or replacement of device for intrathecal or epidural drug infusion; programmable pump, including preparation of pump, with or without programming		
62350	Implantation, revision, or repositioning of tunneled intrathecal or epidural catheter, for long-term medication administration via an external pump or implantable reservoir/infusion pump; without laminectomy	NA	414.45
62362	Implantation or replacement of device for intrathecal or epidural drug infusion; programmable pump, including preparation of pump, with or without programming	NA	397.87
62367	Electronic analysis of programmable, implanted pump for intrathecal or epidural drug infusion (includes evaluation of reservoir status, alarm status, drug prescription status); without reprogramming or refill	41.08	25.95
62368	Electronic analysis of programmable, implanted pump for intrathecal or epidural drug infusion (includes evaluation of reservoir status, alarm status, drug prescription status); with reprogramming	56.58	36.40
62369	Electronic analysis of programmable, implanted pump for intrathecal or epidural drug infusion (includes evaluation of reservoir status, alarm status, drug prescription status); with reprogramming and refill	120.37	36.40
62370	Electronic analysis of programmable, implanted pump for intrathecal or epidural drug infusion (includes evaluation of reservoir status, alarm status, drug prescription status); with reprogramming and refill (requiring skill of a physician or other qualified health care professional)	125.06	47.93

Table 2 CPT codes applicable to epidural spinal injections

Code	Description	Medicare payment	
		Non-facility	Facility
62320	Injection(s), of diagnostic or therapeutic substance(s) (e.g., anesthetic, antispasmodic, opioid, steroid, other solution), not including neurolytic substances, including needle or catheter placement, interlaminar epidural or subarachnoid, cervical or thoracic, *WITHOUT IMAGING GUIDANCE* (previous code—62310)	168.66	102.71
62321	62320 WITH IMAGING GUIDANCE (i.e., fluoroscopy or CT)	259.12	110.64
62322	Injection(s), of diagnostic or therapeutic substance(s) (e.g., anesthetic, antispasmodic, opioid, steroid, other solution), not including neurolytic substances, including needle or catheter placement, interlaminar epidural or subarachnoid, lumbar or sacral (caudal), *WITHOUT IMAGING GUIDANCE* (previous code **62311**)	157.13	88.66
62323	62322 WITH IMAGING GUIDANCE (i.e., fluoroscopy or CT)	256.24	102.35
62324	Injection, including indwelling catheter placement, continuous infusion or intermittent bolus, of diagnostic or therapeutic substance(s) (e.g., anesthetic, antispasmodic, opioid, steroid, other solution), not including neurolytic substances, interlaminar epidural or subarachnoid, cervical or thoracic, *WITHOUT IMAGING GUIDANCE* (previous code 62318)	148.48	93.7
62325	WITH IMAGING GUIDANCE (i.e., fluoroscopy or CT)	240.38	111.0
62326	Injection, including indwelling catheter placement, continuous infusion or intermittent bolus, of diagnostic or therapeutic substance(s) (e.g., anesthetic, antispasmodic, opioid, steroid, other solution), not including neurolytic substances, interlaminar epidural or subarachnoid, lumbar or sacral (caudal), *WITHOUT IMAGING GUIDANCE* (previous code 62319)	154.25	92.26
62327	62326 WITH IMAGING GUIDANCE (i.e., fluoroscopy or CT)	241.1	100.19

Table 3 CPT codes applicable to trigger point injections

Code	Description	Medicare payment	
		Non-facility	Facility
20550	Injection(s); single tendon sheath, or ligament, aponeurosis (e.g., plantar "fascia")	54.42	40.72
20551	Injection(s); single tendon origin/insertion	55.14	41.44
20552	Injection(s); single or multiple trigger point(s), 1 or 2 muscle(s)	56.58	39.28
20553	Injection(s); single or multiple trigger point(s), 3 or more muscles	65.23	44.69

Table 4 CPT codes applicable to transforaminal epidural injections

Code	Description	Medicare payment	
		Non-facility	Facility
64480	Injection(s), anesthetic agent, and/or steroid, transforaminal epidural, with imaging guidance (fluoroscopy or CT); cervical or thoracic, each additional level (list separately in addition to code for primary procedure)		
64479	Injection(s), anesthetic agent, and/or steroid, transforaminal epidural, with imaging guidance (fluoroscopy or CT); cervical or thoracic, single level	250.47	135.51
64480	Injection(s), anesthetic agent, and/or steroid, transforaminal epidural, with imaging guidance (fluoroscopy or CT); cervical or thoracic, each additional level (list separately in addition to code for primary procedure)	123.25	64.87
64483	Injection(s), anesthetic agent, and/or steroid, transforaminal epidural, with imaging guidance (fluoroscopy or CT); lumbar or sacral, single level	232.09	114.96

Table 5 CPT codes applicable to facet joint injections

Code	Description	Medicare payment	
		Non-facility	Facility
64490	Injection(s), diagnostic or therapeutic agent, paravertebral facet (zygapophyseal) joint (or nerves innervating that joint) with image guidance (fluoroscopy or CT), cervical or thoracic; single level	194.25	109.2
64491	Injection(s), diagnostic or therapeutic agent, paravertebral facet (zygapophyseal) joint (or nerves innervating that joint) with image guidance (fluoroscopy or CT), cervical or thoracic; second level (list separately in addition to code for primary procedure)	96.58	61.99
64493	Injection(s), diagnostic or therapeutic agent, paravertebral facet (zygapophyseal) joint (or nerves innervating that joint) with image guidance (fluoroscopy or CT), lumbar or sacral; single level	176.95	92.98
64494	Injection(s), diagnostic or therapeutic agent, paravertebral facet (zygapophyseal) joint (or nerves innervating that joint) with image guidance (fluoroscopy or CT), lumbar or sacral; second level (list separately in addition to code for primary procedure)	89.74	53.7
64495	Injection(s), diagnostic or therapeutic agent, paravertebral facet (zygapophyseal) joint (or nerves innervating that joint) with image guidance (fluoroscopy or CT), lumbar or sacral; third and any additional level(s) (list separately in addition to code for primary procedure)	89.74	54.42

Table 6 CPT codes applicable to radiofrequency ablations

Code	Description	Medicare payment	
		Non-facility	Facility
64634			
64633	Destruction by neurolytic agent, paravertebral facet joint nerve(s), with imaging guidance (fluoroscopy or CT); cervical or thoracic, single facet joint	428.5	231.73
64634	Destruction by neurolytic agent, paravertebral facet joint nerve(s), with imaging guidance (fluoroscopy or CT); cervical or thoracic, each additional facet joint (list separately in addition to code for primary procedure)	192.45	70.28
64635	Destruction by neurolytic agent, paravertebral facet joint nerve(s), with imaging guidance (fluoroscopy or CT); lumbar or sacral, single facet joint	423.82	228.49
64636	Destruction by neurolytic agent, paravertebral facet joint nerve(s), with imaging guidance (fluoroscopy or CT); lumbar or sacral, each additional facet joint (list separately in addition to code for primary procedure)	174.79	61.63
64999[a]	Unlisted procedure, nervous system	0.0	0.0
77003	Fluoroscopic guidance and localization of needle or catheter tip for spine or paraspinous diagnostic or therapeutic injection procedures (epidural or subarachnoid) (list separately in addition to code for primary procedure)	99.83	NA

[a]64999 is used for pulsed radiofrequency ablation

Table 7 CPT codes applicable to spinal cord stimulators

Code	Description	Medicare payment	
		Non-facility	Facility
63650	Percutaneous implantation of neurostimulator electrode array, epidural	1657.08	425.98
63655	Laminectomy for implantation of neurostimulator electrodes, plate/paddle, epidural	NA	868.54
63685	Insertion or replacement of spinal neurostimulator pulse generator or receiver, direct or inductive coupling	NA	374.81
63688	Revision or removal of implanted spinal neurostimulator pulse generator or receiver	NA	386.7
95970	Electronic analysis of implanted neurostimulator pulse generator/transmitter (e.g., contact group[s], interleaving, amplitude, pulse width, frequency [Hz], on/off cycling, burst, magnet mode, dose lockout, patient selectable parameters, responsive neurostimulation, detection algorithms, closed-loop parameters, and passive parameters) by physician or other qualified healthcare professional; with brain, cranial nerve, spinal cord, peripheral nerve, or sacral nerve, neurostimulator pulse generator/transmitter, without programming	19.46	19.10
95971	Electronic analysis of implanted neurostimulator pulse generator/transmitter (e.g., contact group[s], interleaving, amplitude, pulse width, frequency [Hz], on/off cycling, burst, magnet mode, dose lockout, patient selectable parameters, responsive neurostimulation, detection algorithms, closed-loop parameters, and passive parameters) by physician or other qualified healthcare professional; with simple spinal cord or peripheral nerve (e.g., sacral nerve) neurostimulator pulse generator/transmitter programming by physician or other qualified healthcare professional	51.90	42.17
95972	Electronic analysis of implanted neurostimulator pulse generator/transmitter (e.g., contact group[s], interleaving, amplitude, pulse width, frequency [Hz], on/off cycling, burst, magnet mode, dose lockout, patient selectable parameters, responsive neurostimulation, detection algorithms, closed-loop parameters, and passive parameters) by physician or other qualified healthcare professional; with complex spinal cord or peripheral nerve (e.g., sacral nerve) neurostimulator pulse generator/transmitter programming by physician or other qualified healthcare professional	58.38	42.89

Table 8 Comparison reimbursements of typical interventional pain management procedures versus that of intrathecal drug delivery system placement and ongoing management

Interventional pain procedure	Annual reimbursement per patient
Pump and catheter implantation (CPT 62350, 62362) $397.87 + $414.45 *Reprogramming and refills* (CPT 62370, 6 refills/year): Min: In facility = $47.93 × 6 refills/year Max: Non-facility participating provider = $125.06 × 6 refills/year Year 1: *Pump and catheter implantation + reprogramming and refills* Years 2–7: *Reprogramming and refills only*	$812.32 (year 1 only) $287.58–$750.36 Total reimbursement Year 1: **$1099.90–$1562.68/year** Total reimbursement years 2–7: **$287.58–$750.36/year** **7-year annual average: $198.21–$330.43/year**
Trigger point injections (CPT 20551, 3 injections/year): Facility: $41.44 × 3 injections/year Non-facility: $55.14	$124.32–$155.42
Lumbar ESI (CPT 62323, 3 injections/year): Facility: $102.35 × 3 injections/year Non-facility: $256.24	$307.05–$768.72
Cervical ESI (CPT 62325, 3 injections/year): Facility: $111 × 3 injections/year Non-facility: $240.38	$333–$721.14
Lumbar transforaminal (CPT 64483, 3 injections/year) Facility: $114.96 × 3 injections/year Non-facility: $232.09	$344.88–$696.27
Cervical transforaminal (CPT 64479, 3 injections/year) Facility: $135.51 × 3 injections/year Non-facility: $250.47	$406.53–$751.41
Lumbar facet joint injection (CPT 64493, 3 injections/year) Facility: $92.98 × 3 injections/year Non-facility: $176.95	$278.94–$530.85
Cervical facet joint injection (64490, 3 injections/year) Facility: $109.2 × 3 injections/year Non-facility: $194.25	$327.6–$582.75
Lumbar RFA (64635, 2/year) Facility: $228.49 × 2/year Non-facility: $423.82	$456.98–$847.64
Cervical RFA (64633, 2/year) Facility: $231.73 × 2/year Non-facility: $428.50	$463.46–$857

Table 9 Reimbursement comparison for intrathecal drug delivery versus neuromodulation

Intrathecal drug delivery	Neuromodulation
(Calculations taken from Table 11.3.1) **Year 1:** $1099.9–$1562.68 **Year 2–7:** $287.58–$750.36 **7-year total: $2825.38–$6064.84**	DCS implantation (percutaneous leads, 63650): $425.98 DCS implantation (laminectomy, 63655): 868.54 Quarterly reprogramming (95972): $42.89 **Year 1:** $597.54–$1040.10 **Year 2–10**: $42.89 × 4 = $171.56/year **7-year total: $1626.90–$2069.46**

3   2019 Current Procedural Terminology (CPT) Codes and Medicare Physician Payment Schedule Payment Information

The figures presented below are for informational purposes and are based on 2019 CPT codes and Medicare Physician Payment Schedule payment data. Medicare payments for facility include hospitals (inpatient, outpatient, and emergency department), ambulatory surgical centers, and skilled nursing facilities. Medicare payments for non-facility include all other settings. The following information was taken from the American Medical Association (AMA) Medicare Payment Search, and the tables below show the AMA National average payment.

The following lists of CPT Codes are for references purposes only and may not be all inclusive.

4   Comparison of Reimbursements for IDD Versus Other Interventional Pain Procedures

4.1   Annual Reimbursement Per Patient for Interventional Pain Procedures

The following calculations seen in Table 8 are just examples of typical reimbursements seen for IDD treatment as compared to typical interventional pain management procedures. The injection reimbursements are based on performing the procedure on a single level for ESI and TFESI and for a single facet joint only.

4.2   Intrathecal Drug Delivery Versus Neuromodulation Reimbursements Per Patient

A 7-year total cost was used as this is the maximum expected battery life for the most commonly placed intrathecal pump. The 7-year cost

would be more if the IDD was replaced or revised earlier than 7 years.

5   Conclusion

Intrathecal drug delivery incurs lower cost compared to conventional medical management despite the larger upfront cost as a result of decreased medical utilization post-implant. A recent trend is for earlier use of IDD rather than to utilize this treatment only as a salvage therapy. When considering a patient for IDD, the appropriate patient selection should be based on the patient's underlying condition and the effectiveness of the various treatments of other choice compared with the efficacy and durability of IDD. There are reimbursements associated with all aspects of IDD ranging from the initial placement to the ongoing management and any required system revisions. These reimbursements not only provide a sustainable treatment strategy when compared to other interventional pain management procedures and neuromodulation, but they may even be more optimal for the clinician and the facility providing this type of treatment for their patients.

References

Bolash R, Udeh B, Saweris Y et al (2015) Longevity and cost of implantable intrathecal drug delivery systems for chronic pain management: a retrospective analysis of 365 patients. Neuromodulation 18(2):150–156. https://doi.org/10.1111/ner.12235

Deer TR, Pope JE, Hayek SM, Bux A, Buchser E, Eldabe S et al (2017) The polyanalgesic consensus conference (PACC): recommendations on intrathecal drug infusion systems best practices and guidelines. Neuromodulation 20(2):96–132. https://doi.org/10.1111/ner.12538

Guillemette S, Witzke S, Leier J, Hinnenthal J, Prager JP (2013) Medical cost impact of intrathecal drug delivery for noncancer pain. Pain Med 14(4):504–515. https://doi.org/10.1111/j.1526-4637.2013.01398.x)

Kumar K, Hunter G, Demeria D (2006) Spinal cord stimulation in treatment of chronic benign pain: challenges in treatment planning and present status, a 22-year experience. Neurosurgery 58:481–496

Kumar K, Taylor RS, Jacques L et al (2007) Spinal cord stimulation versus conventional medical management for neuropathic pain: a multicentre randomised controlled trial in patients with failed back surgery syndrome. Pain 132:179–188

North RB, Kidd DH, Farrokhi F, Piantadosi SA (2005) Spinal cord stimulation versus repeated lumbosacral spine surgery for chronic pain: a randomized, controlled trial. Neurosurgery 56:98–106; discussion 106–107. http://www.ncbinlm.nih.gov/pubmed/15617591

Pope JE, Deer TR, McRoberts WP (2015) Intrathecal therapy: the burden of being positioned as a salvage therapy. Pain Med 16:2036–2038

Stearns LJ, Hinnenthal JA, Hammond K, Berryman E, Janjan NA (2016) Health services utilization and payments in patients with cancer pain: a comparison of intrathecal drug delivery vs. conventional medical management. Neuromodulation 19(2):196–205. https://doi.org/10.1111/ner.12384. Epub 2016 Jan 27. PMID: 26816205; PMCID: PMC5066649

Stearns LJ, Narang S, Albright RE Jr et al (2019) Assessment of health care utilization and cost of targeted drug delivery and conventional medical management vs conventional medical management alone for patients with cancer-related pain. JAMA Netw Open 2:e191549

Interventional Pain Management in Palliative Care

Pippa Hawley

Contents

Abstract

There is widespread misperception of what modern palliative care actually offers and interventional pain management providers may not be always aware that what they are

P. Hawley (✉)
UBC Division of Palliative Care, and BC Cancer Pain and Symptom Management/Palliative Care Program, Vancouver, BC, USA
e-mail: phawley@bccancer.bc.ca

© The Author(s), under exclusive license to Springer Nature Switzerland AG 2022
D. P. Beall et al. (eds.), *Intrathecal Pump Drug Delivery*, Medical Radiology Diagnostic Imaging,
https://doi.org/10.1007/978-3-030-86244-2_12

doing is part of a palliative approach to care. This chapter aims to place interventional pain management into the context of whole-person care. This type of care can be categorized as the care that is rendered throughout the whole patient journey including from the time of diagnosis to the final stages of the disease process. It provides a model for communication about the role for palliative care alongside disease-modifying treatments. It then describes some non-interventional treatment options that may be able to relieve suffering without the need for invasive treatments. It also outlines the potential role for a selection of minimally invasive palliative procedures which may be able to achieve the similar outcomes as more invasive therapies, such as intrathecal infusions. These interventions can enhance patients' functional capacity and optimize their independence and dignity. This is important regardless of whether death is the expected outcome of the illness or where there is still a possibility of survivorship, either living long-term with controlled disease or being cured. A brief review of the need for impeccable inter-and intradisciplinary communication and collaboration in complex patients care is also presented. This emphasizes the use of case conferences and concludes with three case examples to illustrate how these interventions can be applied in practice.

1   Intrathecal Infusions in Palliative Care

When pain is not sufficiently responsive to non-invasive management, the benefits regarding improved pain control and reduction in side effects from opioids and other analgesics given intrathecally can be dramatic. All patients living with serious illnesses that cause severe pain should ideally have access to all varieties of interventional pain management techniques. Although only a small proportion of the patients will need these techniques, they are a very helpful adjunct

to help patients along with good medical management. That comparatively smaller patient group is, however, the group that suffers the most and consumes the most healthcare resources. Their suffering also has a secondary negative impact on the people who care for them by instilling a fear of suffering that comes from witnessing unrelieved and unremitting suffering. Healthcare professionals can also experience negative impact from this suffering, most commonly a feeling of inadequacy that contributes to professional burnout. The original three-step WHO Pain ladder did not include interventional pain management, but there is clearly a "Step 4" for the most difficult pain syndromes in which intrathecal infusions could prove enormously helpful.

2   Collaboration with the Palliative Care Team

People with progressive serious illnesses are complex in different ways compared to patients with that suffer from chronic pain but do not have a life-threatening condition. These patients will also have disease-generated needs that extend well beyond analgesia. Despite the enormous potential for improved pain management, having an intrathecal pump does add complexity to patient care by requiring recurrent visits to specialty centre for pump refills and dose adjustments. This has to be understood prior to initiating intrathecal therapy so as not to create a situation that is burdensome and unsustainable. Having a home death may also necessitate home-based pump refills, and this is optimally planned prior to the time that it is needed.

When patients have progressive disease and a high probability of clinical change and decreasing functional capabilities, it is important to understand the aspects of care that people need other than managing their pain and the context in which this additional care is provided. People referred for interventional pain management very often have complex needs requiring a multiple healthcare professionals and multidisciplinary approach. If the underlying illness is life-threatening, a specialist palliative care team may already be involved in their care. The palliative care team is usually responsible for patient referrals, the choice of which interventional service to refer to, and for looking after much of the ongoing care before and after an intervention. When interacting with such people, it is important for the interventionalist to recognize that they become part of this palliative care team. Being able to work effectively with the other people involved in caring for patients and their families requires a thorough understanding of modern palliative care, a clear understanding of the team members' roles and responsibilities, and the ability to communicate using correct terminology.

3   History of Palliative Care

The term "palliative care" was coined in the 1980s by Montreal urologist Balfour Mount, who set up the first palliative care unit in in Canada after visiting Cicely Saunders' St Christopher's Hospice in London, England. In francophone culture, the term "hospice" was traditionally associated with lepers and unwed mothers, and initially "palliative care" was synonymous with "hospice". Over the last 40 years, it has become associated with care that improves the quality of life of patients who are facing the difficulties of a life-threatening illness. It has also become clear from clinical experience and multiple studies that the benefits of palliative care are maximized when palliative care is provided early in the course of illness, rather than waiting until the person is sure that they are dying (Ferrell et al. 2017). In 2013, the World Health Organization changed their definition of palliative care from including the term "life-limiting" to using the term "life-threatening" (World Health Organization 2013). This has transformed the understanding of modern palliative care from focusing primarily on dying to focusing on living as well as possible up to the point of death and including rehabilitation and survivorship programs as well as through hospice and bereavement care (Hawley 2014).

The evolution of palliative care from Dame Saunders' founding of St. Christopher's to the modern day can be more clearly illustrated by the three most widely used visual models of palliative care (Figs. 1, 2, and 3).

The most important feature of the bow tie model (Fig. 3) is the inclusion of the possibility of survivorship.

This is not only reflective of modern medical treatment options such as transplantation for organ failure, gene therapies for some inherited diseases, and new very promising cancer treatments, but it also recognizes that people with serious illness spend the vast majority of their time after the diagnosis of a life-threatening illnesses living in the dual reality of acknowledging their mortality yet, at the same time, hoping that they will get better.

This is aptly described as "hope for the best, but plan for the rest". Requiring that a person accepts that they are dying can be a barrier to accessing specialists in palliative care and interventional pain management, especially if locations of care delivery have strict requirements for patient acceptance of "do not resuscitate" orders.

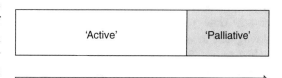

Fig. 1 The traditional dicotomy of curative and palliative care for chronic progressive illness illustrates an abrupt change from active treatment to palliative treatment that is initiated at some well defined point in time

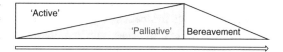

Fig. 2 The integrated model including active and palliative care for progressive illness that focuses on the patient with the illness as opposed to the bereavement segment of the continuum that pertains to the family and caregivers. Note the progressive change in the type of treatment that is emphasized from active to palliative as the disease course advances over time

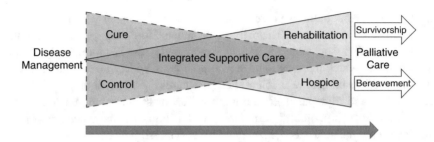

Fig. 3 The palliative care-enhanced model in a format known as a bow tie model with two opposing triangles that intersect. The first triangle represents disease management and the second triangle is palliative care. The base of the palliative care triangle includes both death and survival as possible outcomes. The arrow indicates that this is a dynamic process with a gradual switch in focus. The primary difference between this and traditional models is that survivorship is included as a possible outcome

4 What Is Palliative Care?

The three core components of palliative care are:

- Prevention, assessment, and management of symptoms
- Communication about expectations for disease progress and options for management, including advance care planning
- Coordination of all the services involved in the care of a patient and their family

Palliative care can be provided alongside disease management, whether that treatment is curative or palliative in nature, and should be provided at any time point from the initial diagnosis throughout the entire disease process. Specialist palliative care is provided by teams of specially trained healthcare providers from multiple disciplines, but a palliative approach to care (primary palliative care) may be provided by healthcare professionals of all disciplines, as components of their core professional competencies allow.

When palliative care is provided at (or close to) end of life, it is referred to as "hospice" and focuses on caring for patient and their family through the dying process, including their bereavement.

Palliative care can be provided in any location including at home, in long-term care facilities, in residential hospices, and in acute care hospitals on designated palliative care units or through various consultative services. It can include virtual care support when circumstances require for homebound patients or patients in remote areas and has been widely utilized during the Coronavirus pandemic.

5 The Importance of Correct Terminology

The term "palliative" is a descriptor of a type of care, not a patient type or diagnostic category label. It should never be applied to individuals or groups of patients as a euphemism for a terminal disease or a condition that is inexorably incurable and one should avoid using this label in phrases such as "Is the patient palliative?" or "You're palliative now" (Hawley 2017). Misuse like this is sadly still very common and, unfortunately, can lead to patients avoiding any treatment perceived as palliative and can result in the lack of access to palliative care until very late in the course of illness. Referrals to specialist palliative care services for those with complex needs are often delayed by misunderstandings of the nature of palliative care until that patient has already experienced a substantial amount of suffering that would have been preventable with an earlier referral. When having conversations with patients and families about prognosis and expectations, it is important to use language that is clear and unambiguous, such as "The usual course of this illness means that it will most likely take your life"; "….it will be fatal"; or "….you will most likely die from it at some point". Other useful phrases include "Though we can't yet cure the underlying disease, there is much that we can do to help you live with it as well as possible for as long as possible".

6 Specialist Non-interventional Therapies

6.1 Adjuvant Analgesics

Before considering any procedure, particularly one that is surgical and requires ongoing maintenance, all patients should have had an opportunity to try standard non-interventional analgesic approaches. For neuropathic pain, a tricyclic antidepressant such as nortriptyline, and gabapentin or pregabalin, should be given tried in sufficient doses and for long enough to determine response. Other adjuvants such as cannabinoids for neuropathic pain, baclofen or tizanidine for muscle spasm, and NSAIDs or steroids for those with no contraindications may occasionally provide sufficient comfort so that a procedure is not required.

6.2 Methadone

All opioids are not equal. Failure to either tolerate or get analgesia from one opioid does not mean that all other opioids will have the same results. Methadone has a special place in management of severe pain, as it has some unique features that set it apart from other opioids. It can often be much more effective and/or much better tolerated than other opioids, especially over long periods of time where tolerance might lead to dose escalation in the absence of disease progression as would be expected with other opioids. It may be appropriate for some patients to be given the opportunity to try it before considering a significant procedure. A "start low-go slow" method for methadone initiation is safe and effective in patients experiencing cancer-related pain which is poorly responsive to other opioids and adjuvant analgesics (Methadone for Pain in Palliative Care 2020).

6.3 Sublingual Sufentanil

Severe incident pain can have a much more devastating impact on quality of life than continuous pain, partly because of its impact on function and partly because of the challenge of titrating short-acting opioids without causing intolerable sedation in between incident pain episodes. Like methadone, sublingual sufentanil is another relatively underused treatment modality that can be extremely helpful for incident pain and can allow patients to avoid intrathecal delivery. It has very rapid transmucosal absorption with onset of effect within 5 min. It is rapidly cleared between doses, with little potential for accumulation and no active metabolites, which makes it very unlikely to cause delirium.

6.4 Lidocaine Infusion

Another intervention which is a little more challenging to deliver but can be dramatically effective is parenteral lidocaine (Chong and Yeo 2020). Infusions can be effective for about 50% of individuals with opioid-resistant cancer pain and can be given intermittently in low-technology environments provided that simple safety steps are taken in its administration. It has been a much-maligned treatment that has widely and inappropriately been denied to patients because of unjustified fears of cardiac toxicity associated with its use in cardiac arrest protocols. The side effects of lidocaine are blood level-related and quite distinct, with perioral numbness and tingling occurring at blood levels lower than that which could lead to more serious toxicity complications such as cardiac arrhythmias. Determining whether a potentially therapeutic blood level has been reached in a trial can be achieved simply by talking to the patient, and the infusion can be slowed or stopped and restarted to avoid any serious toxicity. When given to conscious patients with no cardiac problems, no electrocardiographic monitoring is required and blood levels do not have to be measured.

Despite lidocaine having a short half-life, the analgesic effects of a single effective infusion can last for days or even weeks, especially if there has been a lot of secondary sensitization prior to the infusion. Doses range from 5 to 10 mg/kg that is given intravenously over 1 h. Longer duration intermittent infusions may lead to an even longer response, but more care needs to be taken during the longer the infusion, and this should not continue when the patient is asleep unless they are in a specialist unit with appropriate monitoring. Continuous infusions are generally used only in patients with a short life expectancy or who are too sick for a more invasive intervention.

6.5 Ketamine

Ketamine can be administered intravenously either by intermittent dosing or continuous infusion and can also be compounded into an oral medication and delivered via capsules or in a strongly flavoured drink to disguise the unpleasant taste of the solution. Ketamine can also be administered by nasal inhalation for rapid onset of effect, similar to how sufentanil is used for incident pain. Despite being widely used in palliative care units worldwide for pain crises, there is a lack of good clinical trial evidence as a basis for using ketamine as an analgesic. Although effective for pain, ketamine is a difficult drug to use clinically because of significant perceptual side effects including hallucinations that often require concurrent benzodiazepine administration. Using ketamine chronically also carries a risk of the patient developing haemorrhagic cystitis (Middela and Pearce 2011).

6.6 "Total Pain"

It is also important to understand that pain may be a subconscious expression of nonphysical forms of suffering and can present as something known as "total pain". In addition to investigating the physiologic needs, the psychological, social, and spiritual needs of patients presenting with complex pain or total body pain should always be explored. Total pain should also always

be considered if pain expression does not seem to fit with patterns expected from the underlying condition. For example, if the same treatment seems to produce different effects at different times or if pain expression seems to be more closely associated with the patient's psychological or social circumstances than to physical phenomena, then complex or total pain should be strongly considered. All potential causes of suffering should be assessed by way of routine care pathways where possible, but if there is doubt about the extent or location of the pain generator(s), the non-physiologic needs of the patient must be addressed in order to avoid disappointing results from more advanced interventional therapies designed to treat physiologic pathologies.

7 Interventional Pain Management Options

Though people with serious illnesses other than cancer are becoming more commonly referred to specialist palliative care programs, the majority of patients referred for interventional pain management from palliative care programs have pain conditions related to an underlying neoplastic disorder. The most appropriate method of interventional pain management depends on the disease, the patient, the patient's comorbidities, and the treatment goals. An intrathecal infusion may be the right choice from a disease-related perspective but can fail if the other factors are not taken into consideration such as the pain location, the aetiology of the pain, and the patient's anatomy. It is important to be aware of all the choices available for a particular pain problem and to select the most appropriate based on all these factors (Chou et al. 2020). Different procedures may be required at different times.

7.1 Cementoplasty ± Cryoablation

For destructive primary or metastatic bone lesions which have caused (or are at risk of causing) fractures, particularly of the pelvis or vertebrae, acrylic cement can be injected percutaneously into the lesion with immediate fracture stabilization and resulting analgesia. A degree of local cancer control can also occur due to the chemical effect of the cement and the exothermic reaction that occurs with the polymerization of the cement. Cementoplasty can be combined with cryoablation or radiofrequency ablation for enhanced tumour control. Large soft tissue lesions can also be treated with cryoablation alone for the purpose of debulking, providing the mass does not involve major nerves or blood vessels that would be ablated along with the rest of the tissue in the ablation zone. Though only available in select centres, these procedures can provide very durable analgesia and markedly improved function (Hong and Andren-Sandberg 2007). There are also a number of other ablative modalities that can be effective including microwave and focused ultrasound, and other techniques such as chemo-embolization and electroporation that are used to target cancers in specific locations. There may be a wide variation between centres in how a particular kind of problem may be approached, and there also may be a number of different approaches that are perfectly acceptable depending on the available equipment and skills. Moving or transferring the patient to be able to access these procedures, even if inconvenient, can be very worthwhile.

Cryoablation can be repeated for tumour regrowth, and cementoplasties can be done in different bones as the underlying disease progresses. Multiple myeloma is an example of a condition where multiple cementoplasties may be required over the course of a protracted illness and skeletal failure. Cementoplasty can provide analgesia following fractures but can also be done in anticipation of future fractures where the imaging studies suggest a high risk of fracture. The prophylactic cementoplasty can serve to prevent such adverse anatomic derangements as progressive kyphosis, facet joint distraction, spinal cord and/or nerve root compression, and the adverse consequences of vertebral height loss on the patient's respiratory and abdominal capacity.

As with intrathecal pump placement, cryoablation and cementoplasty are contraindicated in irreversible coagulopathy and where there is ongoing risk of bacteraemia which might seed the cement. In patients on myelotoxic chemother-

apy, the procedure may need to be timed to make sure there is an adequate neutrophil count. Some newer kinds of anticancer therapies cause impaired wound healing, and the timing of a procedure may need to be adjusted to allow for sufficient time after the last dose to avoid wound breakdown. Patients must also be fit enough to tolerate the anaesthesia for cryoablation and/or pelvic cementoplasty, and overnight hospital admission is typically required following the post-procedure. Alternatively, some of the cementation procedures such as vertebroplasty are commonly performed as an outpatient procedure and may be completed under conscious sedation or even local anaesthesia if necessary.

Acrylic cement is very resistant to fracture by compressive forces but is not especially resistant to shear forces. This means that bone cement is not a good option for fractures in long bones where forces involved in function of the native bone have significant shear and torsional components. Sternal cementoplasty can be effective and durable but structurally compromising lesions of long bones such as the humerus and femur are better dealt with through a combination of instrumentation fixation plus cement or with robust instrumentation alone.

7.2 Nerve Blocks

A local anaesthetic and steroid injection around a nerve can offer good analgesia which can often be temporary but sometimes can last months or more. The blocks are straightforward to perform, can be repeated when they wear off with very little morbidity, and are typically done by interventional radiologists, anaesthetists, or physiatrists.

7.3 Neurolytic Procedures

For patients who do not live close enough to a major centre or a facility that can provide ongoing care for intrathecal drug delivery, neurolytic procedures may provide prolonged periods of maintenance-free analgesia. For those with a life expectancy of less than a year, the risk of neural regrowth and procedure-induced pain is low, but

nerve regrowth can often occur in those with longer survival so if the neurolytic procedure being
considered is associated with any prominently
negative long-term outcomes, this should be
avoided in patients with unclear or a possibly
prolonged life expectancy. In these situations, an
intrathecal pump placed for targeted drug delivery would be preferable.

Percutaneous cordotomy is very useful for unilateral pain. It is achieved with radiofrequency
ablation and the patient conscious during the procedure so they can acknowledge when the spinothalamic tract has been reached by reporting a
sensation of pain or warmth in the distribution of
their pain. Once accurate placement of the probe
is confirmed, radiofrequency ablation disables
pain and temperature sensation from the contralateral side of the body below the level of the ablation while preserving the other sensory functions.

Midline myelotomy can be done in the cervical spine and functions to block the pain signals
from reaching the brain. This is done by creating
a small radiofrequency lesion in the midline of
the dorsal column of the spinal cord. This has
been shown to be effective in the treatment of
otherwise intractable abdominal and pelvic cancer pain (Hong and Andren-Sandberg 2007).

Any nerves that can be temporarily blocked
can also be destroyed by various ablative substances such as alcohol or phenol or by thermal
techniques such as radiofrequency ablation or
cryoablation. The choice of which type of ablative technique to use primarily depends on the
anatomical location of the target nerve or plexus.
Celiac plexus blocks can either be a traditional
nerve block or can be a neurolytic procedure that
is frequently done for severe upper abdominal
pain, especially from pancreatic cancer.
Trigeminal neuralgia can often respond to nerve
ablation, though a potential for the loss of the
corneal reflex or other more severe complications
such as anaesthesia dolorosa requires an expert
knowledge of the anatomy and performance of
the ablation with fastidious technique. Dorsal
horn rhizotomy can be more effective than temporary nerve root blocks but can also occasionally result in an unpleasant deafferentation pain
syndrome so this technique is generally reserved

for situations where a temporary procedure is not
practical to repeat and the patient's life expectancy is short.

There are also many other potentially useful
neurolytic procedures, including central destruction of neural tissue such as that seen with a thal-
amotomy as well as neurolysis procedures of the
peripheral nerves including the superior hypo-
gastric plexus, intercostal nerves, sympathetic
plexus, and the medial branches of the dorsal
ramus. Close collaboration with interventional
radiology and anaesthesia is needed to ensure
that each and every procedure that is performed
has the best chance of success.

7.4   Spinal Cord Stimulation

When pain is in the upper body or arms, intrathecal infusions can be somewhat more complex,
and the amount of pain relief is often less in the
upper extremities than in the low back and legs.
Often the patient will have focal pain that affects
a single portion of the spine (i.e., cervical or lumbar) along with the associated extremities adjacent to the affected spinal segment. In these
situations, a spinal cord stimulator may provide
good analgesia safely and with less frequent need
for follow-up visits than would be required for an
intrathecal pump (Peng et al. 2015). There are
many devices that are rechargeable and can
provide low maintenance analgesia for long periods of time, including in survivorship. For example, patients with severe chronic regional pain
syndrome following a resection of a soft tissue
neoplasm from an extremity may benefit from
long-term spinal cord stimulation.

8   Case Conferencing

It can be very difficult to ensure that all the people involved in a complex case of treating a
patient's pain are communicating and collaborat-
ing effectively and in a timely fashion, especially
if the pain and discomfort is refractory to early
treatment. Every patient is different and has complexities that may need attention from a diverse

selection of care providers. One way of facilitating coordinated care is to have a regular case conference where challenging patient problems are discussed and a management plan developed. The British Columbia Cancer Minimally Invasive Palliative Procedures Conference is an example. The ability to have regular scheduled discussions allows for attendance by a wide range of clinicians and for the attendees to be exposed to the treatment options offered for patents other than the referrers' own patients, thereby enhancing their knowledge and ability to care for future challenging cases (Chu et al. 2015).

9 Case Examples

The following three case descriptions are based on real patients.

9.1 "David"

A 57 year old professional musician was diagnosed with a gastrointestinal stromal cancer, treated surgically followed by post-operative radiotherapy and Imatinib systemic therapy.

One year later he developed low back pain and was found to have developed lytic metastases in the sacrum and asymptomatic lung metastases. He had more radiotherapy to the sacrum but had persistent severe incident pain despite regular long-acting hydromorphone for resting pain and sufentanil for weight-bearing, and his function gradually declined. He became wheelchair-bound. After developing sacral fractures, he underwent cryoablation and cementoplasty of the sacrum with excellent pain control (Figs. 4 and 5).

A few weeks later David walked his daughter down the aisle for her wedding, and his cognitive function had improved back to normal. Part of the reason for that was that he was also able to dramatically reduce his need for opioids to deal with his pain which also had the added benefit of far less opioid related side effects.

David's cancer treatment was changed to the targeted anti-cancer treatment sunitinib, with a partial response that lasted for approximately 9 months, but the cancer started to progress again. Soft tissue expansion of the disease in the pelvis started to involve the lumbosacral plexuses bilaterally. This produced neuropathic pain that radiated down both of his legs. He was

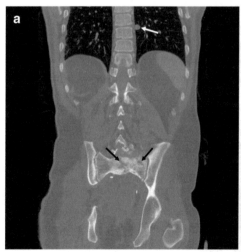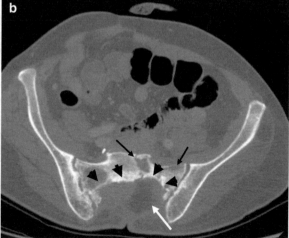

Fig. 4 (**a** and **b**) Coronal CT reconstruction showing metastatic disease involving the central and left alar potion of the sacrum (black arrows in **a** and **b**) along with a large soft tissue met just posterior to the central and left sacrum (white arrow in **b**) that is eroding into the posterior portion of the sacrum (black arrowheads in **b**). A metastatic lesion to the patient's left lung is also seen adjacent to the thoracic spine (white arrow in **a**)

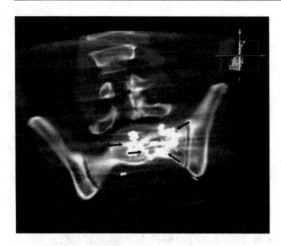

Fig. 5 Coronal CT reconstruction obtained after percutaneous sacroplasty shows polymethylmethacrylate in the central portion of the sacrum and left sacral ala (black arrows) filling the region of the sacrum that were invaded by the metastases

unable to tolerate a tricyclic antidepressant (nortriptyline) because of the lack of pain relief and the medication caused him to have nightmares. Similarly, gabapentin was increased to the point of dose-limiting side-effects with minimal benefit and significant tremor. His opioid therapy was changed to methadone, with much improved pain control which lasted for approximately 6 months.

Disease progression then required a gradual increase in methadone dose until his cognitive function again became impaired. Lidocaine infusions were utilized and these gave good pain control but required repeating every 2 weeks and this was unable to be performed in the community where he lived. An intrathecal infusion trial went well and a pump was implanted with excellent results. He found the breakthrough pain bolus delivery feature with the external activator to be particularly helpful for planned incident pain episodes associated with movement. He survived for an additional 5 months and died comfortably at home a few days after a pump refill visit.

This case study illustrates the need for patients to have access to a range of palliative procedures. There is very often more than one way to approach a difficult pain syndrome. Having all the pain relief techniques available and the clinicians to deploy them can make sure the patient is offered the most appropriate procedure(s) at the most appropriate time.

9.2   "Karen"

A 44 year old horse-breeder was diagnosed with renal cell carcinoma following an episode of hematuria. She had a nephrectomy of the involved kidney but a year later developed a metastasis in the left side of the sacrum that had a significant soft tissue component. It was treated with radiotherapy with some initial response, and she also underwent systemic therapy to which the tumour initially responded after a period of about 2 years, however, the tumor progressed and caused a mixed nociceptive and neuropathic severe pain syndrome affecting the left buttock, perineum and leg. Some of her activity restrictions including not being able to ride her horse were especially troubling for her. Cryoablation of the tumor was performed twice, both times with good benefit. The tumor then progressed in size wrapping around the sciatic nerve and other nerves so that additional cryoablation was not advised as it would most likely cause permanent nerve damage with significant loss of motor function and/or continence. The patient also developed lung metastases but these were asymptomatic and she declined further systemic therapy. Oral analgesic therapy was optimized with very high doses of opioids, including methadone and hydromorphone. Gabapentin and nortriptyline were also titrated to maximum tolerated doses, with some benefit, but her pain responded best to steroid therapy. After some time on the steroid therapy she started to become Cushingoid. An intrathecal infusion pump was considered, but she would have had to travel 5 h by car to the nearest specialist centre to have pump refills. Karen lived in a rural area and her primary goal was to spend as much time as possible at home, particularly to be able to ride her horse for as long as possible.

As her pain was unilateral, she was offered percutaneous cordotomy and had the procedure done under the shared supervision and care of the specialist centre's neurosurgical *and palliative care teams. Following the proce-dure her opioid doses were able to be rapidly titrated down, and the nortriptyline stopped. Ten days after the procedure she was dis-charged home on a tapering dose of predni-sone, and low doses of methadone and gabapentin. Over the next 2 months the predni-sone was tapered then discontinued and the methadone and gabapentin were maintained at very low doses by her family doctor with no side-effects. Hydromorphone was used only in low doses before certain activities. She enjoyed a period of excellent quality of life with very good pain control even able to ride her horse for short periods of time before succumbing 4 months later to progressive pulmonary involvement and hypercalcemia.*

This case illustrates the need to adapt the patient-centred management plan to fit with the individual's goals of care and to have all team members working together to meet these goals.

9.3 "Malcolm"

This 65 year old man had metastatic prostate cancer and had pain from bone disease through-out the entire axial skeleton. His pain was con-trolled with a combination of long-acting and short-acting oral morphine with the occasional use of sublingual sufentanil as it was not possi-ble to anticipate incident episodes of increased pain. He required assistance for bathing and dressing but was able to walk short distances with a wheeled walker. He was admitted to hos-pital with a pain crisis and was given rapidly escalating doses of morphine which soon resulted in some confusion and myoclonus. Malcolm described his pain as present through-out his low back, hips and legs. Cross sectional imaging investigations did not show any new fractures in the pelvis or vertebrae, and there was no spinal cord compression. His calcium level was normal and he did not have urosepsis or a fecal impaction. The opioid was changed to hydromorphone with resolution of the myoclo-nus and confusion, but no improvement in pain. Breakthrough hydromorphone dosing seemed

ineffective and the patent became tearful and anxious. A referral was made for consideration of an intrathecal pain pump.

A medical student happened to be on the ward in the evening when Malcolm's wife visited. His wife asked to speak with the student and inquired about how long Malcolm might be able to be kept in the hospital as she had planned to visit her mother who was unwell in another city and had arranged for a friend to look after Malcolm whilst she was away. When Malcolm was asked about this the next morning, he confided that he was very frightened of being left with the friend. He acknowledging that, although she was well-meaning and kind, he was very uncomfortable having to depend on her for his personal hygiene. He understood his wife needed to visit her mother and had not told her of his fear of embarrass-ment, not wanting to be a burden to her. A plan was made for Malcolm to be admitted to a local hospice for respite care for the duration of his wife's upcoming absence, and his pain resolved rapidly. The referral to anesthesia was cancelled and over the next 3 days his dose of long-acting hydromorphone was reduced by 30% without loss of analgesia. His use of breakthrough medi-cation returned to the pre-crisis once a day planned dosing in the morning and he continued to do well with this regimen up to the time of discharge.

This case illustrates the importance of identi-fying psychosocial triggers for pain expression and the need to use all available collateral sources of information in order to provide the best possi-ble care.

References

Chong P, Yeo Z (2020) Parenteral lidocaine for complex cancer pain in the home or inpatient hospice setting: a review and synthesis of the evidence. Lidocaine review Accessed 31 Dec 2020

Chou C, Hopkins T, Badiola I et al (2020) Top ten tips pal-liative care clinicians should know about interventional pain and procedures. J Palliat Med 23(10):1386–1391

Chu L, Hawley P, Munk P, Mallinson P, Clarkson P (2015) Minimally invasive palliative procedures in oncology: a review of a multidisciplinary collaboration. Support Care Cancer 23(6):1589–1596

Ferrell B, Temel J, Temin S et al (2017) Integration of palliative care into standard oncology care: American Society of Clinical Oncology clinical practice guideline update. J Clin Oncol 35(1):96–112

Hawley P (2014) The bow tie model of 21st century palliative care. J Pain Symptom Manag 47(1):e2–e5. https://doi.org/10.1016/j.jpainsymman

Hawley P (2017) Barriers to access to palliative care. Palliative care and social practice. Barriers article Accessed 31 Dec 2020

Hong D, Andren-Sandberg A (2007) Punctate midline myelotomy: a minimally invasive procedure for the treatment of pain in inextirpable abdominal and pelvic cancer. J Pain Symptom Manag 33:99–109

Methadone for Pain in Palliative Care, Canadian Virtual Hospice. Open access at Methadone4pain.ca. Accessed 31 Dec 2020

Middela S, Pearce I (2011) Ketamine-induced vesicopathy: a literature review. Int J Clin Pract 65(1):27–30. https://doi.org/10.1111/j.1742-1241.2010.02502.x. PMID: 21155941.

Peng L, Min S, Zejun Z, Wei K, Bennett MI (2015) Spinal cord stimulation for cancer-related pain in adults. Cochrane Database of Systematic Reviews 6, CD009389. https://doi.org/10.1002/14651858. CD009389.pub3. Cochrane SCS Review 2015. Accessed 31 Dec 2020

World Health Organization definition of palliative care 2013. WHO definition of palliative care (2013). Accessed 30 Dec 2020

The Use of Ziconotide in Intrathecal Drug Therapy

David A. Lindley

Contents

D. A. Lindley (✉)
Pain Management Physician, Pain Clinic of Norman
Dozier MD, Abilene, TX, USA
e-mail: drlindley@mdofficemail.com

© The Author(s), under exclusive license to Springer Nature Switzerland AG 2022
D. P. Beall et al. (eds.), *Intrathecal Pump Drug Delivery*, Medical Radiology Diagnostic Imaging,
https://doi.org/10.1007/978-3-030-86244-2_13

Abstract

The medications used in targeted drug delivery primarily consist of opioids and anesthetics, but a novel medication derived from a marine animal has been adapted for use in patients with chronic pain. Ziconotide was synthesized from the cone snail which is a calcium channel inhibitor that is up to 1000 times stronger than morphine. It has a small molecular mass and inhibits N-type voltage-sensitive calcium channels. By doing this, it inhibits the transmission of noxious signals from the first-order neuron to the second-order neuron. As a peptide, ziconotide would be quickly digested by gastrointestinal enzymes, but it is water soluble and is effective when given intrathecally. The medication is a nonnarcotic analgesic and useful for treatment of refractory pain. Although ziconotide has been FDA approved for intrathecal use since 2004, adoption into common use has been slow primarily because it has been difficult for various investigators to determine the optimal dosing regimen. This process of discovering effective dosing strategies is still evolving, and this chapter will discuss the history of the drug and examine the evolution of dosing strategies from trial dosing to maintenance dosing. Traditionally, the dose response relationships have been difficult to determine due to the heterogeneity of the different studies in regards to the study design, patient population, and underlying conditions. The therapeutic window for ziconotide is relatively narrow compared to other intrathecal medications, and a general trend of fewer side effects is seen with lower medication doses. The intrathecal infusion from the implanted pump can be done via a continuous infusion, through bolus dosing or through a combination of the two, and studies have indicated that bolus dosing may result in higher efficacy for relieving pain. The commercially available concentrations have tended to produce less optimal results than the studies that have used diluted concentrations, and patient-controlled bolus dosing also improves pain relief nearly as well as programmed bolus dosing but with

less side effects. Also the tendency for optimal segmental spread of ziconotide may account for pain relief even when the catheter tip is anatomically far from the location of pain which can give more leniency with placement of the catheter tip during permanent pump and catheter implantation. Overall ziconotide is a nonaddictive, nonnarcotic very effective analgesic that plays an important role in the treatment of chronic pain conditions of many types.

Abbreviations

AE   Adverse event
AIDS   Acquired immune deficiency syndrome
IT   Intrathecal
PTM   Patient therapy manager

1 History of the Use of Ziconotide for Intrathecal Therapy

Cone snails are a large group of predatory venomous snails found in Atlantic and Pacific oceans. Numerous species of cone snail exist and produce venom which is typically a conglomerate of about 50 different toxins (Olivera and Teichert 2007a). A marine natural products laboratory at University of Utah run by Baldomero Olivera has studied various conotoxins. With the help from the undergraduate student, Michael McIntosh, Olivera, and McIntosh discovered one particular conotoxin that has a paralytic motor effect in fish (Brookes et al. 2017). The toxin found in the cone snail *Conus magus* was an omega conotoxin that inhibited N-type voltage-dependent calcium channels, and because these calcium channels are related to pain sensitivity, it produced pain relief at a potency 100–1000 stronger than morphine (McIntosh et al. 1982). The toxin was then successfully developed as a synthetic form of the omega conotoxin which acts as a pain medication for humans (McIntosh et al. 1982).

2   Characteristics of the Medication Ziconotide

2.1   Structure of the Medication

Conus magus injects its fish prey by way of a proboscis with a very small volume of venom (Fig. 1). Although the volume of venom injected is very small, it has extraordinarily rapid effect, pacifying and paralyzing the prey almost instantaneously. How does such a small volume induce such a rapid effect? The conotoxins themselves have a relatively small molecular mass (Olivera and Teichert 2007b). Instead of a protein consisting of hundreds or thousands of residues, conotoxins are peptides containing only 20 to 30 residues (Olivera and Teichert 2007b). Typically,

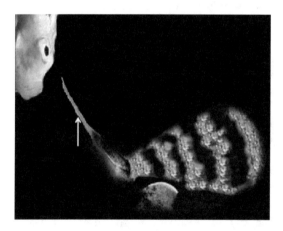

Fig. 1 The cone snail, *Conus magus*, extends its proboscis (white arrow) towards its prey to inject its venomous concoction. One of approximately 50 neuropharmacologically active peptides in the cone snail venom has been developed into a pain relieving intrathecal drug called ziconotide

proteins contain hundreds or thousands of residues which allow for a stable quaternary structure which maintains protein-receptor interactions. Conotoxins have overcome this need for large primary structures by using a high proportion of cysteine bonds which serve to keep the appropriate quaternary structure to maintain peptide-receptor interaction (Chi et al. 2004). Ziconotide has only 25 residues but has 3 cysteine bonds, and the 25-residue peptide is also highly soluble in water (Fig. 2) (McGivern 2007).

2.2   Mechanism of Action

As mentioned above, the mechanism of action of ziconotide is an inhibition of the N-type voltage-sensitive calcium channel (Fig. 3). Different types of calcium channels affect different types of nerves (McGivern 2007). For example, in humans, vascular structures utilize the L-type voltage-sensitive calcium channel, whereas N-type voltage-sensitive calcium channels are involved with pain fiber transmission. In fact, both ziconotide and mu-agonists (opioids) inhibit the N-type voltage-sensitive calcium channel, although ziconotide is not an opioid (McGivern 2007). Ziconotide is a direct inhibitor of the N-type voltage-sensitive calcium channel, whereas opioids inhibit this same receptor indirectly by way of activating a mu-receptor which then inhibits the N-type voltage-sensitive calcium channel by way of a G-protein mechanism (Fig. 3) (McGivern 2007).

By inhibiting preganglionic N-type voltage-sensitive calcium channels, the transmission of the noxious signal from the first-order neuron to

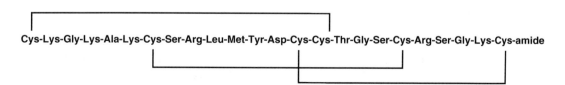

Cys-Lys-Gly-Lys-Ala-Lys-Cys-Ser-Arg-Leu-Met-Tyr-Asp-Cys-Cys-Thr-Gly-Ser-Cys-Arg-Ser-Gly-Lys-Cys-amide

Fig. 2 Peptide structure of ziconotide. Most polyamides use hundreds or thousands of residues to achieve a stable quarternary "lock and key" interaction with their binding site. In contrast, ziconotide has only 25 residues, and utilizes three cysteine bonds to maintain a stable structure. Compare to hemoglobin, which contains over 550 residues

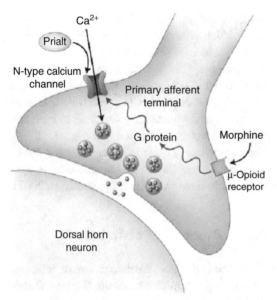

Fig. 3 Mechanism of Action of Ziconotide. Ziconotide's mechanism of action is by pre-synaptic inhibition of the N-Type Voltage Sensitive Calcium Channel. Note the direct binding and inhibition of the N-Type Voltage Sensitive Calcium Channel by ziconotide as compared to the indirect mechanism of action of opioids. Mu opioid receptors utilize a G-protein intermediary system which then inhibits the N-Type Voltage Sensitive Calcium Channel (Adapted from: Lawson, E.F., Wallace, M.S. Current Developments in Intraspinal Agents for Cancer and Noncancer Pain. *Curr Pain Headache Rep* **14**, 8–16 (2010). https://doi.org/10.1007/s11916-009-0092-z)

the second-order neuron is inhibited at the level of the spinal cord (Wallace et al. 2006). As a peptide, ziconotide would be subject to digestive enzymes and would quickly be rendered ineffective by way of oral ingestion. This water-soluble molecule, however, is both potent and effective when given by intrathecal infusion.

2.3 Select Literature Review of Ziconotide

Literature reviews are typically published as a review manuscript in the medical literature, but the clinical trials and other publications on ziconotide have been focused on evaluating this medication specifically for intrathecal use, and it is unique and unlike all other medications for pain. Additionally, clinical trials for ziconotide

have traditionally been at a higher dose and concentration than in common clinical use, and lower concentrations have evolved over time. Given the unique nature of the medication and the evolution of the optimal clinical dosing, a literature review is presented below, and several dosing studies are reviewed in chronological order. After reviewing the medication usage background, a general trend of benefits and adverse effects can be appreciated and applied to clinical use.

2.4 Ziconotide for Chronic Nonmalignant Pain: Wermeling 2003 (Wermeling et al. 2003)

Twenty-two patients with chronic nonmalignant pain were given an infusion of either 1, 5, 7.5, or 10 mcg over 1 h. The total fluid volume and rate of delivery were not reported other than a statement that all groups received equal volumes. The patients were monitored for side effects, and the medication was evaluated for efficacy of pain relief for the following 48 h. Most of the adverse effects that were seen were not severe. The only side effects considered severe were dizziness, headache, and myasthenia, and these occurred only in the group that received the 10 mcg infusion over 1 h. As for efficacy, there was a dose-related improvement in pain which lasted through the 48-h observation time for all groups except the 1 mcg dose. Possible explanations for the lack of efficacy with the smallest dose include that it was too small of a dose to provide pain relief or that the placement of a large bore needle for catheter insertion is more analgesic than the analgesic benefit of the 1 mcg ziconotide infusion given over 1 h.

2.5 Ziconotide Versus Placebo for Pain in Cancer or AIDS: Staats 2003 (Staats et al. 2003)

This randomized control trial contained 111 Cancer or AIDS pain subjects across three continents randomized to either ziconotide IT infusion or placebo. The cancer etiologies and body locations were numerous and widespread. The intrathecal ziconotide used had a concentration of 100 mcg/mL. The ziconotide was titrated for 5–6 days followed by a maintenance dose for 5 days. Crossover was allowed during the maintenance phase of the medication dosing. Although this was a prospective randomized controlled trial, the initial dosing strategy for the ziconotide varied. Early patients received a weight-based dose which equated to 8.4 mcg/day for a 70 kg patient. The dosing was then changed to a starting dose of 9.6 mcg/day and then changed again to 2.4 mcg/day or less with titrations allowed every 24 h. The maximum allowed dose after titration was 57.6 mcg/day. After the medication was appropriately titrated, mean pain scores improved 53% in the ziconotide group versus 18.1% in the placebo group. The reduction in patient opioid use was significantly greater in the ziconotide group as compared to the placebo group. Although there was a significant reduction of pain with intrathecal ziconotide, at the doses given in the trial, 97.2% of patients experienced side effects (compared to 72.2% in placebo group) and 30.6% of patients experienced serious adverse effects (compared to 10% in the placebo group). The most common side effect in the ziconotide group was dizziness, whereas the most common side effect in the placebo group was headache.

2.6 Ziconotide Versus Placebo: Rauck 2006 (Rauck et al. 2006)

Two hundred twenty patients with chronic severe pain were randomized to either ziconotide or placebo. The treatment group initiated the IT ziconotide infusion at 2.4 mcg/day and titrated the dose gradually over 3 weeks. At the end of the 3-week titration, the average dose in the treatment group was 6.96 mcg/day, and the average improvement in pain was 14.7% for the treatment group versus 7.2% for the placebo group. Side effects in the treatment group included dizziness, confusion, ataxia, abnormal gait, and memory

impairment. Interestingly, both the ziconotide and the placebo group had similar discontinuation rates due to adverse effects. The concentration of the medication was not reported and therefore may have been the standard concentration of 25 mcg/mL.

2.7 External Catheter Evaluation of Ziconotide for Malignant and Nonmalignant Pain: Ver Donck 2008
(Ver Donck et al. 2008)

This was an external catheter study in patients with both malignant and nonmalignant pain. An intrathecal ziconotide infusion was started at an average dose of 2.304 mcg/day and titrated to an average dose of 4.032 mcg/day by day 28. The patients reported pain scores improved 29% at day 28. There was a high rate of adverse events (AEs) with 90% of patients experienced an AE during the titration, most commonly dizziness or headache. Other AEs were related to failure of the external catheter or the device or difficulties with placement of the catheter. The concentration was not reported and therefore may have been the standard concentration.

2.8 High- and Low-Dose Ziconotide Trialing: Abramoff 2014
(Abramoff and Shaw 2014)

The authors trialed 5 mcg and 2 mcg ziconotide bolus doses sequentially in 15 patients with chronic nonmalignant pain. They found a greater efficacy in pain reduction with the larger dose as compared to the smaller dose, and one third of the patients had improvements sufficient enough to warrant pump implantation. These patients were followed after implantation, and all five patients were noted to have improved pain. In this trial, the authors utilized a drug holiday for any patients with adverse effects, and this was utilized in one of the five patients with implanted pumps.

2.9 Nocturnal Flex Dosing: Pope 2015 (Pope and Deer 2015)

A case series of 16 patients reported a nocturnal flex dosing strategy. The patients were trialed with an IT bolus of 2 mcg of ziconotide, and then a 2 mcg ziconotide nocturnal flex dose was programmed into the pump and was initiated to start the night following the implant. The ziconotide concentration in the pump was 5 mcg/mL. At a follow-up time that averaged 5.8 months after pump implantation, the average total daily dose of ziconotide was found to be 2.77 mcg/day, but by this time, 30% of the patients had dropped out due to side effects of the medication. The average time it took the patients who left the study to drop out was 4.25 months, and the average daily ziconotide dose for those patient dropping out of the study was 3.825 mcg/day at the time of their exit. Urinary retention and visual hallucinations were most commonly reported side effects associated with the patient's decision to discontinue the study. No serious adverse events or unresolved side effects were reported. The average pain score decreased 79.5% from 9.06 out of 10 to a 1.8, and the average opioid reduction was profound with the patients reporting a mean decrease of 91.5%.

2.10 Open-Label Observational Study: Deer 2018 (Deer et al. 2018)

An open-label observational study enrolled 93 patients, 51 of whom received ziconotide as initial intrathecal therapy and 42 of whom were weaned from their prior intrathecal therapy and switched to intrathecal ziconotide. The concentration of the ziconotide solution used was 25 mcg/mL, and patients were started at an average of 1.6 mcg/day then titrated incrementally as needed. By week 12, the mean daily dose was 3.2 mcg/day. Due to various factors previously stated identifying the reasons for patient attrition, there were only 25 patients that remained in the study at the 12-month time point. At 12 months follow-up, the mean daily dose in the ziconotide as an initial treatment group was lower as compared to the patient group that had previous nonziconotide intrathecal medication treatment. At the 12-month follow-up, 14 of the 25 patients (56%) had at least 30% relief, whereas 9 of 25 (36%) had less than 30% relief. In the ziconotide first group, pain relief varied from 19.2% to 32.7% from month 3 to month 12. In the ziconotide after other intrathecal medication group, pain relief varied from 4.3 to 22.3% between months 3 and 12. Seventy-one percent of the patients reported adverse effects with the most common being nausea, confusion, and dizziness. The adverse effects leading to discontinuation of therapy happened in four patients, and five patients reported serious adverse effects.

2.11 Ziconotide for Axial Nonmalignant Pain: Lindley 2019 (Lindley 2019)

A case series of 17 patients with axial nonmalignant neck and back pain was reported in 2019. All patients discontinued opioids prior to undergoing an intrathecal medication trial with ziconotide and remained off of their systemic opioids until the time of their pump implantation. A dilute concentration of 0.5 mcg/mL of ziconotide was initiated at the lowest programmable rate of 0.024 mcg/day. The patient therapy manager (PTM) was started at dose of 0.25 mcg which was allowed up to three times per day. The medication concentration and dose were titrated as needed. After a follow-up interval of 4.7 months on the average, the mean medication concentration used was 1 mcg/mL with an average basal rate of 0.19 mcg/day, an average PTM dose of 0.27 mcg, and an average total daily ziconotide dose of 0.736 mcg. The mean pain relief was 71%, and the median pain relief was 75% at the time of the last follow-up, and, at this time, 94% of patients remained on the therapy.

2.12 The Use of Ziconotide in Patients with Spinal Cord Injury: Brinzeu 2019 (Brinzeu et al. 2019)

A prospective cohort of 20 spinal cord injury patients underwent an intrathecal medication trial, and, if they met the appropriate criteria for improvement in pain and tolerance to the medication, they were implanted. The trialing method was a series of IT bolus injections with an escalating dose characterized by a sequence of 0.5 mcg/2 mL, 1 mcg/2 mL, and 1.5 mcg/2 mL with each dose being given at 72-h intervals. If the patient failed the bolus test, a continuous catheter trial was performed. The continuous catheter test involved placing an intrathecal catheter which was tunneled subcutaneously and attached to a reservoir with an external pump. The continuous infusion was started at 2 mcg/day, and every 3 days, the infusion could be increased by 1 mcg until a maximum dose of 10 mcg/day was reached. Overall pain relief of 40% was considered a positive test. Ten of 19 patients had a positive lumbar puncture bolus test, and 3 of 8 continuous infusion tests were positive. Three of the 13 patients tested had unacceptable side effects and dropped out. Eleven of 20 patients went on to pump implantation. Of the patients who had positive trials and went on to implantation, 15% dropped out of chronic therapy while 85% continued the chronic therapy. The average follow-up at the end of the study was 3.59 years, and the average daily dose at the final follow-up was 5.36 mcg/day. The average pain score decreased 45% from 7.9 to 4.31. The concentration of drug used after implant and during chronic therapy was not reported.

2.13 The Distal Segmental Spread of Intrathecal Ziconotide: Staub 2019 (Staub et al. 2019)

Although this is a single patient case study, there is a paucity of information on this topic, and this article highlights the distal segmental spread that

has been observed clinically with intrathecal ziconotide. The patient was given a lumbar intrathecal bolus trial at the L3–4 level using 2.5 mcg ziconotide in 2.5 mL volume that resulted in drastic reduction of the patient's chronic severe facial pain for approximately 9 h. At the time of pump implantation, the catheter was inserted at the L4/5 into intrathecal space with the catheter tip placed 17 cm from the skin's surface. This describes an implanted catheter tip well inferior to the mid- to upper thoracic spine. With this distal catheter tip placement, the patient nonetheless experienced complete or near-complete relief of their facial pain over the 22-month follow-up period. At the end of 22 months, the patient was still having 100% relief at a relatively low dose of 2.0 mcg/day. The concentration used for the pump reservoir infusion was not reported.

3 Study-Based Discussion of the Clinical Use of Ziconotide

3.1 Trial Dosing

The studies discussed above utilized both bolus trialing techniques and continuous infusion techniques. From the Wermeling 2003 study, one may conclude that bolus trialing doses should be greater than 1 mcg/day and less than 10 mcg/day, and in 2014, Abramoff utilized 2 mcg and 5 mcg bolus doses. Similar to the Abramoff trial, the consensus recommendation recommends bolus doses ranging from 1 to 5 mcg (Deer et al. 2017). While cardiovascular side effects are rarely observed, other side effects such as confusion and dizziness are possible, and if using trial bolus doses approaching 10 mcg, these side effects become much more common.

3.2 Dose-Efficacy Comparisons

It is difficult to determine dose-response relationships based on the available studies.

Some studies demonstrate increased efficacy with higher doses, but when comparisons are made across studies, a general trend of less efficacy and more AEs may be noted with higher doses. One explanation is that this could be due to the more rigorous study design and/or more serious nature of the pain etiology in higher-dose studies. The Staats 2003 study demonstrated a 53% mean pain score improvement which most clinicians would consider optimal especially given the pain etiology of the participants and the fact that only refractory pain subjects were included in this study (Staats et al. 2003). The Rauck study in 2006 reported "a lot" or "complete" relief in 28.4% of participants, and this was also in a refractory population in which most of the participants had already failed other intrathecal therapies (Rauck et al. 2006). The Pope et al. and Lindley et al. reports consisted of much smaller populations, mostly nonmalignant conditions, and the latter study consisted of nonmalignant pain patients and titrated the patients off of opioids prior to the IT medication trial and pump implantation, and both of these studies demonstrated more optimal levels of pain relief (Pope and Deer 2015; Lindley 2019). This was in contrast to the Staats et al. study that selected patients with refractory cancer pain and pain related to complications from AIDS (Staats et al. 2003). These examples illustrate that different methods of patient selection and heterogeneous study methodologies make it difficult to generate consistent dose-efficacy conclusions based on the existing literature.

3.3 Dose-Adverse Effects Comparisons

The therapeutic window for ziconotide is relatively narrow compared to most other IT medications. Studies using a higher dose of ziconotide (Staats et al., Rauck et al., and Ver Donck et al) reported medication side effects in the 70% to 95% range. Studies using lower doses (Pope et al., Lindley et al., and Brinzeu) reported side effects in the 6% to 45% range. The 2018 study by Deer et al. was a low-dose study but utilized a high concentration of ziconotide and reported side effects in 71% of the patients. As one might expect, the literature shows a general trend of fewer side effects that are seen with lower medication doses.

3.4 Comparison of Bolus Dosing Versus Continuous Infusion

Traditionally in the intrathecal drug delivery literature, it has been recommended that bolus dosing should represent 10% of the basal rate so if the basal rate of intrathecal ziconotide is 1 mcg/day, then the patient administered bolus dose of 0.1 mcg should be programmed. There are other bolus dosing strategies that may be effective, and the inverse of the traditional 10% of basal rate bolus dose has also been shown to be effective. In regards to the timing of the boluses, both the PTM bolus dosing strategy and the nocturnal flex dose strategy effectively utilized bolus delivery techniques with efficacy reported in the >70% range (Pope and Deer 2015; Lindley 2019). Studies utilizing continuous infusion techniques (Staats et al. 2003; Rauck et al. 2006; Ver Donck et al. 2008; Deer et al. 2018) reported generally lower efficacy levels in the 15–30% range. One possibility for this discrepancy is that the bolus technique may result in a wider segmental spinal spread and improved efficacy. This concept of differing spinal segmental coverage by way of varying rates of infusion is supported by a comparison of baclofen and bupivacaine intrathecal delivery in a pig study (Bernards 2006).

3.5 Comparison of High Versus Low Concentration Infusion

Ziconotide is commercially available in 25 mcg/mL and 100 mcg/mL concentrations. It is interesting to note that both studies which utilized diluted concentrations reported similar efficacy

(Pope and Deer 2015; Lindley 2019). In contrast, studies which utilized commercially available concentrations reported somewhat less optimal results. Deer et al. reported pain reduction of 19.2% at month 3 and 30.8% at month 6 in patients beginning with ziconotide as their first IT medication. Although this study used low doses similar to the Pope et al. and Lindley et al. reports, the concentration was a stock 25 mcg/mL solution in the Deer 2018 study compared to a diluted 5 mcg/mL solution in the Pope study and a 0.5 mcg/mL solution in the Lindley report. One possibility for the improved efficacy of the dilute solution may by that a more dilute solution result in a wider segmental spinal spread.

3.6 Programmed Bolus Versus Patient Administered Bolus Techniques

The Pope and Lindley studies both described slightly different bolus techniques (Pope and Deer 2015; Lindley 2019). The former utilized a programmed nocturnal bolus, while the latter employed a patient-controlled bolusing protocol. The study using the programmed nocturnal boluses reported slightly higher daily doses and better pain reduction, but also more side effects and a higher dropout rate. A likely explanation for these differences is the ability of the patient to vary their day-to-day dosage as needed by using the patient administered bolus technique.

3.7 Spinal Segmental Spread of Ziconotide

Studies demonstrate efficacy with ziconotide despite the location of the catheter tip and even when the catheter tip is not near the source of the patient's pain (Staats et al. 2003; Lindley 2019; Staub et al. 2019). In order to further evaluate the initial clinical impression that ziconotide has favorable effect on pain that is located at a distance from the IT catheter tip, one may examine molar solubility. The molar solubility in water of ziconotide is one to two orders of magnitude greater as compared to that of baclofen or bupivacaine. The molar solubility in water of ziconotide is three orders of magnitude greater than morphine. Whether the greater degree of solubility is a causative factor in producing pain relief in regions of the spinal canal distal to the source of pain has not been worked out in detail, but it does explain the clinical observation that ziconotide has extensive spinal segmental spread. The concept of various drugs differing in spinal segment coverage was explored in a pig study comparing intrathecal doses of baclofen and bupivacaine (Bernards 2006).

4 Conclusions

Ziconotide is a natural, non-opioid intrathecal analgesic effective at treating refractory pain. In cases where a patient may be on chronic systemic opioids, ziconotide offers a mechanism of action that is similar to but distinct from opioids and can be effective at relieving pain when opioids are not. Ziconotide is a direct inhibitor of the N-type voltage-sensitive calcium channel and, as such, is not susceptible to the same tolerance mechanisms as mu-agonists. In cases where patients are already tolerant to systemic opioids, intrathecal ziconotide provides an effective alternative. Ziconotide is also an effective choice in cases where the avoidance of opioids is desired. Ziconotide's side effects are largely neurologic, and adverse symptoms such as dizziness or hallucinations may occur if the medication is used at higher doses or concentrations. A low concentration, high volume, low dose, bolus delivery seems to minimize side effects and optimize relief. Clinically, ziconotide seems to have more favorable spinal segmental spread as compared to bupivacaine, baclofen, and morphine. This gives more leniency with catheter tip placement during implantation of the IT catheter. Ziconotide is also nonaddictive but is a very effective analgesic and plays an important role in treatment of both malignant and nonmalignant chronic pain conditions (Table 1).

Table 1 Select literature review of ziconotide

Literature citation	Patient number, type and treatment rendered	Evaluation performed	Results	Conclusions
Ziconotide for Chronic Non-Malignant Pain—Wermeling 2003 (Olivera and Teichert 2007a)	22 pts. with chronic nonmalignant pain given infusion of either 1, 5, 7.5, or 10 mcg over 1 h	Pts monitored for side effects and medication evaluated for efficacy of pain relief for 48 h	Most AEs were not severe. The side effects considered severe were dizziness, headache, and myasthenia and these occurred only in the group that received the 10 mcg infusion over 1 h as for efficacy, there was a dose-related improvement in pain which lasted through the 48-h observation time for all groups except the 1 mcg dose	Possible explanations for the lack of efficacy with the smallest dose include that it was too small to provide pain relief or that the placement of a large bore needle for catheter insertion is more algesic than the analgesic benefit of the 1 mcg ziconotide infusion given over 1 h
Ziconotide versus Placebo for Pain in Cancer or AIDS—Staats 2003 (Brookes et al. 2017)	This RCT had 111 cancer or AIDS pain subjects randomized to either ziconotide or placebo. The IT ziconotide had a concentration of 100 mcg/mL. The ziconotide was titrated for 5–6 days followed by a maintenance dose for 5 days. Crossover was allowed during the maintenance phase. Early pts. received a weight-based dose equal to 8.4 mcg/day for a 70-kg patient dosing was changed to a starting dose of 9.6 mcg/day then changed again to 2.4 mcg/day or less with titrations allowed every 24 h. The maximum allowed dose after titration was 57.6 mcg/day	Pain scores, opioid use, and side effects were evaluated for all patients	After medication titration, mean pain scores improved 53% in the ziconotide group versus 18.1% in the placebo group. The reduction in patient opioid use was significantly greater in the ziconotide group as compared to the placebo group	Although there was a significant reduction of pain with IT ziconotide, at the doses given in the trial, 97.2% of pts. experienced side effects (compared to 72.2% in placebo group) and 30.6% of patients experienced SAEs (compared to 10% in the placebo group). The most common side effect in the ziconotide group was dizziness, and the most common side effect in the placebo group was headache
Ziconotide versus Placebo—Rauck 2006 (McIntosh et al. 1982)	220 patients with chronic severe pain were randomized to either ziconotide or placebo. The treatment group started IT ziconotide infusion at 2.4 mcg/day and titrated the dose gradually over 3 weeks. At 3 weeks, the average dose in the treatment group was 6.96 mcg/day and the average improvement in pain was 14.7% for the treatment group versus 7.2% for the placebo group	Side effects and adverse events	Side effects in the treatment group included dizziness, confusion, ataxia, abnormal gait, and memory impairment. Both ziconotide and the placebo group had similar discontinuation rates due to AEs	Side effects include dizziness, confusion, ataxia, abnormal gait, and memory impairment. Placebo also produces side effects in blinded RCTs

External Catheter Evaluation of Ziconotide for Malignant and Non-malignant Pain— Ver Donck 2008 (Olivera and Teichert 2007b)	This was an external catheter study in pts. with both malignant and nonmalignant pain. IT ziconotide infusion was started at an avg. dose of 2.304 mcg/day and titrated to an average dose of 4.032 mcg/day by day 28	Pain scores and AEs	The patients reported pain scores improved 29% at day 28. There was a high rate of AEs w/90% of pts. experiencing an AE during the titration. Other AEs were related to failure of the external catheter or the device or difficulties with placement of the catheter	The pain reduction was modest, but there was a high rate of AEs. The most common AE was dizziness, and there were a number of AEs related to the external catheter or with difficult in placement of the catheter
High and Low Dose Ziconotide Trialing— Abramoff 2014 (Chi et al. 2004)	The authors trialed 5 mcg and 2 mcg ziconotide bolus doses sequentially in 15 patients with chronic nonmalignant pain	Pain reduction	They found a greater efficacy in pain reduction with the larger dose as compared to the smaller dose and one third of the patients had improvements sufficient enough to warrant pump implantation. All 5 pts. had improved pain. A drug holiday was used in 1 pt. who experienced an AE	The larger dose of ziconotide produced better pain reduction than the smaller dose. A drug holiday may be used in pts. who experience AEs
Nocturnal Flex Dosing— Pope 2015 (McGivern 2007)	Case series of 16 pts. reported a nocturnal flex dosing strategy. The patients were trialed with an IT bolus of 2 mcg of ziconotide, and then a 2 mcg ziconotide nocturnal flex dose was initiated to start the night following the implant. The ziconotide concentration in the pump was 5 mcg/mL	Pain score, AE's and opioid reduction	At the average follow-up time of 5.8 months, the average total daily dose of ziconotide was 2.77 mcg/day with 30% of the patients dropping out due to medication side effects. The avg. time for a pt. to leave the study was 4.25 months, and the avg. daily ziconotide dose for the pts. dropping out was 3.825 mcg/day. Urinary retention and visual hallucinations were the most common AEs. There were no SAEs. The avg. pain score decreased 9.06 out of 10 to a 1.8 and the avg. opioid reduction was 91.5%	The patients experienced a profound reduction of pain with a decrease of nearly 80%, but almost one-third of patients dropped out because of medication side effects. The medication was safe in the dose given with no SAEs noted

(continued)

Table 1 (continued)

Literature citation	Patient number, type and treatment rendered	Evaluation performed	Results	Conclusions
Open Label Observational Study—Deer 2018 (Wallace et al. 2006)	An open-label observational study enrolled 93 patients, 51 received ziconotide as initial intrathecal therapy and 42 were weaned from their prior intrathecal therapy and switched to intrathecal ziconotide. The patients were started at an average of 1.6 mcg/day then titrated incrementally as needed. By week 12, the mean daily dose was 3.2 mcg/day	Pain relief, AEs and mean daily dose of ziconotide	At 12 months, the mean daily dose of ziconotide as an initial treatment group was lower as compared to the group that had previous non-ziconotide IT medication. At 12 months, 14 of the 25 pts. had at least 30% relief, whereas 9 of 25 (36%) had less than 30% relief. In the ziconotide group, pain relief varied from 19.2 to 32.7% from month 3 to month 12. In the ziconotide after other IT medication group, pain relief varied from 4.3% to 22.3% between months 3 and 12. 71% of the pts. reported AEs and 5 pts. reported SAEs	Most of the patients receiving ziconotide had at least 30% pain relief. In both the ziconotide first group and the ziconotide after another IT medication groups, the pain relief improved from month 3 to month 12 but was better overall for the ziconotide first group. Most patients reported AEs and 5 pts. reported SAEs
Ziconotide for Axial Non-malignant Pain—Lindley 2019 (Wermeling et al. 2003)	Case series of 17 pts. with axial nonmalignant neck and back pain. All pts. discontinued opioids prior to IT medication trial with ziconotide and remained off of their systemic opioids. Ziconotide was initiated at 0.024 mcg/day. The PTM was started at dose of 0.25 mcg and allowed up to three times per day	Pain relief off of systemic opioids and medication dose	After a follow-up interval of 4.7 months on the average, the mean medication concentration used was 1 mcg/mL with an average basal rate of 0.19 mcg/day, an average PTM dose of 0.27 mcg, and an average total daily ziconotide dose of 0.736 mcg. The mean pain relief was 71%, and the median pain relief was 75% at the time of the last follow-up and, at this time, 94% of patients remained on the therapy	At relatively low doses of ziconotide and with allowing patient controlled PTM doses the pain relief was substantial with nearly all of the patients remaining on IT ziconotide therapy

Use of Ziconotide in Patients with Spinal Cord Injury—Brinzeu 2019 (Staats et al. 2003)	Prospective cohort of 20 spinal cord injury pts. had IT and was implanted if the trial was positive. The trialing method was a series of IT bolus injections with an escalating dose (sequence of 0.5 mcg/2 mL, 1 mcg/2 mL, and 1.5 mcg/2 mL) with each dose given at 72-h intervals. If the pt. failed the bolus trial, a continuous catheter trial was performed. The continuous infusion was started at 2 mcg/day, and every 3 days the infusion could be increased by 1 mcg until a maximum dose of 10 mcg/day was reached. Overall pain relief of 40% was considered a positive test	Pain relief, trial positivity based on technique, AEs, pump implantation rate after trial	10 of 19 pts. had a positive bolus test and 3 of 8 continuous infusion tests were positive. 3 of 13 pts. had unacceptable side effects and dropped out. 11 of 20 pts. went on to pump implantation. Of the patients who pump implantation, 15% dropped out of chronic therapy. The avg. follow-up at the end of the study was 3.59 years and avg. daily dose was 5.36 mcg/day. The average pain score decreased 45% from 7.9 to 4.31	Most spinal cord injury patients trialed with ziconotide who respond will have a response to escalating bolus doses. A minority. In patients who have a positive trial and undergo pump implantation a distinct minority will autoterminate therapy and the pain relief was moderate at a moderate daily dose
The Distal Segmental Spread of Intrathecal Ziconotide—Staub 2019 (Rauck et al. 2006)	Single patient case study with the pt. was given a lumbar IT bolus trial at the L3–4 level using 2.5 mcg ziconotide in 2.5 mL volume that resulted in drastic reduction of the patient's chronic severe facial pain for 9 h. At pump implantation, the catheter tip was placed at the thoracolumbar junction. This describes an implanted catheter tip well inferior to the mid to upper thoracic spine	Pain relief and catheter tip position	With a distal catheter tip placement, the pt. experienced complete or near-complete relief of their facial pain over the 22-month follow-up period. At the end of 22 months, the patient was still having 100% relief at a relatively low dose of 2.0 mcg/day	The effect of ziconotide occur a substantial distance from the catheter tip position

Pts patients, *AEs* adverse events, *mcg* microgram, *AIDS* acquired immune deficiency syndrome, *RCT* randomized control trial, *IT* intrathecal, *SAEs* significant adverse events, *avg.* average, *PTM* patient therapy manager

[a]Ziconotide should be first choice in patients with >120 morphine equivalents or fast systemic dose escalation, in the absence of history of psychosis

References

Abramoff B, Shaw E Use of double diagnostic high/low dose trialing for ziconotide pump for chronic pain. 18th Annual Meeting of the North American Neuromodulation Society, December 11–14, 2014, Las Vegas, Nevada. . https://www.epostersonline.com/nans2014/node/59

Bernards CM (2006) Cerebrospinal fluid and spinal cord distribution of baclofen and bupivacaine during slow intrathecal infusion in pigs. Anesthesiology 105:169–178

Brinzeu A, Berthiller J, Caillet JB, Staquet H, Mertens P (2019) Ziconotide for spinal cord injury-related pain. Eur J Pain 23(9):1688–1700. https://doi.org/10.1002/ejp.1445. Epub 2019 Aug 29. PMID: 31233255

Brookes ME, Eldabe S, Batterham A (2017) Ziconotide monotherapy: a systematic review of randomized controlled trials. Curr Neuropharmacol 15(2):217–231. https://doi.org/10.2174/1570159x14666160210142056

Chi SW, Kim DH, Olivera BM, McIntosh JM, Han KH (2004) Solution conformation of alpha-conotoxin GIC, a novel potent antagonist of alpha3beta2 nicotinic acetylcholine receptors. Biochem J 380(Pt 2):347–352. https://doi.org/10.1042/BJ20031792. PMID: 14992691; PMCID: PMC1224189

Deer TR, Hayek SM, Pope JE, Lamer TJ, Hamza M, Grider JS, Rosen SM, Narouze S, Perruchoud C, Thomson S, Russo M, Grigsby E, Doleys DM, Jacobs MS, Saulino M, Christo P, Kim P, Huntoon EM, Krames E, Mekhail N (2017) The polyanalgesic consensus conference (PACC): recommendations for trialing of intrathecal drug delivery infusion therapy. Neuromodulation 20(2):133–154. https://doi.org/10.1111/ner.12543. Epub 2017 Jan 2. PMID: 28042906

Deer T, Rauck RL, Kim P, Saulino MF, Wallace M, Grigsby EJ, Huang IZ, Mori F, Vanhove GF, McDowell GC 2nd. (2018) Effectiveness and safety of intrathecal ziconotide: interim analysis of the patient registry of intrathecal ziconotide management (PRIZM). Pain Pract 18(2):230–238. https://doi.org/10.1111/papr.12599. Epub 2017 Jul 14. PMID: 28449352

Lindley D Short-term outcomes of a high volume, high velocity, low concentration bolus (HVLC-B) starting dose technique with ziconotide: a case series. Poster presentation. annual meeting of the American Society of Pain & Neuroscience. July 26–29, 2019, Miami Beach, Florida

McGivern JG (2007) Ziconotide: a review of its pharmacology and use in the treatment of pain. Neuropsychiatr Dis Treat 3(1):69–85. https://doi.org/10.2147/nedt.2007.3.1.69

McIntosh M, Cruz LJ, Hunkapiller MW, Gray WR, Olivera BM (1982) Isolation and structure of a peptide toxin from the marine snail conus magus. Arch Biochem Biophys 218(1):329–334. https://doi.org/10.1016/0003-9861(82)90351-

Olivera BM, Teichert RW (2007a) Diversity of the neurotoxic conus peptides: a model for concerted pharmacological discovery. Mol Interv 7(5):251–260. https://doi.org/10.1124/mi.7.5.7

Olivera BM, Teichert RW (2007b) Diversity of the neurotoxic conus peptides: a model for concerted pharmacological discovery. Mol Interv 7(5):251–260. https://doi.org/10.1124/mi.7.5.7. PMID: 17932414

Pope JE, Deer TR (2015) Intrathecal pharmacology update: novel dosing strategy for intrathecal monotherapy ziconotide on efficacy and sustainability. Neuromodulation 18(5):414–420

Rauck RL, Wallace MS, Leong MD, MineHart M, Webster LR, Charapata SG, Abraham JE, Buffington DE, Ellis D, Kartzinel R (2006) A randomized, double-blind, placebo-controlled study of intrathecal ziconotide in adults with severe chronic pain. J Pain Symptom Manag 31(5):393–406

Staats P, Yearwood T, Charapata S, Presley R, Wallace M, Byas-Smith M, Fisher R, Bryce D, Mangieri E, Luther R, Mayo M, McGuire D, Ellis D (2003) Intrathecal ziconotide in the treatment of refractory pain in patients with cancer or AIDS. JAMA 291:63–70

Staub BP, Casini GP, Monaco EA 3rd, Sekula RF Jr, Emerick TD (2019) Near-resolution of persistent idiopathic facial pain with low-dose lumbar intrathecal ziconotide: a case report. J Pain Res 12:945–949. https://doi.org/10.2147/JPR.S193746. PMID: 30881103; PMCID: PMC6413753

Ver Donck A, Collins R, Rauck RL et al (2008) An open-label, multicenter study of the safety and efficacy of intrathecal ziconotide for severe chronic pain when delivered via an external pump. Neuromodulation 11(2):103–111

Wallace MS, Charapata SG, Fisher R, et al; Ziconotide Nonmalignant Pain Study 96-002 Group (2006) Intrathecal ziconotide in the treatment of chronic non-malignant pain: a randomized, double-blind, placebo-controlled clinical trial. Neuromodulation 9(2):75–86

Wermeling D, Drass M, Ellis D et al (2003) Pharmacokinetics and pharmacodynamics of intrathecal ziconotide in chronic pain patients. J Clin Pharmacol 43(6):624–636

Printed in the United States
by Baker & Taylor Publisher Services